OVARIAN CANCER IMMUNOTHERAPY

OVARIAN CANCER IMMUNOTHERAPY

EDITED BY

Samir A. Farghaly, MD, PhD

PROFESSOR OF OBSTETRICS AND GYNECOLOGY

JOAN AND SANFORD I. WEILL MEDICAL COLLEGE

THE GRADUATE SCHOOL OF MEDICAL SCIENCES

NEW YORK PRESBYTERIAN HOSPITAL

WEILL CORNELL UNIVERSITY MEDICAL CENTER

SANDRA AND EDWARD MEYER CANCER CENTER

CORNELL UNIVERSITY

NEW YORK, NY

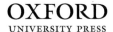

OXFORD
UNIVERSITY PRESS

OXFORD
UNIVERSITY PRESS

Oxford University Press is a department of the University of Oxford. It furthers
the University's objective of excellence in research, scholarship, and education
by publishing worldwide. Oxford is a registered trade mark of Oxford University
Press in the UK and certain other countries.

Published in the United States of America by Oxford University Press
198 Madison Avenue, New York, NY 10016, United States of America.

Library of Congress Cataloging-in-Publication Data
Names: Farghaly, Samir A., editor.
Title: Ovarian cancer immunotherapy / edited by Samir A. Farghaly.
Description: New York, New York : Oxford University Press, Inc., [2018] |
Includes bibliographical references.
Identifiers: LCCN 2018001371 | ISBN 9780190248208 (hardback : alk. paper)
Subjects: | MESH: Ovarian Neoplasms—therapy | Immunotherapy—methods
Classification: LCC RC280.O8 | NLM WP 322 | DDC 616.99/465—dc23
LC record available at https://lccn.loc.gov/2018001371

This material is not intended to be, and should not be considered, a substitute for medical or other professional advice. Treatment for the
conditions described in this material is highly dependent on the individual circumstances. And, while this material is designed to offer accurate information with respect to the subject matter covered and to be current as of the time it was written, research and knowledge about
medical and health issues is constantly evolving and dose schedules for medications are being revised continually, with new side effects
recognized and accounted for regularly. Readers must therefore always check the product information and clinical procedures with the
most up-to-date published product information and data sheets provided by the manufacturers and the most recent codes of conduct and
safety regulation. The publisher and the authors make no representations or warranties to readers, express or implied, as to the accuracy or
completeness of this material. Without limiting the foregoing, the publisher and the authors make no representations or warranties as to
the accuracy or efficacy of the drug dosages mentioned in the material. The authors and the publisher do not accept, and expressly disclaim,
any responsibility for any liability, loss or risk that may be claimed or incurred as a consequence of the use and/or application of any of the
contents of this material.

9 8 7 6 5 4 3 2 1

Printed by Sheridan Books, Inc., United States of America

This book is dedicated to: my beloved children, Raied and Tamer, and the memory of my mother Amina and my father Aly who had a great influence on me and my academic and professional medical career.

Also, to my sisters Sorya and Nadia, my brother Rafat, and their families; and my late siblings: Nabil, Magdy, and their families. In addition: to my late nephew, Islam.

—Samir A. Farghaly, MD, PhD

CONTENTS

PREFACE

Ovarian cancer (OC) is the seventh common cancer in women worldwide, with 239,000 new cases diagnosed in 2012. The American Cancer Society estimates in 2017 about 22, 440 women will receive a new diagnosis of OC. About 14,080 women will die from OC. The five-year survival rate has been reported to range from approximately 30% to 50% effective immune-based cancer treatments to OC patients. Estimated 905 of OC are epithelial in origin. Despite advances in surgery and chemotherapy, only modest progress has been made in improving overall survival in patients with OC. Most women with advanced OC respond to first-line chemotherapy, but most responses are not durable. More than 80% of patients will have a recurrence of their disease after first-line treatment. The poor survival in advanced OC is due to late diagnosis and the lack of effective second-line therapy for patients who relapse. The clinical outcome of these patients is marked by periods of remission and relapse of shortening duration until chemotherapy resistance develops. New treatment options are needed to improve the response rate and survival of women diagnosed with this disease. Current scientific evidence suggests that OC is an immunogenic tumor that can be recognized by the host immune system. Spontaneous anti-tumor immune response is detected in peripheral blood, tumors, and ascites of OC patients in the form of tumor-reactive T cells and antibodies. Tumor-derived or peripheral blood T cells recognize autologous tumor-associated antigens including testis differentiation antigens. However, spontaneous anti-tumor immune response has been reported in about 55% of patients with OC

whose tumors are rich with T-cell infiltrates. Patients with T-cell-rich tumors experience longer progression-free and overall survival. Immune evasion mechanisms in these patients correlate with poor survival. Overall, the relationship of T-cell infiltrates with prolonged survival, and the association of immune escape mechanisms with poor survival, suggest that OC patients may respond to immunotherapy modalities. These modalities are vaccines, adoptive T-cell therapy, or immunomodulatory drug-based such as interleukin-2, antibodies against cytotoxic T lymphocyte-associated protein 4, or programmed cell death 1 co-inhibitory immune receptors. In addition, chemotherapeutic agents and radiotherapy may also have immunomodulatory roles.

The purpose of this book is to provide a broad background of the basic science, clinical, and therapeutic aspects of OC immunotherapy. It provides state-of-the-art information on the molecular genetics, biology, and clinical aspects of immunotherapy for OC. Also, the book chapters provide better understandings of the molecular and cellular events that underlie OC immunology. The contributors to this book are affiliated with several renowned major academic medical institutions in the United States, United Kingdom, Canada, France, Japan, and Romania.

Examples of monoclonal antibodies clinically evaluated for efficacy as OC immunotherapy agents are presented in chapter 1. Emerging serum biomarkers in their use for screening, diagnosis, and monitoring of OC are discussed in chapter 2. Antitumor immune response and immune evasion mechanism of epithelial OC are illustrated in chapter 3. The role of stromal cells associated secreted factors and the immune system on tumor progression in ovarian adenocarcinoma is detailed in chapter 4. An overview of adoptive cell immunotherapy for epithelial OC focusing on HLA-restricted tumor infiltrating lymphocytes and MHC-independent immune effectors is discussed in chapter 5. Development and application in clinical trials of three therapeutic antibodies classes related to OC are reported in chapter 6. Two monoclonal antibodies, RP215 and GHR106, have been studied and developed as anti-OC immunotherapy agents detailed in chapter 7. The biology of dendritic cells, including dendritic cell subsets, development, activation, maturation, and strategies for clinical use in patients with OC is reported in chapter 8. The development of dendritic cell-based vaccine pulsed with tumor antigen as an OC immunotherapy agent is described in chapter 9. The use of immunocheckpoint inhibitors, anti-PD-1, and anti PD-L1 therapies as immunotherapeutic agents for OC is detailed in chapter 10. The role of growth factors such as VEGF, FGFs, and PDGFs and their corresponding receptors in the pathogenesis, progression, and selection of OC immunotherapy is detailed in chapter 11. The fundamental immunologic principles that have guided the development of cancer immunotherapy and the success and limitations of immunotherapy for patients with metastatic OC are reviewed in chapter 12. An overview of OC immunotherapy, important discoveries in OC-related immune dysfunction, recent developments, ongoing clinical trials, and future directions are discussed in chapter 13.

This volume is intended for all clinicians and basic medical scientists caring for women with OC, including attending surgeons and physicians, clinical fellows, and residents in the disciplines of gynecologic oncology, medical oncology, and surgical oncology. It is also useful for PhD students and postdoctoral fellows in basic medical sciences.

I would like to thank Mrs. Andrea Knobloch, senior editor, and Ms. Tiffany Lu, assistant editor, at Oxford University Press for their efficiency and valuable help in the process of developing, editing, and publishing this book.

I hope that you find this book very useful and benefit from the extensive experience of the knowledgeable team of contributors who have authored its contents.

Samir A. Farghaly, MD, PhD

CONTRIBUTORS

Eman Abdulfatah, MD
Resident
Division of Pathology
Detroit Medical Center
Detroit, MI

Hiroyuki Abe, MD, PhD
Director of Abe Cancer Clinic
Tokyo, Japan

Minako Abe, MD
Abe Cancer Clinic
Tokyo, Japan

Scott I. Abrams, PhD
Professor of Oncology
Department of Immunology
Roswell Park Cancer Institute
Buffalo, NY

Yousef Alharbi, MS
Doctoral Candidate
Endocrinology and Reproductive Physiology
   Graduate Program
Department of Obstetrics and Gynecology
University of Wisconsin–Madison
Madison, WI

Rouba Ali-Fehmi, MD
Professor
Director of the GYN Oncology Tissue
   Procurement Program
Director of Surgical Pathology Fellowship
   Program
Department of Pathology
Wayne State University School of Medicine
Detroit, MI

Heather J. Bax, PhD
St. John's Institute of Dermatology
Division of Genetics and Molecular
   Medicine
Division of Cancer Studies
Faculty of Life Sciences and Medicine
King's College London and NIHR
   Biomedical Research Centre
Guy's and St. Thomas' Hospital
King's College London
London, United Kingdom

Florian Cabillic, MCUPH
Cytogenetics and Cell Biology Laboratory
Rennes University Hospital Center
Rennes, France

Anca Maria Cimpean, MD, PhD
Department of Microscopic Morphology/
   Histology
Angiogenesis Research Center
Victor Babes University of Medicine and
   Pharmacy
Timisoara, Romania

Curtis A. Clark, MS
MD/PhD Candidate
Department of Microbiology, Immunology,
   and Molecular Genetics
University of Texas Health Science Center
San Antonio, TX

Tyler J. Curiel, MD, MPH
Department of Medicine
Department of Cell Systems and Anatomy
School of Medicine
Cancer Therapy and Research Center
University of Texas Health Science Center
San Antonio, TX

Brian J. Czerniecki, MD, PhD
Chair and Senior Member
Department of Breast Oncology
Moffitt Cancer Center
Tampa, FL
Emeritus Professor CE of Surgery
Department of Surgery
University of Pennsylvania Perelman School
   of Medicine
Philadelphia, PA

Justin M. Drerup, BS
MD/PhD Candidate
Department of Cell Systems and Anatomy
School of Medicine
University of Texas Health Science Center
San Antonio, TX

Fabrice Foucher, MD
Department of Gynecology
Rennes University Hospital Center
Rennes, France

Amy Harper, MD
Department of Obstetrics, Gynecology and
   Reproductive Sciences
University of Maryland Medical Center
Baltimore, MD

Sébastien Henno, MD
Anatomy and Pathology Cytology
   Department
Rennes University Hospital Center
Rennes, France

Andreea Adriana Jitariu, PhD
Assistant Professor
Department of Microscopic Morphology/
   Histology
Angiogenesis Research Center
Victor Babes University of Medicine and
   Pharmacy
Timisoara, Romania

**Debra H. Josephs, BSc, MBChB,
   MRCP, PhD**
NIHR Academic Clinical Lecturer in
   Medical Oncology
King's College London and NIHR
   Biomedical Research Centre
Guy's and St. Thomas' Hospital
London, United Kingdom

Sophia N. Karagiannis, PhD
Reader in Translational Cancer Immunology
Head of Cancer Antibody Discovery and
   Immunotherapy
King's College London and NIHR
   Biomedical Research Centre
Guy's and St. Thomas' Hospital
London, United Kingdom

Vincent Lavoué, MD, PhD
Department of Gynecology
Rennes University Hospital Center
Rennes, France

Gregory Lee, PhD
Professor Emeritus
University of British Columbia
Vancouver Coastal Health Research Institute
Vancouver, Canada

Patrick Legembre, PhD
Research Director
Oncogenesis Stress Signaling Lab
Rennes University Hospital Center
Rennes, France

Jean Levêque, MD, PhD
Head of Gynecological Service
Surgeon of the Oncological Surgical Unit of
   Rennes CLC
Rennes University Hospital Center
Rennes, France

Sarah Lynam, MD
Gynecologic Oncology Fellow
Roswell Park Cancer Institute
Buffalo, NY

Maya Matheny, PhD
Division of Gynecologic Oncology
University of Maryland Medical Center
Baltimore, MD

Michelle N. Messmer, PhD
Senior Fellow
Department of Immunology
University of Washington Seattle
Seattle, WA

Scott Moerdler, MD
Department of Microbiology and
  Immunology
Albert Einstein College of Medicine
Department of Pediatrics
Montefiore Medical Center
New York, NY

Ana Montes, MD
Consultant for Lung and Gynaecology
Department of Medical Oncology
Guy's and St Thomas' NHS Foundation Trust
London, United Kingdom

Colleen S. Netherby, PhD
Department of Immunology
Roswell Park Cancer Institute
Buffalo, NY

Manish S. Patankar, PhD
Associate Professor
Department of Obstetrics and Gynecology
University of Wisconsin–Madison
Madison, WI

Giulia Pellizzari, MSc
Research Student
King's College London and NIHR
  Biomedical Research Centre
Guy's and St. Thomas' Hospital
London, United Kingdom

Marius Raica, MD, PhD
Department of Microscopic Morphology/
  Histology
Angiogenesis Research Center
Victor Babes University of Medicine and
  Pharmacy
Timisoara, Romania

Gautam Rao, MD
Division of Gynecologic Oncology
University of Maryland Medical Center
Baltimore, MD

Jocelyn Reader, PhD
Division of Gynecologic Oncology
University of Maryland Medical Center
Baltimore, MD

Dana M. Roque, MD
Assistant Professor
Division of Gynecologic Oncology
University of Maryland Medical Center
Baltimore, MD

Amane Sasada, MD
Abe Cancer Clinic
Tokyo, Japan

James F. Spicer, MRCP, PhD, FCRP
Professor of Experimental Cancer
  Medicine
Division of Cancer Studies
Faculty of Life Sciences and Medicine
King's College London
Guy's and St. Thomas' Hospital
London, UK

Caitlin Stashwick, MD
Department of Obstetrics and Gynecology
University of Pennsylvania Health System
Lancaster General Health
Lancaster, PA

Shigeki Tabata, MD
Abe Cancer Clinic
Tokyo, Japan

Janos L. Tanyi, MD, PhD
Department of Obstetrics and Gynecology
University of Pennsylvania
Perelman Center for Advanced Medicine
Philadelphia, PA

Rebecca J. Whelan, PhD
Associate Professor and Chair
Department of Chemistry and Biochemistry
Oberlin College
Oberlin, OH

Xingxing Zang, PhD
Professor, Department of Microbiology and
  Immunology
Professor, Department of Medicine
  (Oncology)
Albert Einstein College of Medicine
New York, NY

OVARIAN CANCER IMMUNOTHERAPY

1.

ANTIBODY THERAPEUTICS FOR OVARIAN CARCINOMA AND TRANSLATION TO THE CLINIC

Debra H. Josephs, Heather J. Bax, Giulia Pellizzari,
James F. Spicer, Ana Montes, and Sophia N. Karagiannis

INTRODUCTION

In 2015, approximately 21,290 American women were diagnosed with ovarian cancer, and just over 14,000 died from the disease.[1] The mainstay of treatment combines maximal surgical cytoreduction with combination chemotherapy (CT) using taxane and platinum agents. However, most patients relapse after primary treatment and succumb to disease progression. Unfortunately, exploration of alternative chemotherapeutic agents,[2-4] novel delivery routes,[5] new dosing schedules,[6] and combinatorial strategies with targeted agents[7,8] have not led to meaningful improvements in cure rates.[9]

Ovarian carcinoma is known to be an immunogenic cancer, with described spontaneous T-cell responses. Indeed, patients with ovarian tumors with high numbers of infiltrating T cells have demonstrated improved five-year overall survival (38%) relative to patients with tumors showing poor T-cell infiltration (4.5%).[10] It is thought that antibody-based therapies, designed to mediate specific anti-tumor immune responses, may harness this immune infiltrate against tumors and thus lead to improved clinical outcomes. Antibody immunotherapy has several proposed advantages over standard cytotoxic therapy. Antibodies demonstrate exquisite specificity and can circumvent primary or acquired resistance to cytotoxic drugs. Moreover, the efficacy of immune-based therapy can be durable due to immunologic memory. In this chapter, we discuss ovarian cancer antibody immunotherapy, including established therapies in current clinical use. We also highlight promising emerging therapeutic strategies able to harness the immune system to improve clinical outcomes.

MONOCLONAL ANTIBODIES FOR THE TREATMENT OF CANCER

THE STRUCTURE AND FUNCTION OF ANTIBODIES

Antibodies or immunoglobulins (Ig) are soluble glycoproteins produced by B-lymphocytes in response to pathogens or foreign antigens and play an important role in the adaptive immune response. Antibodies may act as antigen receptors (the B-cell receptor), bound to the surface membrane of B cells, or they may be secreted as soluble proteins, with each B-cell-producing antibodies with specificity for a single epitope of an antigen.[11]

Antibodies are each composed of two identical heavy (H) and two identical light (L) chains linked by disulfide bonds and non-covalent interactions. They exist as nine major classes and subclasses (or isotypes) known as

IgM, IgD, IgG (IgG1-4), IgE, and IgA (IgA1-2), denoted from differences in their heavy chain structure (Figure 1.1). Although antibody structure is similar among the five Ig classes, there are key differences between these which can be grouped into three main categories: (a) the number of heavy chain domains, (b) the distribution and number of carbohydrate groups, and (c) the number and location of disulfide bonds linking the different domains. Ig heavy chains are comprised of one variable domain (V_H) and multiple constant domains (C_H), three for IgA, IgG, and IgD and four for IgE and IgM (Figure 1.1). Light chains are also composed of one variable domain (V_L); however, in contrast to the heavy chains, they only have a single constant domain (C_L) which is either kappa (κ) or lambda (λ).[11]

Antibodies can be divided into two distinct functional binding units: the fragment of antigen binding (Fab) and the constant fragment (Fc), each having a distinct functional role (Figure 1.1). The Fab region contains the variable domains of each chain (V_H and V_L) and consists of three hypervariable polypeptide loops, termed complementarity-determining regions (CDRs), that form the antigen binding site of the antibody. The CDRs are the key determinants of the specificity and affinity of antigen binding and are supported by four polypeptides in each V_H and V_L called framework regions, which form a structural scaffold for CDR presentation.[11] Antibodies are linked to immune effector mechanisms via their Fc fragment, which engages class-specific Fc receptors (FcR) expressed on immune effector cells. Each antibody class or isotype binds to one or more specific FcR.

Antibodies play an important role in the adaptive immune response against pathogens or foreign antigens. In contrast to the innate immune response which is mediated by natural killer (NK) cells, monocytes/macrophages, eosinophils, basophils, neutrophils, mast cells, and dendritic cells, the adaptive immune response is mediated by only two immune effector cell types, namely B and T cells. In addition to secreting mediators able to drive an adaptive T-cell response, the key role of B cells in adaptive immunity is the production of antibodies specific for foreign antigens, thereby mounting a humoral immune response.[12] These antibodies function to destroy pathogens either by their neutralization or by interaction with cellular and non-cellular components of the innate immune system.[11]

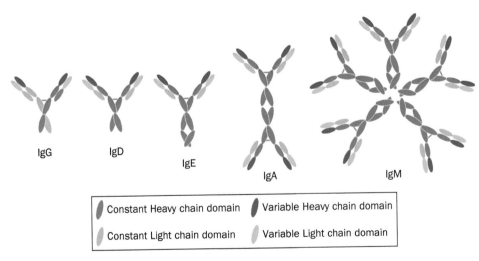

Figure 1.1 Schematic representation of the five immunoglobulin classes. Immunoglobulins are divided into five different classes, distinguished by their heavy chain structure: IgG, IgD, and IgA contain three constant domains (CH1, CH2, and CH3), while IgE and IgM have four (CH1, CH2, CH3, and CH4). IgG, IgD, and IgE are found in monomeric assembled structure, whereas IgA can form dimers and IgM can form pentamers.

MECHANISMS OF ACTION OF MONOCLONAL ANTIBODIES FOR THE TREATMENT OF CANCER

Monoclonal antibodies (mAbs) targeting tumor-associated antigens (TAAs) are able to mediate specific anti-tumor responses through a variety of mechanisms, in order to eliminate cancer cells (Figure 1.2). Antibodies can act via their Fab region (the antigen-binding site), their Fc region (the isotype-specific region), or both regions combined.

Fab-Mediated Mechanisms

By engaging tumor cells through their Fab region, antibodies are able to block vital cell growth signals and intracellular signaling cascades to reduce tumor cell proliferation and engender apoptosis (Figure 1.2).

Antibody therapeutics were first designed to target the mitogenic or prosurvival signal transduction pathways that are activated or differentially overexpressed in cancer cells compared to normal cells. These pathways are mainly triggered through the interaction of extracellular ligands with cell surface molecules, a process which can be interrupted by targeted mAbs. Such antibodies can bind to the ligand itself to prevent its interaction with a cell surface receptor. An example of this concept has been used in the case of bevacizumab, which targets vascular endothelial growth factor (VEGF), and prevents its binding to the VEGF receptor (VEGFR) expressed on the endothelial cells of the tumor-associated vasculature. In binding to the VEGFR, VEGF stimulates new blood vessel formation (angiogenesis), which is a fundamental event in the process of tumor growth and metastatic dissemination.[13]

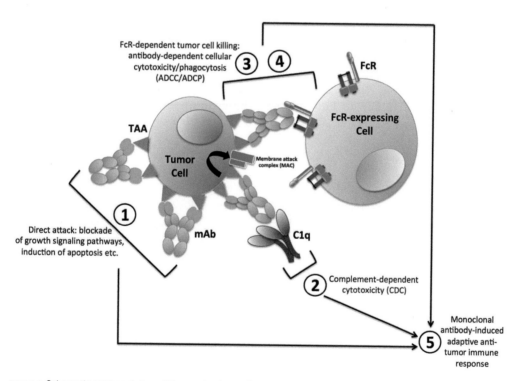

Figure 1.2 Schematic representation of the mechanisms of action of anti-tumor monoclonal antibodies. Antibodies, with specificity to TAAs, may operate through several mechanisms to kill cancer cells. These include: (1) direct attack resulting in blockade of growth signaling pathways, restriction of proliferation and cell differentiation, or induction of apoptosis; (2) CDC; (3) ADCC; or (4) ADCP. In favorable situations, these mechanisms may also lead to the induction of long-lasting adaptive anti-tumor immune responses (5).

Bevacizumab specifically binds to the VEGF protein, thereby potently inhibiting the process of angiogenesis and subsequently inhibiting tumor growth.[14]

Alternatively, mAbs can directly bind to receptors on the tumor cell surface itself. Antibodies acting via this mechanism work by either blocking the access of a ligand to its cell-associated receptor, antagonizing ligand-induced receptor signaling, or allowing ligand binding to occur but sterically inhibiting the subsequent receptor heterodimerization required for signal transduction.[15] These concepts are exemplified by antibodies targeting the epidermal growth factor receptor (EGFR) family, such as those already in clinical use, including trastuzumab, pertuzumab, cetuximab, and panitumumab for the treatment of breast, squamous cell carcinoma of the head and neck, and colorectal cancer, respectively.[16-19] For example, trastuzumab binds to the extracellular domain of the tumor surface-expressed HER2/*neu* receptor, preventing intracellular tyrosine kinase activation and subsequent promotion of cellular proliferation and survival,[20] and pertuzumab binds HER2, preventing heterodimerization with HER1 (EGFR) or HER3. In contrast, cetuximab and panitumumab bind specifically and selectively to EGFR, preventing binding of activating ligands such as the epidermal growth factor and transforming growth factor-α.

Antibodies targeting such functional tumor antigens were principally designed to achieve their effects through Fab-mediated mechanisms. However, antibodies can also be conjugated to drugs such as immunotoxins, radioisotopes, or toxin-containing liposomes, or enzymes followed by a prodrug in the case of antibody-directed enzyme prodrug therapy, to specifically deliver these agents to targeted cancer cells.[21-24] Such antibodies are known as antibody-drug conjugates. Potential advantages of radioisotope-conjugated antibodies include the "bystander effect," which causes adjacent tumor cells to be destroyed in addition to the targeted cells. Furthermore, with radioisotope-conjugated antibodies, it is possible to visualize the distribution of the therapeutic agent and ensure target delivery.[21,22] In addition to their Fab-mediated mechanisms, mAbs can also act by additional mechanisms via their Fc domain, recruiting components of the host immune system to trigger tumor cell death.

Fc-Mediated Mechanisms

Therapeutic antibodies bound to tumor cell surface antigens also have the potential to elicit immune-mediated tumor cell death, either by engaging cells of the innate immune system or by activating the complement cascade (Figure 1.2). Antibody-dependent cellular cytotoxicity (ADCC) and antibody-dependent cellular phagocytosis (ADCP) are dependent on interactions between immune cellular FcRs and the antibody Fc domains. ADCC involves recruitment of immune effector cells such as NK cells, neutrophils, and monocytes/macrophages, which become activated as a result of antibody binding to their FcRs. Activation of these cells has several consequences; for example, NK cells can kill cancer cells directly by a variety of means, including local release of granzymes and perforins or release of cytokines and chemokines that can inhibit cell proliferation and also tumor-related angiogenesis.[25] Similarly, ADCP involves recruitment of phagocytic cells (e.g., macrophages) by virtue of their FcR expression, culminating in phagocytosis and death of the target cell (Figure 1.2). In addition, ADCP by cells with antigen-presenting capacity also has the potential to engage the adaptive immune system. This concept is again exemplified by trastuzumab, which functions not only through cell signaling inhibition by direct targeting of cell surface HER2/neu but also by initiating immunological pathways, whereby it targets tumor cells for elimination via ADCC and ADCP.[26-28] Indeed a study in which FcγR knockout mice were unable to arrest tumor growth in vivo following treatment with trastuzumab highlights the importance of

Fc-mediated immune mechanisms of action of therapeutic antibodies.[29]

Activation of the classical complement system is another strategy employed by mAbs to induce tumor cell death. Antibody-mediated complement-dependent cytotoxicity (CDC) is triggered when C1q, the initiating component of the classical complement pathway, is fixed to the Fc portion of target-bound antibodies. This triggers a cascade leading to the formation of C3 convertase and C5 convertase and the assembly of a "membrane attack complex" in the target cell membrane, which triggers the direct killing of tumor cells through tumor cell lysis.[30] Alternatively, antibody-mediated CDC can be conducted via neutrophils in a process termed complement-dependent neutrophil-mediated cytotoxicity.[31]

Engaging the Adaptive Immune System

Engagement of the adaptive immune system against tumor antigens represents a longstanding goal in cancer therapy. The concept that therapeutic mAbs not only trigger early anti-tumor events such as direct effects on tumor cells or innate immune-mediated cell killing mechanisms but that they also allow the host immune system to mount an anti-tumor response through the development of a long-lasting adaptive immunity has emerged over the past decade (Figure 1.2).[32]

Supporting the hypothesis that anti-tumor adaptive immunity might play a crucial role in long-term mAb therapeutic efficacy in vivo, MUC1 and HER2/neu-specific T-cell responses have been reported in cancer patients treated with either an anti-MUC1 mAb or trastuzumab, respectively.[33,34] This suggests that specific anti-tumor T-cell immunity can be triggered by mAb therapy, at least in some situations.[33,34] It is thought that this T-cell–mediated anti-tumor protection is initiated by antigen-presenting cell (APC) presentation of TAAs to T cells following endocytosis of TAA-antibody immune complexes by APCs and/or tumor

cell phagocytosis by these cells. Indeed, pioneering work from Selenko et al. revealed that the anti-CD20 mAb rituximab promoted antigen capture and DC maturation in vitro leading to the generation of specific anti-tumor cytotoxic T lymphocytes.[35,36] Thus, the therapeutic mAb paradigm has changed from a passive immunotherapy approach to also being considered as an active modulation of tumor immunity.

Engaging Anti-Tumor Immunity

More recently, another mechanism by which therapeutic mAbs can function to actively modulate anti-tumor immunity has been discovered. This involves targeting negative regulators of the immune system, so-called immunological checkpoints, which have been found to play important roles in restraining otherwise effective anti-tumor immunological responses.[37] MAbs that target these negative regulator checkpoints, such as those directed against cytotoxic T lymphocyte-associated antigen 4 (CTLA-4; ipilimumab, tremelimumab) and PD-1/PD-L1 (nivolumab, pembrolizumab), have demonstrated promising clinical results in a number of tumor types.[37] CTLA-4 is a member of the CD28:B7 immunoglobulin superfamily. T cells mediate immune responses, via (a) recognition and binding of the T-cell receptor to antigen bound-major histocompatibility complex molecules presented by APCs and (b) the co-stimulatory interaction of CD28 on T cells with B7 family ligands on APCs.[38] However, CTLA-4 acts as a CD28 homologue and binds B7 ligands on antigen-presenting cells.[39,40] While CD28 signals act to stimulate T-cell activation and survival, the alternative T cell-APC interaction via CTLA-4 signaling inhibits T-cell responses, preventing the release of IL-2 and leading to cytotoxic T-cell-cycle arrest and attenuation of effector functions.[39–41] Antibodies that target CTLA-4 prevent the attenuating function of CTLA-4 and thereby enhance anti-tumor T-cell function. In addition, these antibodies have the ability to deplete tumor-associated Tregs possibly by triggering ADCC against these cells in the tumor microenvironment (TME).[42] These findings highlight the importance of FcR-mediated mechanisms of action of mAbs alongside their immunomodulatory mechanisms.

The programmed cell death 1 (PD-1) receptor is another immune checkpoint and highly promising therapeutic target. PD-1 is expressed on T cells, B cells, and myeloid cells after activation, and its ligands, PD-L1 (B7-H1) and PD-L2 (B7-DC), are expressed on tumor cells, APCs, and other cells in the TME.[43] The interaction of PD-1 with its ligand is thought to function as an immunological checkpoint that tumors may use to defend themselves against antitumor immune responses through multiple immunosuppressive pathways, including the induction of T-cell anergy and apoptosis. The interaction of PD-1 on T cells and PD-L1 on tumor cells may additionally render tumor cells more resistant to T-cell–mediated apoptosis.[43] Therefore, antibodies that target the PD-1/PD-L1 interaction also act by enhancing antitumor T-cell functions.

MONOCLONAL ANTIBODIES FOR THE TREATMENT OF OVARIAN CANCER

A number of mAbs have been clinically evaluated for efficacy in ovarian cancer. Here we summarize examples of established monoclonal antibodies and those demonstrating most promise in late clinical trials. These antibodies are described in the following sections and in Table 1.1.

CATUMAXOMAB

Catumaxomab is a bispecific trifunctional antibody: the Fab portion of the antibody binds to EpCAM on tumor cells, and the CD3 antigen expressed on T-cells. The Fc portion of the antibody is recognized by type I, IIa, and III Fcγ receptors expressed on accessory cells (Figure 1.3). The simultaneous binding of target cells, T-cells, and FcγR positive cells is the key to catumaxomab's anti-tumor activity via T-cell–mediated lysis, ADCC, and ADCP.

The development of catumaxomab arose from the concept of engaging two different anti-tumor cell types (T cells and accessory

TABLE 1.1 MONOCLONAL ANTIBODIES FOR OVARIAN CANCER IN CURRENT CLINICAL USE OR UNDER DEVELOPMENT

Name	Target	Isotype	Mechanism of Action	Approval Status
Avelumab	PD-L1	IgG1	Blockade of PD-L1, ADCC	Not approved
Bevacizumab	VEGF-A	IgG1	Inhibition of angiogenesis	Approved (FDA, EMA)
BMS-936559	PD-L1	IgG4	Blockade of PD-L1	Not approved
Catumaxomab	EpCAM, CD3	IgG2a-IgG2b	ADCC, ADCP, apoptosis	Approved (EMA)
Farletuzumab	FR-α	IgG1	Inhibition of FR-α pathway	Not approved
Ipilimumab	CTLA-4	IgG1	T cell activation	Not approved
Nivolumab	PD-1	IgG4	Blockade of PD-1 receptor	Not approved
Pembrolizumab	PD-1	IgG4	Inhibition of PD-L1-PD-L2 interaction	Not approved
Tremelimumab	CTLA-4	IgG2	T cell activation	Not approved

NOTE: FDA = US Food and Drug Administration; EMA = European Medicines Agency.

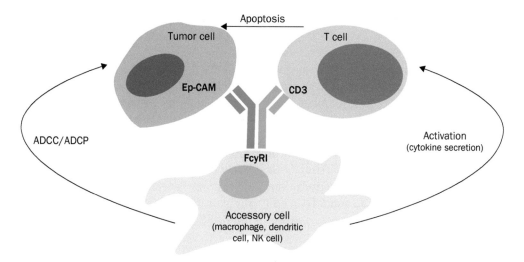

Figure 1.3 Catumaxomab: Structure and mechanism of action. Catumaxomab is a bispecific trifunctional antibody: the Fab portion binds to EpCAM on tumor cells, and the CD3 antigen expressed on T cells. The Fc portion is recognized by type I, IIa, and III Fcγ receptors expressed on accessory effector cells. The simultaneous binding of target cells, T cells, and FcγR positive cells promotes T-cell-mediated lysis, ADCC, and ADCP of EpCAM-expressing tumor cells.

cells) through one single antibody. The efficient recruitment of T cells represented an outstanding improvement in cancer immunotherapy, since T cells represent the most potent cytotoxic tool in the immune system.[44]

A Phase I/II dose-escalating study in 2007 assessed the tolerability and efficacy of catumaxomab administered intraperitoneally in ovarian cancer patients with ascites containing EpCAM positive tumor cells. Patients were treated with four to five infusions of catumaxomab of 5–200 μg in a period of 9 to 13 days. Minimal adverse effects (AEs) were observed, and catumaxomab administration led to significant reduction of ascites. Furthermore, monitoring of tumor cells in ascites revealed an important reduction of EpCAM-positive malignant cells, defining catumaxomab as a valid treatment option in ovarian cancer patients with malignant ascites.[45]

In 2010 a two-arm, randomized, Phase II/III trial was performed in patients with symptomatic malignant ascites requiring therapeutic paracentesis. Patients were randomized to receive paracentesis plus catumaxomab (catumaxomab) or paracentesis only (control) and divided by tumor type (129 ovarian and 129 non-ovarian). Intraperitoneal infusions of catumaxomab were performed on days 0, 3, 7, and 10 at doses of 10, 20, 50, and 150 μg. The efficacy endpoints of the study were puncture-free survival, time to next paracentesis, ascites signs and symptoms, and overall survival (OS). Puncture-free survival was significantly prolonged in patients treated with catumaxomab (median = 46 days) compared to control patients (median = 11 days). The second efficacy endpoint, time to next paracentesis, was also improved in catumaxomab patients, characterized by a median of 77 days compared to that of 13 days for the control patients. Catumaxomab-treated patients showed fewer signs and symptoms of ascites compared to patients on the control arm, and OS was characterized by a positive trend in treated patients, demonstrating that catumaxomab may be of real clinical benefit in patients with malignant ascites secondary to epithelial tumors.[46]

Catumaxomab was approved in 2009 in the European Union for the treatment of malignant ascites in patients with EpCAM-positive carcinomas, representing the first drug to be approved worldwide for the specific treatment of this clinical condition.[45]

FARLETUZUMAB

Farletuzumab (MORab003) is a fully humanized monoclonal IgG1 antibody specific for folate receptor-α (FRα). This antibody does not prevent binding of folate to its receptors, nor does it inhibit the transport of folate into the cell via the folate receptor. In vitro studies have demonstrated a number of modes of anti-tumor activity of farletuzumab against FRα-expressing tumor cells, including tumor cell killing by ADCC and CDC, sustained autophagy of tumor cells, and reduction of intracellular growth signaling by blockade of FRα-lyn kinase interactions.[47–51]

In a Phase I trial, farletuzumab was given as monotherapy to 25 patients with platinum-resistant epithelial ovarian cancer (EOC). No dose-limiting toxicities (DLTs) were observed, and dose escalation was continued to the maximum 400 mg/m^2 dose.[52] A subsequent Phase Ib study demonstrated safety of farletuzumab in combination with carboplatin and pegylated liposomal doxorubicin in patients with platinum-sensitive EOC.[53]

In a single-arm Phase II study, improved overall response rates compared to historical controls were observed in patients with platinum-sensitive ovarian cancer given farletuzumab combined with carboplatin and a taxane, followed by farletuzumab maintenance therapy. Farletuzumab was well tolerated as a single agent without additive toxicity when combined with CT.[54]

These promising results led to a large Phase III trial in patients with platinum-sensitive recurrent ovarian cancer, in which farletuzumab, in combination with carboplatin and a taxane, was compared to carboplatin/taxane treatment alone. Unfortunately, the primary endpoint of improved progression-free survival (PFS) was not met; however, subsequent analyses of the data suggested an improved PFS in some patient subgroups given higher doses and in those with lower CA125.[55,56] A second Phase III study compared treatment with paclitaxel alone, or in combination with farletuzumab in patients with platinum-resistant ovarian cancer; however, this trial was discontinued when the prespecified criteria for continuation were not met.

In 2014 the manufacturer of farletuzumab announced the development of a diagnostic assay to identify patients with high FRα expression. It is thought that these patients may demonstrate greater benefit from farletuzumab therapy than those with low levels of FRα expression, suggesting that, in the future, farletuzumab trials may involve the stratification of patients based on their tumor FRα expression.[57]

Furthermore, a Phase II study comparing farletuzumab, combined with carboplatin and paclitaxel, or with carboplatin and pegylated liposomal doxorubicin in patients with low CA125 platinum sensitive ovarian cancer, is currently recruiting (NCT02289950). In addition, a novel approach to targeting FRα has recently entered the clinical arena. MOv18 IgE, a chimeric IgE antibody specific to FRα,[58] was developed to investigate the hypothesis that IgE antibodies may offer advantages over their IgG counterparts as immunotherapeutic agents against cancer.[59,60] A first-in-class Phase I clinical trial of MOv18 IgE in patients with advanced FRα-expressing cancer, including ovarian cancer, has recently opened (NCT02546921).

BEVACIZUMAB

Bevacizumab is a recombinant humanized monoclonal IgG1 antibody that targets all biologically active forms of VEGF-A. Therefore, bevacizumab represents an inhibitor of angiogenesis, which plays a major role in promoting growth and progression of ovarian cancer by increasing ascites formation and metastatic spread.[61] Antibodies against VEGF for the treatment of ovarian carcinoma were initially tested in animals models, where the blocking of VEGF signaling resulted in the inhibition of ascites formation and tumor growth.[61] Moreover, VEGF-specific antibodies are used in combination with CT: normalization of tumor vasculature and decreases in interstitial fluid pressure were observed, resulting in an enhanced delivery of chemotherapeutic drugs.[62]

A Phase I trial and pharmacokinetics study was conducted in 2008 in pediatric patients refractory to standard treatment for solid tumors: patients were infused with bevacizumab on days 1 and 15 of a 28-day course with a starting dose of 5mg/kg, with cohort escalations to 10 and 15 mg/kg. No DLTs were observed and an maximum tolerated dose (MTD) was not defined.[63]

A Phase II trial was conducted to assess the efficacy and the tolerability of bevacizumab as a single agent for the treatment of persistent or recurrent EOC and primary peritoneal cancer (PPC). In this study bevacizumab was administered 15mg/kg i.v. every 21 days, unless a prohibitive toxicity or a progression of the disease was observed. Among 62 patients, two complete responses (CRs) and 11 partial responses (PRs) were observed, while 25 patients were progression-free for at least six months after treatment.[64]

Multiple Phase III trials have been performed to assess bevacizumab efficacy as a single agent or in combination with CT. In 2010 bevacizumab was tested for the primary treatment of advanced EOC, PPC, and fallopian tube cancer (FTC) in 1,873 newly diagnosed patients who did not receive previous CT. This study represented the first randomized Phase III trial demonstrating the efficacy and safety of adding bevacizumab with first-line CT for ovarian cancer. In this study patients were randomized to one of three different arms: (a) CT (paclitaxel and carboplatin) + placebo cycles 2-22; (b) CT + concurrent bevacizumab 15 mg/kg + placebo courses 7–22; (c) CT + concurrent bevacizumab + maintenance bevacizumab during courses 7–22. In terms of PFS, there was no difference between the control arm (a) and the concurrent one (b). The comparison between arms 1 and 3 instead showed a statistically significant difference with a hazard ratio of 0.77 ($p < 0.0001$). Moreover, arm c patients showed an increased PFS of 3.8 months, but no difference in OS was observed. The major AEs were observed during the CT part of the treatment and the overall rate of gastrointestinal (GI)-related events was <3%, comparable to previous studies in GI cancers, showing that the treatment was well-tolerated and that CT with concurrent and maintenance bevacizumab should be considered as standard option for this group of patients.[65] Two more Phase III trials were conducted, ICON7 in 2010 and AURELIA in 2014. The third Phase III randomized trial, ICON7 was conducted by the UK Medical Research Council Clinical Trials Unit on 1,528 women with high-risk, early-stage, or advanced EOC, PPC, or FTC; 90% of them had EOC. Patients were randomly assigned to carboplatin and paclitaxel, given every three weeks for six cycles, or to the same regimen with bevacizumab (7.5mg/kg) administered concurrently every three weeks for five or six cycles and continued until progression of disease. In this study bevacizumab improved the PFS in women with EOC, and the benefits were greater in patients with a higher risk for progression of disease.[66] The AURELIA Phase III trial was started in 2009 and represents the first trial to combine bevacizumab with CT in platinum-resistant ovarian cancer: patients who relapse within six months after platinum-based therapy are considered to have platinum-resistant ovarian cancer. Patients were selected for CT with paclitaxel, pegylated liposomal doxorubicin or topotecan either alone or in combination with bevacizumab 10 mg/kg every two weeks. The study demonstrated a significant improvement in PFS when bevacizumab was added to CT: the median PFS of CT was 3.4 months compared to 6.7 months with bevacizumab.[67]

IMMUNE CHECKPOINT INHIBITORS

Immunotherapy of cancer targeting the immune-checkpoint receptors CTLA4 or PD1 and PDL1 are transforming cancer treatment. In particular, anti-PD1/PDL1 antibodies have demonstrated clinical activity in more than 15 cancer types.[68]

In contrast to the aforementioned therapeutic mAbs that target tumor cells directly, antibodies that block immune checkpoints target lymphocyte receptors or their ligands to enhance endogenous antitumor activity. A key feature of immune checkpoint inhibitors given as monotherapy is their ability to induce durable responses in 10% to 15% of the patients treated.[69-72] This supports the concept that immunotherapies take time to re-educate the immune system, and their tumor-suppressive activity persists long after treatment has ceased.

Anti-CTLA-4 Antibodies

In the immunosuppressive TME, blocking CTLA-4 has the potential to directly activate T cells, leading to tumor clearance. In several preclinical tumor models, the administration of an anti-CTLA-4 antibody induced tumor rejection.[73] Clinically, to date, the majority of data comes from studies in patients with melanoma. Data from these studies formed the basis of the 2011 Food and Drug Administration approval of the first fully human IgG1 anti-CTLA-4 mAb, ipilimumab, to treat metastatic or unresectable melanoma.[74] Experience in ovarian cancer is still in its infancy; however, data are promising (Table 1.2).

In the Phase I/II trial of ipilimumab by Hodi et al., anti-tumor effects were seen in 11 patients with stage IV ovarian carcinoma who had previously either received CT or had been vaccinated with granulocyte-macrophage colony-stimulating factor modified irradiated autologous tumor cells.[75,76] Ipilimumab was generally well tolerated with the exception of grade 3 inflammatory toxicities. Significant anti-tumor effects were noted in one ovarian cancer patient who showed a dramatic fall of serum CA125 levels during treatment with a substantial regression of a large hepatic metastasis, mesenteric lymph nodes, and omental cake.[76] Moreover,

generation of antibody responses to NY-ESO-1 was detectable, and this correlated with the observed therapeutic effects. Another ovarian cancer patient had a reduction in pain and ascites, which correlated with stabilization of CA125 levels. Four other patients had stable disease (SD) as assessed by blood CA125 levels and imaging. Tumor regression correlated with the CD8+/Treg ratio, suggesting that other forms of therapy that target Treg depletion might have a synergistic effect when combined with the tumor vaccine and CTLA-4 antibody molecules. A Phase II study of ipilimumab monotherapy in patients with platinum-sensitive ovarian cancer is ongoing (NCT01611558).

Another antibody targeting CTLA-4 is tremelimumab, a fully human IgG2 mAb. The combination of tremelimumab and poly (ADP-ribose) polymerase inhibition is currently being studied in a Phase I–II study of patients with BRCA-deficient recurrent ovarian cancer (NCT02571725). Furthermore, the combination of tremelimumab and a PD-1 inhibitor (see later discussion) is currently being evaluated in two Phase I clinical trials, both in patients with advanced solid tumors including ovarian cancer (NCT02261220; NCT019755831).[77]

Anti-PD-1 and PD-L1 Antibodies

Conversely to CTLA-4, which regulates T cells at their initial activation, PD-1 regulates immunity at a number of stages, including exerting its effect on effector T-cell activity in peripheral tissues. Specifically in ovarian cancer, expression of PD-L1 on patient blood monocytes and in ascites correlates with poor clinical outcome.[78] In addition, PD-L1 overexpression on murine ovarian cancer ID8 cells has been shown to inhibit cytotoxic T lymphocyte (CTL) degranulation and reduced CTL-mediated tumor lysis, an effect that was reversed on PD-L1 blockade. Several mAbs have been developed that block the PD-1 synapse, either by interactions with

TABLE 1.2 CLINICAL TRIALS OF CHECKPOINT INHIBITOR MONOCLONAL ANTIBODIES FOR OVARIAN CANCER

Name	Phase I	Phase II	Phase III	References
Anti-CTLA4 antibodies				
Ipilimumab	Anti-tumor effects observed in 11 patients with stage IV OC	Ongoing: Ipilimumab monotherapy in patients with platinum-sensitive OC (NCT01611558)	N/A	Hodi et al., 2003[75] Hodi et al., 2008[76]
Tremelimumab	Ongoing: Tremelimumab + PARP-inhibition combination in patients with BRCA-deficient recurrent OC (NCT02571725).	N/A	N/A	-
Anti-PD-1 antibodies				
Nivolumab	Anti-tumor effects observed in 4/17 patients with OC	Single agent nivolumab in platinum-resistant OC: response rate 15%, disease control rate 45%.	NA	Topalian et al., 2012[69] Hamanishi et al., 2015[79]
Pembrolizumab	KEYNOTE-028: PD-L1 expressing advanced OC. Response rate 11.5%, disease control rate 34.6%.	NA	NA	Varga et al., 2015[80]
Anti-PD-L1 antibodies				
Avelumab	Ongoing: Avelumab in patients with recurrent or refractory ovarian cancer (NCT01772004). Anti-tumor effects observed in 15/23 patients	NA	Ongoing: Avelumab vs. avelumab + pegylated liposomal doxorubicin vs. pegylated liposomal doxorubicin in patients with platinum resistant or refractory OC (NCT02580058).	Disis et al., 2015[82]
BMS-936559	Anti-tumor effects observed in 4/17 patients with OC	NA	NA	Brahmer et al., 2012[70]

NOTE: OC = ovarian carcinoma; PARP = poly (ADP-ribose) polymerase.

the PD-1 receptor or with its specific ligands (Table 1.2).

Nivolumab is a fully human IgG4 mAb that targets PD-1. The IgG4 subtype was selected in order to prevent ADCC of T cells. The first Phase I trial of nivolumab in patients with advanced cancer included 17 patients with ovarian cancer.[69] In this study, patients with melanoma achieved the highest rates of objective responses (17.3%). Of the ovarian cancer patients, 1 of 17 (6%) had a PR, and 3 (18%) had SD lasting at least 24 weeks.[69] The first Phase II clinical trial of nivolumab in platinum-resistant ovarian cancer was published in 2015.[79] Twenty patients were treated with nivolumab given i.v. every two weeks at a dose of 1 or 3 mg/kg for up to six cycles. The response rate for the overall study population was 15% (2 CRs and 1 PR), and the disease control rate was 45%. Median PFS was short at 3.5 and 3.0 months in the 1-mg/kg and 3-mg/kg cohorts, respectively. Median OS was 16.1 months in the low-dose arm, but OS data were not yet mature for those treated with the higher dose. The median OS for the total population was 20 months.[79] Interestingly, one of the two patients to experience a CR had a clear cell tumor, which is known to have a worse prognosis than the more common serous ovarian adenocarcinoma and for which there are few effective therapies for recurrent disease.

To identify predictive biomarkers for nivolumab in patients with ovarian cancer, the expression of PD-L1 in ovarian cancer tissues was examined. However, unfortunately, no significant correlation between clinical response and PD-L1 expression was identified.[79]

Another anti-PD-1 antibody evaluated in patients with ovarian cancer is pembrolizumab, a humanized IgG4 mAb, highly selective against PD-1 and designed to block its interaction with PD-L1 and PD-L2. Interim results from a Phase Ib study of pembrolizumab in patients with PD-L1 expressing advanced ovarian cancer (part of KEYNOTE-028) were presented at ASCO 2015.[80] Pembrolizumab 10 mg/kg was given

every two weeks for up to two years or until confirmed progression or unacceptable toxicity. Twenty-six evaluable patients were treated with pembrolizumab, with a confirmed response rate of 11.5% (one patient achieved a CR and two patients experienced PR). Additionally, six patients (23.1%) had SD, for a disease control rate of 34.6%. At the time of analysis, all of the three patients who achieved a response remained in remission with a duration of response ≥ 24 weeks.[80]

In addition to antibodies targeting PD-1, several different anti-PD1-L1 mAbs, including BMS-936559, MSB0010718C, MPDL3280A, and MEDI4736, have also been developed and evaluated in patients with ovarian cancer.

BMS-936559 is a fully human IgG4 mAb that binds PD-L1 and blocks its binding to its two known receptors PD-1 and CD8. In a Phase I trial of BMS-936559 that included 17 patients with ovarian cancer, only those treated at the maximum dose of 10mg/kg achieved objective responses: one (6%) with a PR and three (18%) with SD lasting more than 24 weeks.[70]

MSB0010718C, known as avelumab, is a fully human IgG1 mAb targeting PD-L1. In contrast to other PD-L1 targeting agents, however, avelumab has a functional Fc region by virtue of its IgG1 isotype, enabling ADCC of tumor cells. In a Phase I trial,[81] 27 patients with refractory malignancies, including ovarian cancer, were treated with avelumab twice weekly. In pharmacodynamics studies, at the 3 and 10mg/kg doses, the drug was found to inhibit 93.8% and 93.2% of the PD-L1 receptor on peripheral blood leukocytes, respectively.[81] At the time the study was reported, the data was too immature to comment on efficacy of avelumab. Results from a cohort of patients with recurrent or refractory ovarian cancer in an ongoing Phase Ib study of avelumab (NCT01772004) were reported at ASCO 2015.[82] Patients were given avelumab at 10 mg/kg every two weeks. Of the 23 patients evaluable for efficacy, 4 (17.4%) achieved a PR within 30 weeks of commencing treatment, and 11 (47.8%) had SD.[82] The median PFS was 11.9 weeks. Drug-related AEs were reported in 18 patients, 2 of whom experienced grade ≥ 3 drug-related AEs. The authors concluded that avelumab was clinically active in this heavily pretreated ovarian cancer patient population.[82] Indeed, a Phase III study comparing avelumab alone to avelumab plus pegylated liposomal doxorubicin or to pegylated liposomal doxorubicin alone in patients with platinum resistant or refractory ovarian cancer is currently in setup (NCT02580058).

Other molecules, such as MPDL3280A and MEDI4736, are currently under investigation in Phase I trials including ovarian cancer patients (NCT01375842; NCT02431559; NCT01938612).

Overall, results from larger Phase III studies in patients with ovarian cancer are still required in order to validate the outcomes for checkpoint inhibition described here, particularly with regard to the duration of response seen with these agents. Furthermore, work is needed to evaluate predictive biomarkers and effective combination strategies.

CONCLUSION

In advanced ovarian cancer, optimal debulking surgery is the most important determinant of survival.[83] Over the past 50 years, paclitaxel- and platinum-based CT have produced only incremental improvements in clinical outcomes. Targeted therapies such as monoclonal antibodies and antibody immunotherapy approaches are now emerging and may constitute highly promising approaches to ovarian cancer therapy. However, despite some successes in early- to mid-phase clinical trials, only a single antibody (bevacizumab) has achieved approval for clinical use in ovarian cancer. Further research and new targeted therapeutic approaches are therefore needed to improve patient stratification and target selection, perhaps through discovery of novel biomarkers and predictors of response to treatment. Importantly, emerging

successes in cancer immunotherapy mandate a deeper understanding of patient immune responses to ovarian carcinoma and the mechanisms associated with tumor immune escape.

REFERENCES

1. Cancer Stat Facts: Ovarian Cancer. http://seer.cancer.gov/statfacts/html/ovary.html. Accessed January 25, 2016.
2. Bookman MA, Brady MF, McGuire WP, et al. Evaluation of new platinum-based treatment regimens in advanced-stage ovarian cancer: a Phase III Trial of the Gynecologic Cancer Intergroup. J Clin Oncol. Mar 20 2009;27(9):1419–25.
3. McGuire WP, Hoskins WJ, Brady MF, et al. Cyclophosphamide and cisplatin compared with paclitaxel and cisplatin in patients with stage III and stage IV ovarian cancer. N Engl J Med. Jan 4 1996;334(1):1–6.
4. Ozols RF, Bundy BN, Greer BE, et al. Phase III trial of carboplatin and paclitaxel compared with cisplatin and paclitaxel in patients with optimally resected stage III ovarian cancer: a Gynecologic Oncology Group study. J Clin Oncol. Sep 1 2003;21(17):3194–200.
5. Armstrong DK, Bundy B, Wenzel L, et al. Intraperitoneal cisplatin and paclitaxel in ovarian cancer. N Engl J Med. Jan 5 2006;354(1):34–43.
6. Katsumata N, Yasuda M, Isonishi S, et al. Long-term results of dose-dense paclitaxel and carboplatin versus conventional paclitaxel and carboplatin for treatment of advanced epithelial ovarian, fallopian tube, or primary peritoneal cancer (JGOG 3016): a randomised, controlled, open-label trial. Lancet Oncol. Sep 2013;14(10):1020–26.
7. Aghajanian C, Blank SV, Goff BA, et al. OCEANS: a randomized, double-blind, placebo-controlled phase III trial of chemotherapy with or without bevacizumab in patients with platinum-sensitive recurrent epithelial ovarian, primary peritoneal, or fallopian tube cancer. J Clin Oncol. Jun 10 2012;30(17):2039–45.
8. Ledermann J, Harter P, Gourley C, et al. Olaparib maintenance therapy in platinum-sensitive relapsed ovarian cancer. N Engl J Med. Apr 12 2012;366(15):1382–92.
9. Huang L, Cronin KA, Johnson KA, Mariotto AB, Feuer EJ. Improved survival time: what can survival cure models tell us about population-based survival improvements in late-stage colorectal, ovarian, and testicular cancer? Cancer. May 15 2008;112(10):2289–300.
10. Zhang L, Conejo-Garcia JR, Katsaros D, et al. Intratumoral T cells, recurrence, and survival in epithelial ovarian cancer. N Engl J Med. Jan 16 2003;348(3):203–13.

11. Janeway CTP, Walport M, Shlomchik M. *Immunobiology: the immune system in health and disease*. New York: Garland; 2005.

12. Lund FE, Randall TD. Effector and regulatory B cells: modulators of CD4+ T cell immunity. *Nat Rev Immunol*. Apr 2010;10(4):236–47.

13. Hurwitz H. Integrating the anti-VEGF-A humanized monoclonal antibody bevacizumab with chemotherapy in advanced colorectal cancer. *Clin Colorectal Cancer*. Oct 2004;4(Suppl. 2):S62–S68.

14. Hicklin DJ, Ellis LM. Role of the vascular endothelial growth factor pathway in tumor growth and angiogenesis. *J Clin Oncol*. Feb 10 2005;23(5):1011–27.

15. Franklin MC, Carey KD, Vajdos FF, Leahy DJ, de Vos AM, Sliwkowski MX. Insights into ErbB signaling from the structure of the ErbB2-pertuzumab complex. *Cancer Cell*. Apr 2004;5(4):317–28.

16. Romond EH, Perez EA, Bryant J, et al. Trastuzumab plus adjuvant chemotherapy for operable HER2-positive breast cancer. *N Engl J Med*. Oct 20 2005;353(16):1673–84.

17. Bonner JA, Harari PM, Giralt J, et al. Radiotherapy plus cetuximab for squamous-cell carcinoma of the head and neck. *N Engl J Med*. Feb 9 2006;354(6):567–78.

18. Van Cutsem E, Kohne CH, Lang I, et al. Cetuximab plus irinotecan, fluorouracil, and leucovorin as first-line treatment for metastatic colorectal cancer: updated analysis of overall survival according to tumor KRAS and BRAF mutation status. *J Clin Oncol*. May 20 2011;29(15):2011–19.

19. Gibson TB, Ranganathan A, Grothey A. Randomized Phase III trial results of panitumumab, a fully human anti-epidermal growth factor receptor monoclonal antibody, in metastatic colorectal cancer. *Clin Colorectal Cancer*. May 2006;6(1):29–31.

20. Hudis CA. Trastuzumab—mechanism of action and use in clinical practice. *N Engl J Med*. Jul 5 2007;357(1):39–51.

21. Dancey G, Begent RH, Meyer T. Imaging in targeted delivery of therapy to cancer. *Target Oncol*. Sep 2009;4(3):201–17.

22. Meyer T, Gaya AM, Dancey G, et al. A phase I trial of radioimmunotherapy with 131I-A5B7 anti-CEA antibody in combination with combretastatin-A4-phosphate in advanced gastrointestinal carcinomas. *Clin Cancer Res*. Jul 1 2009;15(13):4484–92.

23. Junutula JR, Flagella KM, Graham RA, et al. Engineered thio-trastuzumab-DM1 conjugate with an improved therapeutic index to target human epidermal growth factor receptor 2-positive breast cancer. *Clin Cancer Res*. Oct 1 2010;16(19):4769–78.

24. FitzGerald DJ, Wayne AS, Kreitman RJ, Pastan I. Treatment of hematologic malignancies with immunotoxins and antibody-drug conjugates. *Cancer Res*. Oct 15 2011;71(20):6300–9.

25. Iannello A, Ahmad A. Role of antibody-dependent cell-mediated cytotoxicity in the efficacy of therapeutic anti-cancer monoclonal antibodies. *Cancer Metastasis Rev*. Dec 2005;24(4):487–99.

26. Nahta R, Esteva FJ. Trastuzumab: triumphs and tribulations. *Oncogene*. May 28 2007;26(25):3637–43.

27. Karagiannis P, Singer J, Hunt J, et al. Characterisation of an engineered trastuzumab IgE antibody and effector cell mechanisms targeting HER2/neu-positive tumour cells. *Cancer Immunol Immunother*. Jun 2009;58(6):915–30.

28. Lazar GA, Dang W, Karki S, et al. Engineered antibody Fc variants with enhanced effector function. *Proc Natl Acad Sci U S A*. Mar 14 2006;103(11):4005–10.

29. Clynes RA, Towers TL, Presta LG, Ravetch JV. Inhibitory Fc receptors modulate in vivo cytotoxicity against tumor targets. *Nat Med*. Apr 2000;6(4):443–46.

30. Wang SY, Weiner G. Complement and cellular cytotoxicity in antibody therapy of cancer. *Expert Opin Biol Ther*. Jun 2008;8(6):759–68.

31. Kaul TN, Faden H, Baker R, Ogra PL. Virus-induced complement activation and neutrophil-mediated cytotoxicity against respiratory syncytial virus (RSV). *Clin Exp Immunol*. Jun 1984;56(3):501–8.

32. Abes R, Teillaud JL. Modulation of tumor immunity by therapeutic monoclonal antibodies. *Cancer Metastasis Rev*. Mar 2011;30(1):111–24.

33. de Bono JS, Rha SY, Stephenson J, et al. Phase I trial of a murine antibody to MUC1 in patients with metastatic cancer: evidence for the activation of humoral and cellular antitumor immunity. *Ann Oncol*. Dec 2004;15(12):1825–33.

34. Taylor C, Hershman D, Shah N, et al. Augmented HER-2 specific immunity during treatment with trastuzumab and chemotherapy. *Clin Cancer Res*. Sep 1 2007;13(17):5133–43.

35. Selenko N, Maidic O, Draxier S, et al. CD20 antibody (C2B8)-induced apoptosis of lymphoma cells promotes phagocytosis by dendritic cells and cross-priming of CD8+ cytotoxic T cells. *Leukemia*. Oct 2001;15(10):1619–26.

36. Selenko N, Majdic O, Jager U, Sillaber C, Stockl J, Knapp W. Cross-priming of cytotoxic T cells promoted by apoptosis-inducing tumor cell reactive antibodies? *J Clin Immunol*. May 2002;22(3):124–30.

37. Ribas A. Releasing the brakes on cancer immunotherapy. *N Engl J Med*. Oct 15 2015;373(16):1490–92.

38. Harris NL, Ronchese F. The role of B7 costimulation in T-cell immunity. *Immunol Cell Biol*. Aug 1999;77(4):304–11.

39. Bellati F, Napoletano C, Gasparri ML, et al. Monoclonal antibodies in gynecological cancer: a critical point of view clinical and developmental immunology. *Clin Dev Immunol*. 2011;2011(9):1–16.

40. Leone Roberti Maggiore U, Bellati F, Ruscito I, et al. Monoclonal antibodies therapies for ovarian cancer. *Expert Opin Biol Ther*. May 2013;13(5):739–64.

41. Greenwald RJ, Freeman GJ, Sharpe AH. The B7 family revisited. *Annu Rev Immunol*. 2005;23:515–48.

42. Yang A, Kendle RF, Ginsberg BA, Roman R, Heine AI, Pogoriler E. CTLA-4 blockade with ipilimumab

increases peripheral CD8+ T cells: correlation with clinical outcomes. *J Clin Oncol.* 2010;28:2555.

43. Hirano F, Kaneko K, Tamura H, et al. Blockade of B7-H1 and PD-1 by monoclonal antibodies potentiates cancer therapeutic immunity. *Cancer Res.* Feb 1 2005;65(3):1089–96.

44. Hoffmann P, Hofmeister R, Brischwein K, et al. Serial killing of tumor cells by cytotoxic T cells redirected with a CD19-/CD3-bispecific single-chain antibody construct. *Int J Cancer.* May 20 2005;115(1):98–104.

45. Burges A, Wimberger P, Kumper C, et al. Effective relief of malignant ascites in patients with advanced ovarian cancer by a trifunctional anti-EpCAM x anti-CD3 antibody: a Phase I/II study. *Clin Cancer Res.* Jul 1 2007;13(13):3899–905.

46. Heiss MM, Murawa P, Koralewski P, et al. The trifunctional antibody catumaxomab for the treatment of malignant ascites due to epithelial cancer: results of a prospective randomized Phase II/III trial. *Int J Cancer.* Nov 1 2010;127(9):2209–21.

47. Ebel W, Routhier EL, Foley B, et al. Preclinical evaluation of MORAb-003, a humanized monoclonal antibody antagonizing folate receptor-alpha. *Cancer Immun.* 2007;7:6.

48. Lin J, Spidel JL, Maddage CJ, et al. The antitumor activity of the human FOLR1-specific monoclonal antibody, farletuzumab, in an ovarian cancer mouse model is mediated by antibody-dependent cellular cytotoxicity. *Cancer Biol Ther.* Nov 2013;14(11):1032–38.

49. Thomas A, Maltzman J, Hassan R. Farletuzumab in lung cancer. *Lung Cancer.* Apr 2013;80(1):15–18.

50. Wen Y, Graybill WS, Previs RA, et al. Immunotherapy targeting folate receptor induces cell death associated with autophagy in ovarian cancer. *Clin Cancer Res.* Jan 15 2015;21(2):448–59.

51. Kamen BA, Smith AK. Farletuzumab, an anti-folate receptor alpha antibody, does not block binding of folate or anti-folates to receptor nor does it alter the potency of anti-folates in vitro. *Cancer Chemother Pharmacol.* Jul 2012;70(1):113–20.

52. Konner JA, Bell-McGuinn KM, Sabbatini P, et al. Farletuzumab, a humanized monoclonal antibody against folate receptor alpha, in epithelial ovarian cancer: a Phase I study. *Clin Cancer Res.* Nov 1 2010;16(21):5288–95.

53. Kim KH, Jelovac D, Armstrong DK, et al. Phase 1b safety study of farletuzumab, carboplatin and pegylated liposomal doxorubicin in patients with platinum-sensitive epithelial ovarian cancer. *Gynecol Oncol.* Feb 2016;140(2):210–14.

54. Armstrong DK, White AJ, Weil SC, Phillips M, Coleman RL. Farletuzumab (a monoclonal antibody against folate receptor alpha) in relapsed platinum-sensitive ovarian cancer. *Gynecol Oncol.* Jun 2013;129(3):452–58.

55. Vergote I, Armstrong D, Scambia G, Fujiwara K, Gorbunova V, Schweizer C. Phase III double-blind, placebo-controlled study of weekly farletuzumab with carboplatin/taxane in subjects with platinum-sensitive ovarian cancer in first relapse. *Int J Gynecol Cancer.* 2013;23(8 Suppl. 1):11.

56. Vergote IB, Marth C, Coleman RL. Role of the folate receptor in ovarian cancer treatment: evidence, mechanism, and clinical implications. *Cancer Metastasis Rev.* Mar 2015;34(1):41–52.

57. Marchetti C, Palaia I, Giorgini M, et al. Targeted drug delivery via folate receptors in recurrent ovarian cancer: a review. *Onco Targets Ther.* 2014;7:1223–36.

58. Gould HJ, Mackay GA, Karagiannis SN, et al. Comparison of IgE and IgG antibody-dependent cytotoxicity in vitro and in a SCID mouse xenograft model of ovarian carcinoma. *Eur J Immunol.* Nov 1999;29(11):3527–37.

59. Karagiannis SN, Josephs DH, Karagiannis P, et al. Recombinant IgE antibodies for passive immunotherapy of solid tumours: from concept towards clinical application. *Cancer Immunol Immunother.* Sep 2012;61(9):1547–64.

60. Josephs DH, Spicer JF, Karagiannis P, Gould HJ, Karagiannis SN. IgE immunotherapy: a novel concept with promise for the treatment of cancer. *MAbs.* Jan-Feb 2014;6(1):54–72.

61. Byrne AT, Ross L, Holash J, et al. Vascular endothelial growth factor-trap decreases tumor burden, inhibits ascites, and causes dramatic vascular remodeling in an ovarian cancer model. *Clin Cancer Res.* Nov 15 2003;9(15):5721–28.

62. Jain RK. Antiangiogenic therapy for cancer: current and emerging concepts. *Oncology.* Apr 2005;19(4 Suppl. 3):7–16.

63. Glade Bender JL, Adamson PC, Reid JM, et al. Phase I trial and pharmacokinetic study of bevacizumab in pediatric patients with refractory solid tumors: a Children's Oncology Group Study. *J Clin Oncol.* Jan 20 2008;26(3):399–405.

64. Burger RA, Sill MW, Monk BJ, Greer BE, Sorosky JI. Phase II trial of bevacizumab in persistent or recurrent epithelial ovarian cancer or primary peritoneal cancer: a Gynecologic Oncology Group Study. *J Clin Oncol.* Nov 20 2007;25(33):5165–71.

65. Burger RA. Role of vascular endothelial growth factor inhibitors in the treatment of gynecologic malignancies. *J Gynecol Oncol.* Mar 2010;21(1):3–11.

66. Perren TJ, Swart AM, Pfisterer J, et al. A Phase 3 trial of bevacizumab in ovarian cancer. *N Engl J Med.* Dec 29 2011;365(26):2484–96.

67. Pujade-Lauraine E, Hilpert F, Weber B, et al. Bevacizumab combined with chemotherapy for platinum-resistant recurrent ovarian cancer: the AURELIA open-label randomized Phase III trial. *J Clin Oncol.* May 1 2014;32(13):1302–08.

68. Smyth MJ, Ngiow SF, Ribas A, Teng MW. Combination cancer immunotherapies tailored to the tumour microenvironment. *Nat Rev Clin Oncol.* Mar 2016;13(3):143–58.

69. Topalian SL, Hodi FS, Brahmer JR, et al. Safety, activity, and immune correlates of anti-PD-1 antibody in cancer. *N Engl J Med.* Jun 28 2012;366(26):2443–54.

70. Brahmer JR, Tykodi SS, Chow LQ, et al. Safety and activity of anti-PD-L1 antibody in patients with advanced cancer. *N Engl J Med.* Jun 28 2012;366(26):2455–65.

71. Schadendorf D, Hodi FS, Robert C, et al. Pooled analysis of long-term survival data from Phase II and Phase III trials of ipilimumab in unresectable or metastatic melanoma. *J Clin Oncol.* Jun 10 2015;33(17):1889–94.

72. Eroglu Z, Kim DW, Wang X, et al. Long term survival with cytotoxic T lymphocyte-associated antigen 4 blockade using tremelimumab. *Eur J Cancer.* Nov 2015;51(17):2689–97.

73. Egen JG, Kuhns MS, Allison JP. CTLA-4: new insights into its biological function and use in tumor immunotherapy. *Nat Immunol.* Jul 2002;3(7):611–18.

74. Hodi FS, O'Day SJ, McDermott DF, et al. Improved survival with ipilimumab in patients with metastatic melanoma. *N Engl J Med.* Aug 19 2010;363(8):711–23.

75. Hodi FS, Mihm MC, Soiffer RJ, et al. Biologic activity of cytotoxic T lymphocyte-associated antigen 4 antibody blockade in previously vaccinated metastatic melanoma and ovarian carcinoma patients. *Proc Natl Acad Sci U S A.* Apr 15 2003;100(8):4712–17.

76. Hodi FS, Butler M, Oble DA, et al. Immunologic and clinical effects of antibody blockade of cytotoxic T lymphocyte-associated antigen 4 in previously vaccinated cancer patients. *Proc Natl Acad Sci U S A.* Feb 26 2008;105(8):3005–10.

77. Callahan MK, Ott PA, Odunsi K, et al. A Phase 1 study to evaluate the safety and tolerability of MEDI4736, an anti–PD-L1 antibody, in combination with tremelimumab in patients with advanced solid tumors. *J Clin Oncol.* 2014;32(5s):Abstract TPS3120.

78. Maine CJ, Aziz NH, Chatterjee J, et al. Programmed death ligand-1 over-expression correlates with malignancy and contributes to immune regulation in ovarian cancer. *Cancer Immunol Immunother.* Mar 2014;63(3):215–24.

79. Hamanishi J, Mandai M, Ikeda T, et al. Safety and antitumor activity of anti-PD-1 antibody, nivolumab, in patients with platinum-resistant ovarian cancer. *J Clin Oncol.* Dec 1 2015;33(34):4015–22.

80. Varga A, Piha-Paul SA, Ott PA. Antitumour activity and safety of pembrolizumab in patients (pts) with PD-L1 positive advanced ovarian cancer: interim results from a Phase Ib study. *J Clin Oncol.* 2015;33:Abstract 5510.

81. Heery CR, Coyne GH, Madan RA, et al. Phase I open-label, multiple ascending dose trial of MSB0010718C, an anti-PD-L1 monoclonal antibody, in advanced solid malignancies. *J Clin Oncol.* 2014;32:5s (Abstract 3064).

82. Disis ML, Patel MR, Pant S, et al. Avelumab (MSB0010718C), an anti-PD-L1 antibody, in patients with previously treated, recurrent or refractory ovarian cancer: A Phase Ib, open-label expansion trial. *J Clin Oncol.* 2015;33(15 Suppl.):5509.

83. Bristow RE, Gossett DR, Shook DR, et al. Recurrent micropapillary serous ovarian carcinoma. *Cancer.* Aug 15 2002;95(4):791–800.

2.

BIOLOGICAL ASPECTS AND CLINICAL APPLICATIONS OF SERUM BIOMARKERS IN OVARIAN CANCER

Rouba Ali-Fehmi and Eman Abdulfatah

INTRODUCTION

Ovarian carcinoma is the most aggressive gynecological malignancy, with 22,280 new cases and 14,240 deaths estimated in the United States in 2015,[1] accounting for 4% of all cancers diagnosed and 4.2% of all cancer deaths in women worldwide.[2] According to the cancer statistics of 2016, ovarian carcinoma ranks fifth among the most lethal cancers.[1] At early-stage disease, patients are mostly asymptomatic which results in the majority of the cases presenting at advanced stage with metastatic disease. Over 70% of women are diagnosed with International Federation of Gynecology and Obstetrics (FIGO) stages III to IV at presentation. The dualistic model of ovarian carcinogenesis established on the basis of the molecular profile divides this tumor into two broad subtypes, defined as type I and type II. Type I consists of low-grade serous, low-grade endometrioid, clear cell, mucinous, and Brenner tumors (Figure 2.1). Tumors under this category are less aggressive with early-stage disease confined within the ovaries and harbor multiple somatic mutations such as PTEN, KRAS, BRAF, CTNNB, PIK3CA, PPP2R1A, ARID1A, and rarely P53.[3,4] Type II tumors include high-grade serous, high-grade endometrioid, malignant mixed mullerian tumor, and undifferentiated carcinoma.

These tumors show more aggressive behavior and harbor P53 gene mutations in more than 95% of cases.[5] A five-year overall survival rate of less than 20% has been reported in advanced-stage disease; however, surgery and chemotherapy can cure up to 90% of patients if diagnosed in stage I. Therefore, diagnosis at an early stage is the most important determinant of survival. The current diagnostic tools used in clinics show limited success in early detection and hence the need for new diagnostic biomarkers. A biomarker is a measurable or assessable entity that provides prognostic, diagnostic, or treatment response information that can drive patient care. The National Cancer Institute's Early Detection Research Network described a five-step system for biomarker discovery and evaluation: preclinical exploration to identify promising candidate biomarkers, a clinical assay to determine the ability of the test to detect the disease, a retrospective determination of the biomarker's ability to detect preclinical disease, a prospective screening to identify the extent and characteristics of disease detected by the test, and the impact of screening on reducing burden of disease on the population.[6] Ideally, biomarker-based screening tests must have several key characteristics: the test used must be easy to administer; the biomarker should be present in accessible specimens including body fluids, urine, blood, or serum;

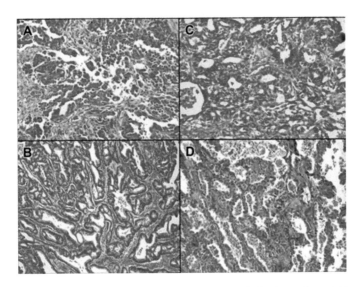

Figure 2.1 (A) Ovarian serous carcinoma. (B) Ovarian mucinous carcinoma. (C) Ovarian endometrioid carcinoma. (D) Ovarian clear cell carcinoma. (H and E stain, 20x).

and the test must be sensitive and specific. However, because of the low prevalence of ovarian carcinoma, screening tests with the highest specificity would have a low positive predictive value and a high false positive rate. This may indicate the need for targeting the screening for high-risk populations. With the advance of techniques in genomic and proteomics, numerous biomarkers are emerging which may serve as a platform for early detection of ovarian cancer.

CURRENT SERUM BIOMARKER IN CLINICAL USE: CA-125

EARLY DETECTION OF OVARIAN CARCINOMA

CA-125, the most commonly used serum biomarker for the evaluation of women presenting with pelvic mass, is a high molecular weight glycoprotein produced primarily by mesothelial cells lining the peritoneum, pleural, and pericardial cavities. The CA-125 antigen complex contains two major domains, A and B. A portion of the extracellular domain binds OC125 and M11 monoclonal antibodies. The original CA125 reacts with OC125 and the new CA125 II

reacts with both moieties. While serum levels of CA-125 are elevated in almost 80% of patients with ovarian carcinoma, elevations can be also seen in common benign conditions including endometriosis, pelvic inflammatory diseases, pregnancy, and leiomyomas as well as liver cirrhosis and peritonitis. Furthermore, serum levels vary according to the menopausal status; premenopausal women show higher levels.[7,8] Moreover, CA-125 can be elevated in other cancers involving the endometrium, breast, pancreas, gastrointestinal system, and lung. Therefore, the sensitivity and specificity for screening and early detection of ovarian carcinoma is low when used alone. The cutoffs used may range from 20 to 200 U/ml with the commonly used ones being ≤ 35 and < 20 for CA125 and CA125 II, respectively. A metanalysis of six studies using the cutoff of < 35U/ml for CA125 showed a sensitivity of 50% to 74% and 69% to 87%, and a specificity of 69% to 78% and 81% to 93% in premenopausal and menopausal patients, respectively. The lower specificity and sensitivity in premenopausal may be secondary to other factors (as listed previously) causing elevated CA125 in this age group. Hence, the American College of Obstetricians and

Gynecologists recommends using a higher cutoff (>200) for the premenopausal age group for referral to a gynecologic oncologist. To augment its value for screening, CA-125 has been combined with transvaginal ultrasonography. Using the CA125 level, ultrasound findings and the patient's age, a Risk of Malignancy Index is created (a product of the three factors) and if ≥ 200, the patient should be referred to a gynecologic oncologist. Studies have also shown that combining CA125 with additional biomarkers is more effective.[9,10] For example, CA125 is combined with Human Epididymis 4 (HE4) in a Risk of Malignancy Algorithm (ROMA) which was approved by the Food and Drug Administration (FDA) in 2011 for assessing the likelihood of malignancy in patients planning for surgery. A ROMA score of ≥13.1% and 27.7% denotes a higher risk of malignancy in premenopausal and menopausal patients, respectively.

PROGNOSTIC VALUE AND SURVEILLANCE FOR RECURRENCE

The predictive value of preoperative CA-125 levels on prognosis remain controversial. While some studies report no prognostic significance,[11,12] others document a poor prognostic value, independent of tumor stage.[13,14] Changes in CA-125 levels can also correlate with progression of the disease in the majority of the cases.[15] In addition, serum CA-125 concentrations have been useful in monitoring chemotherapy responses. A decline during chemotherapy treatment is considered a favorable prognosis, and serial measurements of CA-125 levels is an indicator of therapeutic outcomes and for assessing disease stabilization.[16,17]

INFLAMMATORY MARKERS AND OVARIAN CARCINOMA

The role of inflammation in ovarian carcinogenesis has been proposed in the ovulation theory. During ovulation, rupture of ovarian surface epithelium leads to an inflammatory reaction with subsequent cell damage, proliferation, and increased potential for aberrant DNA repair, tumor-suppressor gene inactivation, and eventually mutagenesis.[18]

Tumor-promoting inflammation has been recently established as a hallmark of cancer.[19] Cytokine levels in the serum have been investigated as prognostic and diagnostic markers in ovarian carcinoma. Ascitic fluids from women with advanced-stage ovarian serous carcinoma serves as an inflammatory milieu that is rich in inflammatory promoting factors such as proinflammatory cytokines, chemokines, and growth factors.[20] Such inflammatory environment results in drug resistance. A recent multiplex cytokine profiling in the ascitic fluid of patients with ovarian carcinomas revealed several inflammatory markers including interleukin-6 (IL-6), IL-6R, IL-8, IL-10, leptin, and urokinase plasminogen activator.[21] Furthermore, IL-6 has been shown to be an independent prognostic factor for worse outcome by contributing to disease progression through increased migration and invasion, stimulation of angiogenesis and cell proliferation, and inhibition of apoptosis.

C-reactive protein (CRP) is an inflammatory marker that is believed to be associated with increased risk for epithelial cancers including liver, lung, colon, and endometrium. CRP is synthesized in the liver under the influence of Il-6 which induces cell proliferation and hinders apoptosis in breast, colon, and prostate cell lines.[22] Associations of inflammatory markers with ovarian cancer risk varies between histologic subtypes. Studies have shown that inflammation particularly may be strongly associated with tumors of serous histology that may arise from the fallopian tube fimbriae, induced by chronic intratubal inflammation.[23] Additionally, these associations vary between type I and type II tumor, with high-grade serous carcinomas being linked to inflammatory markers.[24]

BIOMARKERS AND HISTOLOGIC SUBTYPES OF OVARIAN CANCER

Several cancer biomarkers specific to different ovarian carcinoma histologic subtypes have been described. CA-125 is mostly associated with high-grade serous carcinomas, the most prevalent and aggressive subtype, whereas other subtypes show minimal expression.[25,26] Carcinoembryonic antigen, on the other hand, is highly expressed in mucinous carcinomas.[27] Matrix metalloproteinases (MMPs), produced in response to growth factor and cytokines signaling, are found to be associated with serous ovarian carcinomas, particularly MMP-2, MMP-7, and MMP-9.[28,29] Expression of MMP-7 and MMP-14 has been also identified in mucinous and clear cell carcinomas, respectively. Vascular endothelial growth factor was found to be highly expressed in serous and clear cell carcinomas and was proposed as a potential therapeutic target for these tumors.[30]

GENOMICS AND OVARIAN CANCER BIOMARKERS

Ovarian carcinomas are thought to arise from environmental factors, genetic alterations, or a combination of both. While the majority of ovarian cancers occur as a result of accumulation of genetic alterations, the specific genetic pathways for the development of both borderline and malignant ovarian tumors remain unclear. Given the relation between genetic changes and ovarian tumorigenesis, studies at the molecular level (including polymerase chain reaction, sequencing and fluorescent in situ hybridization, among others) yielded potential ovarian cancer biomarkers (Table 2.1).

INHERITED GENETIC ALTERATIONS

It is estimated that between 10% and 15% of ovarian cancers are associated with an underlying hereditary syndrome, with up to 90% of these attributed to BRCA1 and

TABLE 2.1 POTENTIAL GENE-BASED BIOMARKERS FOR OVARIAN CARCINOMA

Biomarkers	
Inherited genetic alterations	BRCA1 and BRCA2
	MMR protein loss (MLH1, PMS2, MSH2, and MSH6)
Gene expression profiles	Prostasin, mesothelin, osteopontin, HE4, epithelial cell adhesion molecule and kallikrein 10, folate receptor 1 (FOLR1), cyclin D1 (CCND1), collagen type XVIII a1 (COL18A1), and claudin 3 (CLDN3)

BRCA2 alterations;[31] almost all of the remainder are attributable to Lynch syndrome/hereditary nonpolyposis colorectal cancer.[32] BRCA1 and BRCA2 are tumor suppressor proteins that play an important role in the repair of damaged DNA. Germline mutations in BRCAs (frameshift or nonsense) confer a high risk of developing breast and ovarian carcinomas. Over the last decade, genetic testing for these mutations has gained importance as diagnostic and biomarker tools as well as a guide for treatment decision-making at the time of cancer diagnosis. Patients with BRCA mutated ovarian carcinomas tend to show better response to platinum- based chemotherapeutic agents.[33] Furthermore, testing for the BRCA genetic status in young women with a positive family history provides valuable information for personalized follow-up recommendations and therapy decisions; regular surveillance with CA125 and transvaginal ultrasound every six months until prophylactic salpingo-oopherectomy is performed at the age of 40 is the currently accepted recommendation.[34]

Platinum-based drugs and paclitaxel are landmarks in the treatment of ovarian carcinoma; however, little progress in the results of first-line treatment has been well documented. Development of maintenance therapy to delay disease progression and retreatment with chemotherapy are new therapeutic strategies. This is particularly achieved through inhibition of angiogenesis[35,36] and DNA repair pathways. The latter is exemplified by poly (ADP-ribose) polymerase (PARP) inhibitors which are crucial enzymes activated in response to single-strand DNA damage. It was originally thought that PARP inhibitors could be used augment chemotherapy; however, it is recently hypothesized that the survival of cells with homozygous BRCA1 and BRCA2 gene mutations is impaired significantly by PARP inhibitors. Several PARP inhibitors are being investigated in ovarian cancer. Olaparib is the first-line therapeutic agent to be licensed for the treatment of recurrent ovarian carcinomas that harbor BRCA1 and BRCA2 gene mutations. Many other PARP inhibitors are now under clinical trials for maintenance therapy in combination with chemotherapy as well as other molecular targeted therapies.

Microsatellites (short tandem repeats) are sequences of DNA made up of repeating units of one to six base pairs in length, distributed throughout the genome, which play an important role in preventing DNA alterations (noncomplementary base match) that occur during DNA replication (i.e., mismatch repair system). Many proteins encoded by genes responsible for microsatellites are involved in this system, but the four most common DNA mismatch repair proteins are hMLH-1, hPMS2, hMSH2, and hMSH6 (Figure 2.2). DNA mismatch repair gene inactivation, either through germ-line mutations in Lynch syndrome or through MLH-1 promoter methylation in sporadic tumors, results in variation in the size of nucleotide repeats throughout the genome, a phenomenon referred to as microsatellite instability (MSI).[37] Women with MSI have a 9% to 12% increased lifetime risk of developing ovarian cancer, as well as a 40% to 60% lifetime increased risk for endometrial cancer.[38] Mismatch repair defect–associated ovarian carcinoma tend to occur in younger females[39] and is significantly higher in endometriosis-associated subtypes, namely endometrioid and clear cell carcinomas. Patients present with low grade and low stage tumors as well as increased incidence of synchronous endometrial carcinomas. Evaluation for the presence of hereditary cancer syndromes provides options for tailored screening and prevention strategies that may reduce morbidity associated with the development of these malignancies. Identifying epithelial ovarian tumors with mismatch repair defects is not only important for early detection of women with Lynch syndrome but may also

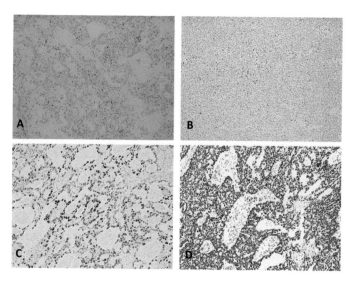

Figure 2.2 Immunohistochemical stain demonstrating: (A) Loss of MSH2 (200X). (B) Loss of MSH6 (200X). (C) Intact MLH 1 (200X). (D) Intact PMS2 (200X).

have treatment implications. Several studies suggest a relation between mismatch repair defects and decreased susceptibility to cisplatin, a common chemotherapeutic agent used to treat ovarian carcinomas.

GENE EXPRESSION PROFILING

By comparing the gene expression between normal and malignant cells, genes that are differentially regulated in cancer development can be identified. Several methods have been used in studying the expression of genes; microarray technology and Serial Analysis of Gene Expression (SAGE) are the most commonly used in ovarian carcinoma. The use of microarray technology enabled the simultaneous detection of expression levels of thousands of genes in a single tissue sample and therefore is promising for tumor diagnosis. Microarray data can be also used to categorize tumors based on their transcriptional profile, providing important prognostic information as well as helping to predict response to therapeutic agents.[40] Several microarray studies have generated a number of potential biomarkers; prostasin,[41] mesothelin,[42] osteopontin,[43] HE4,[44] epithelial cell adhesion molecule,[45] and kallikrein 10.[46]

SAGE represents another technology for quantitative analysis of gene expression in ovarian carcinoma. The advantage of this technology over the traditional microarray is its capability of detecting the expression of novel transcripts and therefore identifying previously uncharacterized genes. These include folate receptor 1 (FOLR1), cyclin D1 (CCND1), collagen type XVIII a1 (COL18A1), and claudin 3 (CLDN3).[47]

Human Epididymis Protein 4

HE4 is a member of the whey acidic four disulfide core family of proteins and is found to be overexpressed in ovarian cancer. Its high sensitivity and specificity when combined with CA125 shows great promise in early detection of ovarian carcinoma.[48] The FDA has approved its use as a tumor marker for monitoring relapse or progression of the disease with the reference range at ≤ 150pM.[49]

In early-stage disease (stage I), HE4 demonstrated the highest sensitivity but was only 45% to 90% specific. As mentioned previously, together with CA125 (ROMA), HE4 comprises a promising biomarker panel for early detection and risk stratification of ovarian cancer.[50,53]

Prostasin

Prostasin, a serine protease, is normally secreted by the prostate gland and was originally isolated from the seminal fluid.[54] Its presence in high levels in the prostate gland and seminal fluid suggests its physiologic role during fertilization; activation of other proteases, and liquefaction of semen. Prostasin is also expressed at a lower level in other organs including liver, kidney, pancreas, salivary gland, lung, bronchus, and colon; however, its functions in these organs are not fully determined. Studies have shown significant high expression of prostasin in epithelial ovarian cancer cells and stroma when compared to normal ovarian tissue.[41] When measured postoperatively, prostasin levels were found to be significantly lower than preoperative levels. When combined with CA125, the sensitivity and specificity for detecting ovarian cancer is 92% and 94%, respectively, and therefore could be used for screening or as a tumor marker, alone or in combination with CA125 in ovarian cancer.

Epithelial Cell Adhesion Molecule

Ep-CAM, a cell adhesion molecule, is involved in the signaling pathway related to differentiation, proliferation, and apoptosis[55] and is found to be low in normal ovarian surface epithelial cells but highly overexpressed in ovarian carcinoma.[56] Using a combination of Ep-CAM autoantibody and CA125 was found to be more specific than using CA125 alone; therefore Ep-CAM autoantibody may be valuable in ovarian cancer screening.

Mesothelin

Mesothelin, a glycoprotein present on mesothelial cells lining the peritoneum, pleura, and pericardium, is overexpressed in most epithelial ovarian cancers and could be a potential target for cancer therapy.[42] Age, BMI, talc usage, and smoking are factors that influence the levels of mesothelin, CA125, and HE4 expression. Studies have shown that mesothelin/CA125 interaction may play a role in peritoneal metastasis of ovarian carcinoma.[57] Combining mesothelin and CA125 provides a greater sensitivity for early detection of ovarian carcinoma.[58]

Kallikreins

The human kallikrein gene family (KLK), present on chromosome 19, is composed of 15 genes that encodes low molecular mass serine proteases, which dysregulate different types of cancers including ovarian carcinomas among others, affecting prognosis. Kallikreins functions in multiple physiologic and pathologic processes, including smooth muscle contractions, hormone regulation, vascular growth/repair, and blood pressure.[59] Their genetic polymorphisms including sequence and splice variants are associated with increased risk for many cancers including ovarian, and therefore may play a potential role as diagnostic, prognostic, and predictive biomarkers.

KLK4-8, KLK10-11, and KLK13-15 were shown to be upregulated in ovarian tissue and serum of patients with ovarian cancer. High levels of KLK4 is associated with the progression of ovarian cancer, particularly late-stage serous carcinomas, and hence KLK4 represents a potential biomarker for diagnosis and prognosis.[60,61] KLK4 and KLK5 tend to be associated with poor outcome in grade 1 and 2 tumors, reflecting their association with aggressive forms of cancer.

KLK6 was reported to be a novel biomarker for ovarian cancer diagnosis as well as association with advanced stage disease, good response to chemotherapy, serous histology, and disease-free survival.[62,63] KLK6 shows better specificity than CA125 for early detection of ovarian carcinoma; however, it is less sensitive as compared to CA125. When used in combination, KLK6 and CA125 show significantly increased sensitivity. Preoperative KLK6 serum levels of > 4.4 ug/L carry worse prognosis than lower preoperative serum levels.

Another important member of the KLK family, KLK7, is a serine protease that has been known to play a role in the desquamation of plantar stratum corneum and catalyzes desmosome degradation in the deeper skin layers during reconstruction, thus displaying a crucial role in cell shedding.[64] Similarly, KLK7, by being present on the surface of cancer cells, suggests its function in shedding of tumor cells and therefore in invasion and early metastasis. The significance of KLK7 in early detection of ovarian carcinoma is related directly to its upregulated levels in ovarian cancer cells.[65]

Folate Receptor 1

FOLR1 is a membrane-bound receptor protein that is involved in the transport of folate into cells and other cellular processes. The expression of FOLR1 is regulated through depletion of extracellular folate levels, accumulation of homocysteine, steroid hormone levels, genetic mutations, certain transcription factors, and cytosolic proteins.[66] FOLR1 overexpression was documented in 69% of uterine serous carcinoma[67] as well as the majority of serous ovarian carcinomas.[68] Moreover, overexpression of FOLR1 has been shown to be a poor prognostic factor with worse disease-free survival and overall survival in serous ovarian carcinoma patients. Furthermore, FOLR1 regulates the expression of bcl-2 and Bax and inhibits cytotoxic drug–induced apoptosis, suggesting that FOLR1 could be a potential biomarker for detection, prognosis, and monitoring chemotherapy responses of ovarian cancer.[68]

Studying the diagnostic and prognostic role of FOLR1 and FOLR3 in cytology fluids of ovarian cancer, breast cancer, and malignant mesothelioma showed significantly higher levels of FOLR1 and FOLR3 in ovarian carcinoma samples compared to breast cancer or mesothelioma. Moreover, high expression of folate receptors in ovarian carcinomas suggests the validity of FOLR1 as drug targets in chemotherapeutic management of ovarian cancer. Clinical trials are currently being performed to evaluate the potential role of FOLR1 as a biomarker for ovarian carcinoma early detection.

PROTEOMICS AND OVARIAN CANCER BIOMARKERS

Gene-based biomarkers have a potential for ovarian carcinoma detection; however, no novel cancer-specific biomarker is currently available in clinics. This stems from the fact that gene levels are not always linked directly to protein levels. The emerging of proteomics as a powerful technology to study large-scale characteristics of proteins including isoforms, modifications, interactions, and functional structures is promising. Proteomics characterizes proteins and the associated protein and peptide modifications that make up the complex signaling networks which play an important role in mediating all processes of cellular activity. Among the major goals of proteomics is the identification of biomarkers for predicting, diagnosing, and prognosticating disease. Application of proteomics for the development and validation of prognostic biomarkers, screening biomarkers, and biomarker panels to predict progression and treatment response is currently underway. Traditionally, protein biomarkers have been identified using crude techniques such as enzyme-linked immunosorbent assays (ELISA), Western blot analysis, and gene array analysis. However, these techniques require knowledge of the target protein before application.

Mass spectrophotometry allows the detection of novel proteins and peptides by their unique signature which may be differentially expressed in the cancerous state as compared with normal or benign states and hence do not require sequence identification. Mass spectrophotometry is the main proteomics technique that supported the discovery of many cancer biomarkers. With mass spectrophotometry, samples are ionized and then detected using an ion detector plate. The time required for the sample to reach the detector plate is a function of the mass-to-charge ratio, which is unique to each individual peptide or protein.[69] Among several different mass spectrophotometry–based proteomics approaches, the two most commonly used methods for new biomarker discovery are the matrix-assisted laser desorption and ionization time-of-flight (MALDI-TOF) and the surface-enhanced laser desorption and ionization time-of-flight (SELDI-TOF).[70]

MALDI-TOF uses a matrix that traps a subset of proteins in the sample, which are subsequently ionized and analyzed by time-of-flight. Conversely, SELDI-TOF uses a commercial chip that is customized with specific bait molecules that either chemically bind protein samples using cationic or hydrophobic interactions or use an antibody to which samples bind followed by a matrix to facilitate ionization.[71] Analysis of spectral images is performed by a software that is capable of segregating different patterns of proteomic peak intensities. Quality control is critical when applying proteomic techniques to patient samples, and, as with all high-throughput technologies that generate large data sets, this approach requires complex bioinformatics methods.[72]

In ovarian carcinoma, application of proteomics for diagnosis have followed two different paths.[73] The first is called "proteomic pattern diagnostics" or "serum proteomic profiling," which is based on mass spectrophotometric differences between samples with and without cancer that are identified by bioinformatics. Proteomic pattern analysis in ovarian carcinoma has the potential of being a highly sensitive diagnostic tool for detecting early-stage disease.[74] However, precise information regarding instrument reproducibility, quality control, and standard operating procedures for specimen collection, handling, and transport remains to be determined.

An alternative proteomic approach to ovarian carcinoma biomarkers is its use for identification of a single, novel biomarker and the subsequent development of new assays.

BIOMARKERS FOR EARLY DETECTION OF OVARIAN CANCER USING PROTEOMIC PROFILING

Recently, many promising biomarkers have been discovered for ovarian cancer diagnosis by proteomic analysis (Box 2.1). A seven biomarker panel that included transferrin,[75] apolipoprotein A1,[76] cleavage fragment of inter-alpha-trypsin inhibitor heavy chain H4,[77] beta-2 microglobulin, transthyretin, hepcidin, and connective tissue activating protein III has been evaluated for early detection of ovarian cancer [77] as well as for distinguishing malignant from benign pelvic masses.

BOX 2.1 POTENTIAL PROTEIN-BASED BIOMARKERS FOR OVARIAN CARCINOMA

Proteomics and Biomarkers

Transferrin,[75] apolipoprotein A1,[76] cleavage fragment of inter-alpha-trypsin inhibitor heavy chain H4,[77] beta-2 microglobulin, transthyretin, hepcidin and connective tissue activating protein III, Afamin, plasma retinol-binding protein precursor (RBP4).

An increase in acute phase proteins (hepcidin, transferrin, and beta-2 microglobulin) is observed in malignant versus benign and healthy samples, which suggests that malignancy is accompanied with inflammatory response. Whether this response is specific to ovarian cancer would require further investigation.

Apolipoprotein A-IV is a member of the ApoA1/C3/A4/A5 gene cluster located on the long arm of human chromosome 11.[78] Members of this cluster are involved in lipid and lipoprotein metabolism and thus are associated with cardiovascular disease; ApoA-IV is a 46-kDA glycoprotein that is almost exclusively produced in intestinal enterocytes and secreted into the lymph. It was first identified as a component of chylomicrons and high-density lipoproteins.[79] In fasting plasma, apoA-IV is found associated primarily with high-density lipoproteins.[80] ApoA-IV plays a central role in many physiologic processes including lipid absorption, transport, and metabolism within the cholesterol pathway and may act as a postprandial satiety signal and antioxidant.[81] Decreased plasma concentrations of ApoA-IV could contribute to a more specific diagnosis of ovarian cancer. Immunoassays for Apo-A1, transthyretin, and inter-alpha-trypsin inhibitor heavy chain H4 in combination with CA125 improved the sensitivity for detection of early-stage disease from 65% with CA125 alone to 74% with the addition of the aforementioned proteins. In a biomarker panel comprising Apo-A1, transthyretin, and connective tissue activating protein III, the sensitivity and specificity for detecting early stage ovarian cancer were 84% and 98%, respectively.

Using a differential proteomics approach, Afamin, a serum glycoprotein was recently identified as a potential novel biomarker for ovarian cancer. Afamin is a member of the albumin multigene family with vitamin E-binding properties.[81] It is expressed predominately in the liver and occurs abundantly in human serum and extravascular fluids such as follicular, seminal, and cerebrospinal fluids. Significantly decreased serum concentrations of Afamin were found in ovarian cancer patients compared to patients with benign gynecologic conditions, borderline ovarian tumors, and healthy controls.

Plasma retinol-binding protein precursor (RBP4) is another novel potential protein biomarker recently discovered for early detection of ovarian cancer. RBP4 is an adipokine secreted by adipose tissue and liver and contributes to insulin resistance.[82] Elevated levels of RBP4 were directly correlated with body mass index, insulin resistance, and impaired glucose hemostasis and were inversely correlated with glucose transporter 4 levels in adipocytes.[83] Moreover, RBP4 stimulates hepatic gluconeogenesis and inhibits insulin signaling in the muscle.[84] In ovarian cancer, proteomic analysis, and ELISA, measurement of the serum RBP4 showed that their levels were significantly higher in ovarian cancer patients that those in healthy individuals and those with benign ovarian tumors and myomas. The potential to use RBP4 as an adjunct marker in combination with CA125 for ovarian cancer diagnosis is still under investigation.

OVA-1

Multivariate index assay (OVA-1) was approved by the FDA in 2009 for assessing the likelihood of malignancy in patients planned to have surgery for an adnexal mass. It examines five biomarkers: apolipoprotein A1, beta 2 microglobulin, transferring, transthyretin, and CA125.

CA125 and beta 2 microglobulin are upregulated and the rest of the biomarkers are downregulated. After these five proteins are measured using two immunoassay platforms, they are interpreted using the propriety OvaCalc software. A score ranging from 0.0 to 10.0 is created and interpreted as high probability of malignancy for OVA-1 score ≥ 5.0 and ≥ 4.4 in premenopausal and postmenopausal patients, respectively, and low probability of malignancy for OVA-1 score < 5.0 and < 4.4 in premenopausal

and postmenopausal patients, respectively. In a prospective multi-institution study including 524 patients, OVA-1 was found to have a higher sensitivity in detecting ovarian carcinoma than clinical assessment and CA125. The sensitivity of OVA-1 compared to CA125 in detecting ovarian carcinoma in premenopausal patients was 96% versus 56% and 100% versus 96% in postmenopausal patients. However, OVA-1 showed a lower specificity and positive predictive value when compared to CA125 (43% vs. 84% and 40% vs. 52%, respectively). Because of the decreased sensitivity of OVA-1, more patients with nonmalignant masses should be referred to gynecologic oncologists.

PROTEOMIC PROFILING FOR TREATMENT OF OVARIAN CANCER

Despite the recent advances in biomarker discovery for early detection of ovarian carcinoma, most cases are still diagnosed at a late stage. Novel tyrosine kinase inhibitors and monoclonal antibodies have now been developed that specifically interrupt cellular signals which drives cancer cell survival, growth, proliferation, invasion, and metastasis. Proteomic analysis of samples obtained during clinical trials using these novel agents addresses the complexity of the signaling events associated with advanced ovarian carcinoma. Questions that need to be addressed when designing therapy using signal transduction inhibitors include presence of the target, if the target is affected by the treatment intervention, and if the target effect is sufficient enough to yield a change in clinical outcome.

Recent technologies using protein microarrays have allowed quantification of multiple end points including expression levels of key proteins and their activated forms that compose critical signaling nodes involved in proliferation, survival, and angiogenesis.[85,86] Protein microarray formats can be divided into two major classes: forward-phase arrays, where antibodies are arrayed and probed with cell lysates, and reverse-phase arrays, where cell lysates are arrayed and probed with antibodies.[87] In contrast to forward-phase arrays, reverse-phase arrays do not require labeling of cellular protein lysates and constitute a sensitive high-throughput platform for marker screening, pathophysiologic studies, and therapeutic monitoring. Furthermore, reverse-phase arrays have the ability to analyze signaling pathways using small numbers of cultured cells or cells isolated by laser-captured microdissection from human tissues procured during clinical trials. In ovarian cancer, the reverse-phase arrays platform has been used to study disease progression and profile signaling pathways, identify therapeutic targets, and suggest prognostic indicators.

MICRORNA-BASED OVARIAN CANCER BIOMARKERS

MICRORNA FOR EARLY DETECTION OF OVARIAN CANCER

MicroRNAs (miRNAs) are a class of small (20–25 nt) non-protein coding RNA molecules that are emerging as important diagnostic and potentially therapeutic tools. miRNAs play roles in a variety of biological processes including organogenesis, development, cell proliferation, differentiation, apoptosis, homeostasis, and metabolism. These molecules negatively regulate mRNA translation into proteins either by degradation of the messenger RNA transcript or by translational repression. About 5% of human genes encode for miRNAs and up to 30% of human protein coding genes are regulated by miRNAs that are unique to each cell type and to the development and differentiation stage of the cell. Increasing evidence has revealed aberrant miRNAs expression in different types of cancers including ovarian cancer, suggesting their role as novel classes of oncogenes or tumor suppressor genes. Given the function of miRNAs in cancer progression, characterizing the regulation of miRNAs will provide opportunities for the development

of biomarkers as well as the identification of new therapeutic targets.

The recent development of microarrays has made it possible to analyze miRNA expression profiles in different oncotypes, and a wide range of miRNA candidates are differentially or aberrantly expressed in ovarian cancers.

Changes in tumor miRNA expression patterns occur through multiple mechanisms including genetic alterations, epigenetic regulations, or altered expression of transcription factors which target miRNA genes. In the last five years, several miRNA expression profiles of ovarian carcinomas have been published, reporting underexpression of a substantial number of miRNAs as compared to normal counterparts.[88]

RNase are present abundantly in the bloodstream. In order to remain stable, some secretory miRNAs are contained in microvesicles or are bound to RNA binding proteins.[89] In addition, miRNA in the serum and saliva are found in tiny membrane vesicles, known as exosomes.[90] Cancer cells can secrete excessive amounts of exosomes as compared with normal cells.[91]

Some miRNAs exhibit negative control over the expression of numerous oncoproteins in normal cells and, consequently, their degradation is believed to be an essential mechanism in cancer development, and progression.[92] miRNAs have distinct patterns of expression that are associated with specific cancer types, and once secreted by cancer cells, they have significant stability in the blood and other body fluids. Due to the significant amount of signal amplification that is associated with nucleic acid serum markers, the identification of "miRNA signatures" associating cancer cell phenotypes with disease outcome and specific risk factor exposures will open new avenues for early cancer diagnosis as well as for the development of novel strategies for cancer prevention and treatment. Because these miRNA signatures can appear in the body fluids in exosomes, they can serve as relatively stable circulating diagnostic biomarkers and have been proven to do so for ovarian carcinoma.[93] Isolation of an exosome fraction also improves the sensitivity of miRNA amplification from biological fluids and reduces the probability of false negative results.[90]

Moving from being merely biomarkers for ovarian cancer to being targets for therapy, the development of strategies that might block the expression or mimic the function of miRNAs could represent new therapeutic strategies. Exosome vesicles can also be used as gene therapy vehicles for delivery of miRNAs with therapeutic effects.[94]

The use of miRNA signatures of tumor-derived serum exosomes as a diagnostic biomarker for ovarian cancer was first described by Taylor and Gercel[95] who showed that the level of tumor-derived miRNA containing exosomes in the serum is strongly increased in women with invasive ovarian carcinomas as compared to those with benign ovarian tumors or healthy women. Additionally, the levels of circulating, tumor-derived exosomes increased in parallel to the stage of the disease. By miRNA microarray profiling they identified 218 miRNAs in tumor samples as well as in circulating exosomes.

The Cancer Genome Atlas Network has recently identified a set of 34 miRNAs that are predictive of overall survival in 487 high-grade serous tumors. miRNAs significantly overexpressed included miRNAs-21, miRNAs-29a, miRNAs-92, miRNAs-93, and miRNAs-126, whereas miRNAs-127, miRNAs-155, and miRNAs-99b were significantly underexpressed in ovarian cancers (Table 2.2).[96]

By the use of custom microarray platform to compare miRNA profiles between 69 ovarian carcinomas and 15 normal ovaries, 29 differentially expressed miRNAs were found. Among them, miRNA-200a, miRNA-200b, miRNA-200c, and miRNA-141 have been found to be overexpressed. On the other hand, miRNA-199a, miRNA-140, miRNA-145, and miRNA-125b1 were among the most underexpressed miRNAs.

More recently, a novel real-time PCR platform detected upregulation of miRNA-21,

TABLE 2.2 POTENTIAL MICRO-RNA-BASED BIOMARKERS FOR OVARIAN CARCINOMA

Biomarkers	
Overexpressed	miRNAs-21, miRNAs-29a, miRNAs-92, miRNAs-93, miRNAs-126, miRNA-200a, miRNA-200b, miRNA-200c and miRNA-141, miRNA-21, miRNA-92, miRNA- 93, miRNA-126, and miRNA-29a
Underexpressed	miRNAs-127, miRNAs-155 and miRNAs-99b, miRNA-199a, miRNA-140, miRNA-145 and miRNA-125b1, miRNA-155, miRNA-127, and miRNA-99b

miRNA-92, miRNA- 93, miRNA-126, and miRNA-29a while miRNA-155, miRNA-127, and miRNA-99b were downregulated. Upregulation of miRNA-21, miRNA-92, and miRNA-93 in the serum of patients with normal CA125 suggests its role as complementary biomarker to the current detection approaches.[97]

Recent recognition of high-grade serous ovarian carcinoma precursor lesions, namely serous tubal intraepithelial carcinoma (STIC), provides a new venue for the study of early genetic changes in high-grade serous carcinomas. Using miRNA profiling analysis, Liu and colleagues[98] demonstrated that miRNA-182 expression was significantly higher in STIC than in matched normal fallopian tube. In addition, the oncogenic properties of miRNA-182 in ovarian cancer were mediated in part by its impaired repair of DNA double-strand breaks and negative regulation of BRCA1 gene expression, as well as its positive regulation of the oncogene high-mobility group AT-hook 2.

Chang and colleagues[99] suggested that miRNA-148b may be one of the dysregulated miRNAs involved in the early stages of ovarian carcinogenesis. They found that miRNA-148b was overexpressed in 92% of the ovarian cancer samples and that the overexpression did not correlate with any of the clinicopathological features.

MICRORNA AND PROGNOSIS

miRNA-100 was reported to be significantly downregulated in ovarian carcinoma; however, the clinical significance of miRNA-100 in ovarian carcinoma remains unclear. A recent study demonstrated that low miRNA-100 expression was found to be closely correlated with advanced FIGO stage, lymph node involvement, and higher CA125 levels.[100] In addition, low miRNA-100 expression is associated with shorter overall survival and is an independent poor prognostic factor.

Furthermore, Bagnoli and colleagues[101] delineated a miRNA signature associated with early relapse in advanced-stage disease. Thirty-two differentially expressed miRNAs in early versus advanced late relapsing patients were identified, eight of which belong to a cluster located on chrXq27.3 and were shown to be downmodulated in early relapsing patients.

MICRORNA AND DRUG RESISTANCE

miRNA-93 is significantly upregulated in cisplatin-resistant ovarian cancer cells and inversely correlates with PTEN expression in cisplatin-resistant and cisplatin-sensitive ovarian cancer tissues.[102] The miRNA-34, miRNA-449a, miRNA-449b, and miRNA-192 family of miRNAs has a strong role in regulating the genotoxic-response p53 pathway in ovarian cancer. Studies have shown that the expressions of miRNA-449a/b, miRNA-34b, and miRNA-34c were 19- to 21-fold elevated after p53 activation by genotoxic agents.[103]

METABOLOMICS AND OVARIAN CANCER BIOMARKERS

Metabolomics is the global quantitative assessment of endogenous metabolites within a biological system. It is an analytic tool used in conjunction with pattern recognition approaches and bioinformatics to detect metabolites and follow their changes in biofluids or tissues.[104,105] Metabolites result from the interaction of the system's genome with its environment. Either individually or grouped as a metabolomics profile, detection of metabolites is usually carried out in cells, tissues, or body fluids by either nuclear magnetic resonance (NMR) spectroscopy or mass-spectrophotometry. With the development of metabolic and molecular imaging technologies, metabolomics can provide a link between the laboratory and the clinic as well as a great role in oncology, including the early detection and diagnosis of cancer and monitoring drug response and drug toxicity.[106] In ovarian cancer diagnosis, NMR spectroscopy showed 100% sensitivity and specificity for detection of ovarian carcinoma at the NMR regions 2.77 and 2.04 parts per million. These findings indicates that NMR metabolomic analysis of serum distinguishes ovarian carcinomas from healthy controls and requires further consideration as a potential novel strategy for the early detection of ovarian cancer.[107] NMR-based metabolomics offers several advantages in a clinical setting; first, it can be carried out on standard preparations of serum, plasma, or urine, circumventing the need for specialist preparations of cellular RNA and protein required for genomics and proteomics, respectively.[108] Second, since cancer is known to be a product of the tumor-host microenvironment, the organ-specific milieu can generate and enzymatically modify multiple proteins, peptides, metabolites, and cleavage products at much higher concentrations than for molecules derived only from tumor cells.

The use of gas chromatography/time-of-flight mass spectrometry showed a significant differentiation between borderline tumors and invasive carcinomas through differences in 51 metabolites.[109]

CONCLUSION

Biomarker-based screening for ovarian carcinoma is expected to expand and advance into clinical practice over the next few years. The use of extratumoral biomarkers and alternative biofluids will most likely result in this advancement. It still remains unclear whether a single biomarker or a panel of biomarkers will provide the most accurate approaches for early detection of ovarian carcinoma. However, the advances in the technologies including next-generation sequencing are promising.

REFERENCES

1. Siegel, R.L., K.D. Miller, and A. Jemal, Cancer statistics, 2016. *CA Cancer J Clin*, 2016. 66(1): p. 7–30.
2. Parkin, D.M., et al., Global cancer statistics, 2002. *CA Cancer J Clin*, 2005. 55(2): 74–108.
3. Shih Ie, M. and R.J. Kurman, Ovarian tumorigenesis: a proposed model based on morphological and molecular genetic analysis. *Am J Pathol*, 2004. 164(5): 1511–18.
4. Jones, S., et al., Frequent mutations of chromatin remodeling gene ARID1A in ovarian clear cell carcinoma. *Science*, 2010. 330(6001): 228–31.
5. Ahmed, A.A., et al., Driver mutations in TP53 are ubiquitous in high grade serous carcinoma of the ovary. *J Pathol*, 2010. 221(1): 49–56.
6. Hayashi, H., et al., Bilateral oophorectomy in asymptomatic women over 50 years old selected by ovarian cancer screening. *Gynecol Obstet Invest*, 1999. 47(1): 58–64.
7. Alagoz, T., et al., What is a normal CA125 level? *Gynecol Oncol*, 1994. 53(1): 93–97.
8. Bon, G.G., et al., Serum tumor marker immunoassays in gynecologic oncology: establishment of reference values. *Am J Obstet Gynecol*, 1996. 174(1 Pt 1): 107–14.
9. Moore, R.G., et al., A novel multiple marker bioassay utilizing HE4 and CA125 for the prediction of ovarian cancer in patients with a pelvic mass. *Gynecol Oncol*, 2009. 112(1): 40–46.
10. Jacobs, I., et al., Sensitivity of transvaginal ultrasound screening for endometrial cancer in postmenopausal women: a case-control study within the UKCTOCS cohort. *Lancet Oncol*, 2011. 12(1): 38–48.
11. Makar, A.P., et al., Prognostic value of pre- and postoperative serum CA 125 levels in ovarian cancer: new aspects and multivariate analysis. *Obstet Gynecol*, 1992. 79(6): 1002–10.
12. Scholl, S.M., et al., Circulating levels of colony-stimulating factor 1 as a prognostic indicator in 82 patients with epithelial ovarian cancer. *Br J Cancer*, 1994. 69(2): 342–46.
13. Nagele, F., et al., Preoperative CA 125: an independent prognostic factor in patients with stage I epithelial ovarian cancer. *Obstet Gynecol*, 1995. 86(2): 259–64.
14. Parker, D., et al., Serum albumin and CA125 are powerful predictors of survival in epithelial ovarian cancer. *Br J Obstet Gynaecol*, 1994. 101(10): 888–93.
15. Gadducci, A., et al., Serum tumor markers in the management of ovarian, endometrial and cervical cancer. *Biomed Pharmacother*, 2004. 58(1): 24–38.
16. Guppy, A.E. and G.J. Rustin, CA125 response: can it replace the traditional response criteria in ovarian cancer? *Oncologist*, 2002. 7(5): 437–43.
17. Bast, R.C., Jr., et al., CA 125: the past and the future. *Int J Biol Markers*, 1998. 13(4): 179–87.
18. Ness, R.B. and C. Cottreau, Possible role of ovarian epithelial inflammation in ovarian cancer. *J Natl Cancer Inst*, 1999. 91(17): 1459–67.
19. Hanahan, D. and R.A. Weinberg, Hallmarks of cancer: the next generation. *Cell*, 2011. 144(5): 646–74.
20. Lane, D., et al., The prosurvival activity of ascites against TRAIL is associated with a shorter disease-free interval in patients with ovarian cancer. *J Ovarian Res*, 2010. 3: 1.
21. Matte, I., et al., Profiling of cytokines in human epithelial ovarian cancer ascites. *Am J Cancer Res*, 2012. 2(5): 566–80.
22. Ghosh, S. and K. Ashcraft, An IL-6 link between obesity and cancer. *Front Biosci* (Elite Ed), 2013. 5: 461–78.
23. Kurman, R.J. and M. Shih Ie, Molecular pathogenesis and extraovarian origin of epithelial ovarian cancer--shifting the paradigm. *Hum Pathol*, 2011. 42(7): 918–31.
24. Salvador, S., et al., The fallopian tube: primary site of most pelvic high-grade serous carcinomas. *Int J Gynecol Cancer*, 2009. 19(1): 58–64.
25. Gocze, P. and H. Vahrson, [Ovarian carcinoma antigen (CA 125) and ovarian cancer (clinical follow-up and prognostic studies)]. *Orv Hetil*, 1993. 134(17): 915–18.
26. Molina, R., et al., CA 125 in biological fluids. *Int J Biol Markers*, 1998. 13(4): 224–30.
27. de Bruijn, H.W., et al., Cancer-associated antigen CA 195 in patients with mucinous ovarian tumours: a comparative analysis with CEA, TATI and CA 125 in serum specimens and cyst fluids. *Tumour Biol*, 1993. 14(2): 105–15.
28. Brun, J.L., et al., Serous and mucinous ovarian tumors express different profiles of MMP-2, -7, -9, MT1-MMP, and TIMP-1 and -2. *Int J Oncol*, 2008. 33(6): 1239–46.
29. Murthi, P., et al., Plasminogen fragmentation and increased production of extracellular matrix-degrading proteinases are associated with serous epithelial ovarian cancer progression. *Gynecol Oncol*, 2004. 92(1): 80–88.
30. Mabuchi, S., et al., Vascular endothelial growth factor is a promising therapeutic target for the treatment of clear cell carcinoma of the ovary. *Mol Cancer Ther*, 2010. 9(8): 2411–22.

31. Bonadona, V., et al., Cancer risks associated with germline mutations in MLH1, MSH2, and MSH6 genes in Lynch syndrome. *JAMA*, 2011. 305(22): 2304–10.

32. Pal, T., et al., Frequency of mutations in mismatch repair genes in a population-based study of women with ovarian cancer. *Br J Cancer*, 2012. 107(10): 1783–90.

33. Alsop, K., et al., BRCA mutation frequency and patterns of treatment response in BRCA mutation-positive women with ovarian cancer: a report from the Australian Ovarian Cancer Study Group. *J Clin Oncol*, 2012. 30(21): 2654–63.

34. Kauff, N.D., et al., Risk-reducing salpingo-oophorectomy in women with a BRCA1 or BRCA2 mutation. *N Engl J Med*, 2002. 346(21): 1609–15.

35. Burger, R.A., Experience with bevacizumab in the management of epithelial ovarian cancer. *J Clin Oncol*, 2007. 25(20): 2902–908.

36. Aghajanian, C., et al., OCEANS: a randomized, double-blind, placebo-controlled phase III trial of chemotherapy with or without bevacizumab in patients with platinum-sensitive recurrent epithelial ovarian, primary peritoneal, or fallopian tube cancer. *J Clin Oncol*, 2012. 30(17): 2039–45.

37. Imai, K. and H. Yamamoto, Carcinogenesis and microsatellite instability: the interrelationship between genetics and epigenetics. *Carcinogenesis*, 2008. 29(4): 673–80.

38. Clarke, B.A. and K. Cooper, Identifying Lynch syndrome in patients with endometrial carcinoma: shortcomings of morphologic and clinical schemas. *Adv Anat Pathol*, 2012. 19(4): 231–38.

39. Watson, P., et al., The clinical features of ovarian cancer in hereditary nonpolyposis colorectal cancer. *Gynecol Oncol*, 2001. 82(2): 223–28.

40. Konstantinopoulos, P.A., D. Spentzos, and S.A. Cannistra, Gene-expression profiling in epithelial ovarian cancer. *Nat Clin Pract Oncol*, 2008. 5(10): 577–87.

41. Mok, S.C., et al., Prostasin, a potential serum marker for ovarian cancer: identification through microarray technology. *J Natl Cancer Inst*, 2001. 93(19): 1458–64.

42. Hassan, R., et al., Localization of mesothelin in epithelial ovarian cancer. *Appl Immunohistochem Mol Morphol*, 2005. 13(3): 243–47.

43. Kim, J.H., et al., Osteopontin as a potential diagnostic biomarker for ovarian cancer. *JAMA*, 2002. 287(13): 1671–79.

44. Schummer, M., et al., Comparative hybridization of an array of 21,500 ovarian cDNAs for the discovery of genes overexpressed in ovarian carcinomas. *Gene*, 1999. 238(2): 375–85.

45. Kim, J.H., et al., Identification of epithelial cell adhesion molecule autoantibody in patients with ovarian cancer. *Clin Cancer Res*, 2003. 9(13): 4782–91.

46. Huddleston, H.G., et al., Clinical applications of microarray technology: creatine kinase B is an up-regulated gene in epithelial ovarian cancer and shows promise as a serum marker. *Gynecol Oncol*, 2005. 96(1): 77–83.

47. Peters, D.G., et al., Comparative gene expression analysis of ovarian carcinoma and normal ovarian epithelium by serial analysis of gene expression. *Cancer Epidemiol Biomarkers Prev*, 2005. 14(7): 1717–23.

48. Hellstrom, I. and K.E. Hellstrom, SMRP and HE4 as biomarkers for ovarian carcinoma when used alone and in combination with CA125 and/or each other. *Adv Exp Med Biol*, 2008. 622: 15–21.

49. Montagnana, M., et al., HE4 in ovarian cancer: from discovery to clinical application. *Adv Clin Chem*, 2011. 55: 1–20.

50. Chang, X., et al., Human epididymis protein 4 (HE4) as a serum tumor biomarker in patients with ovarian carcinoma. *Int J Gynecol Cancer*, 2011. 21(5): 852–58.

51. Li, J., et al., HE4 as a biomarker for ovarian and endometrial cancer management. *Expert Rev Mol Diagn*, 2009. 9(6): 555–66.

52. Molina, R., et al., HE4 a novel tumour marker for ovarian cancer: comparison with CA 125 and ROMA algorithm in patients with gynaecological diseases. *Tumour Biol*, 2011. 32(6): 1087–95.

53. Moore, R.G., et al., The use of multiple novel tumor biomarkers for the detection of ovarian carcinoma in patients with a pelvic mass. *Gynecol Oncol*, 2008. 108(2): 402–8.

54. Heid, C.A., et al., Real time quantitative PCR. *Genome Res*, 1996. 6(10): 986–94.

55. Litvinov, S.V., et al., Ep-CAM: a human epithelial antigen is a homophilic cell-cell adhesion molecule. *J Cell Biol*, 1994. 125(2): 437–46.

56. Wong, K.K., R.S. Cheng, and S.C. Mok, Identification of differentially expressed genes from ovarian cancer cells by MICROMAX cDNA microarray system. *Biotechniques*, 2001. 30(3): 670–75.

57. Rump, A., et al., Binding of ovarian cancer antigen CA125/MUC16 to mesothelin mediates cell adhesion. *J Biol Chem*, 2004. 279(10): 9190–98.

58. McIntosh, M.W., et al., Combining CA 125 and SMR serum markers for diagnosis and early detection of ovarian carcinoma. *Gynecol Oncol*, 2004. 95(1): 9–15.

59. Oikonomopoulou, K., et al., Proteinase-mediated cell signalling: targeting proteinase-activated receptors (PARs) by kallikreins and more. *Biol Chem*, 2006. 387(6): 677–85.

60. Dong, Y., et al., Human kallikrein 4 (KLK4) is highly expressed in serous ovarian carcinomas. *Clin Cancer Res*, 2001. 7(8): 2363–71.

61. Obiezu, C.V., et al., Human kallikrein 4: quantitative study in tissues and evidence for its secretion into biological fluids. *Clin Chem*, 2005. 51(8): 1432–42.

62. Shan, S.J., et al., Transcriptional upregulation of human tissue kallikrein 6 in ovarian cancer: clinical and mechanistic aspects. *Br J Cancer*, 2007. 96(2): 362–72.

63. Emami, N. and E.P. Diamandis, Utility of kallikrein-related peptidases (KLKs) as cancer biomarkers. *Clin Chem*, 2008. 54(10): 1600–607.

64. Talieri, M., et al., Expression analysis of the human kallikrein 7 (KLK7) in breast tumors: a new potential biomarker for prognosis of breast carcinoma. *Thromb Haemost*, 2004. 91(1): 180–86.

65. Kyriakopoulou, L.G., et al., Prognostic value of quantitatively assessed KLK7 expression in ovarian cancer. *Clin Biochem*, 2003. 36(2): 135–43.

66. Kelemen, L.E., The role of folate receptor alpha in cancer development, progression and treatment: cause, consequence or innocent bystander? *Int J Cancer*, 2006. 119(2): 243–50.

67. Dainty, L.A., et al., Overexpression of folate binding protein and mesothelin are associated with uterine serous carcinoma. *Gynecol Oncol*, 2007. 105(3): 563–70.

68. Chen, Y.L., et al., Serous ovarian carcinoma patients with high alpha-folate receptor had reducing survival and cytotoxic chemo-response. *Mol Oncol*, 2012. 6(3): 360–69.

69. Koomen, J., D. Hawke, and R. Kobayashi, Developing an understanding of proteomics: an introduction to biological mass spectrometry. *Cancer Invest*, 2005. 23(1): 47–59.

70. Zhang, B., et al., Proteomics and biomarkers for ovarian cancer diagnosis. *Ann Clin Lab Sci*, 2010. 40(3): 218–25.

71. Simpkins, F., et al., SELDI-TOF mass spectrometry for cancer biomarker discovery and serum proteomic diagnostics. *Pharmacogenomics*, 2005. 6(6): 647–53.

72. Annunziata, C.M., et al., Ovarian cancer in the proteomics era. *Int J Gynecol Cancer*, 2008. 18(Suppl 1): 1–6.

73. Plebani, M., Proteomics: the next revolution in laboratory medicine? *Clin Chim Acta*, 2005. 357(2): 113–22.

74. Petricoin, E.F., et al., Use of proteomic patterns in serum to identify ovarian cancer. *Lancet*, 2002. 359(9306): 572–77.

75. Ahmed, N., et al., Proteomic tracking of serum protein isoforms as screening biomarkers of ovarian cancer. *Proteomics*, 2005. 5(17): 4625–36.

76. Kozak, K.R., et al., Characterization of serum biomarkers for detection of early stage ovarian cancer. *Proteomics*, 2005. 5(17): 4589–96.

77. Zhang, Z., et al., Three biomarkers identified from serum proteomic analysis for the detection of early stage ovarian cancer. *Cancer Res*, 2004. 64(16): 5882–90.

78. Lai, C.Q., L.D. Parnell, and J.M. Ordovas, The APOA1/C3/A4/A5 gene cluster, lipid metabolism and cardiovascular disease risk. *Curr Opin Lipidol*, 2005. 16(2): 153–66.

79. Beisiegel, U. and G. Utermann, An apolipoprotein homolog of rat apolipoprotein A-IV in human plasma. Isolation and partial characterisation. *Eur J Biochem*, 1979. 93(3): 601–8.

80. Ezeh, B., et al., Plasma distribution of apoA-IV in patients with coronary artery disease and healthy controls. *J Lipid Res*, 2003. 44(8): 1523–29.

81. Stan, S., et al., Apo A-IV: an update on regulation and physiologic functions. *Biochim Biophys Acta*, 2003. 1631(2): 177–87.

82. Blaner, W.S., Retinol-binding protein: the serum transport protein for vitamin A. *Endocr Rev*, 1989. 10(3): 308–16.

83. Tschoner, A., et al., Retinol-binding protein 4, visceral fat, and the metabolic syndrome: effects of weight loss. *Obesity*, 2008. 16(11): 2439–44.

84. Kowalska, I., et al., Serum retinol binding protein 4 is related to insulin resistance and nonoxidative glucose metabolism in lean and obese women with normal glucose tolerance. *J Clin Endocrinol Metab*, 2008. 93(7): 2786–89.

85. Davidson, B., et al., Proteomic analysis of malignant ovarian cancer effusions as a tool for biologic and prognostic profiling. *Clin Cancer Res*, 2006. 12(3 Pt 1): 791–99.

86. Paweletz, C.P., et al., Reverse phase protein microarrays which capture disease progression show activation of pro-survival pathways at the cancer invasion front. *Oncogene*, 2001. 20(16): 1981–89.

87. Kolch, W., H. Mischak, and A.R. Pitt, The molecular make-up of a tumour: proteomics in cancer research. *Clin Sci*, 2005. 108(5): 369–83.

88. Iorio, M.V., et al., MicroRNA signatures in human ovarian cancer. *Cancer Res*, 2007. 67(18): 8699–707.

89. Kosaka, N. and T. Ochiya, Unraveling the mystery of cancer by secretory microRNA: horizontal microRNA transfer between living cells. *Front Genet*, 2011. 2: 97.

90. Gallo, A., et al., The majority of microRNAs detectable in serum and saliva is concentrated in exosomes. *PLoS One*, 2012. 7(3): e30679.

91. Kharaziha, P., et al., Tumor cell-derived exosomes: a message in a bottle. *Biochim Biophys Acta*, 2012. 1826(1): 103–11.

92. Krutovskikh, V.A. and Z. Herceg, Oncogenic microRNAs (OncomiRs) as a new class of cancer biomarkers. *Bioessays*, 2010. 32(10): 894–904.

93. Kuhlmann, J.D., et al., MicroRNA and the pathogenesis of ovarian cancer--a new horizon for molecular diagnostics and treatment? *Clin Chem Lab Med*, 2012. 50(4): 601–15.

94. Lasser, C., Exosomal RNA as biomarkers and the therapeutic potential of exosome vectors. *Expert Opin Biol Ther*, 2012. 12(Suppl 1): S189–97.

95. Taylor, D.D. and C. Gercel-Taylor, MicroRNA signatures of tumor-derived exosomes as diagnostic biomarkers of ovarian cancer. *Gynecol Oncol*, 2008. 110(1): 13–21.

96. Creighton, C.J., et al., Integrated analyses of microRNAs demonstrate their widespread influence on gene expression in high-grade serous ovarian carcinoma. *PLoS One*, 2012. 7(3): e34546.

97. Resnick, K.E., et al., The detection of differentially expressed microRNAs from the serum of ovarian cancer patients using a novel real-time PCR platform. *Gynecol Oncol*, 2009. 112(1): 55–59.

98. Liu, Z., et al., MiR-182 overexpression in tumourigenesis of high-grade serous ovarian carcinoma. *J Pathol*, 2012. 228(2): 204–15.

99. Chang, H., et al., Increased expression of miR-148b in ovarian carcinoma and its clinical significance. *Mol Med Rep*, 2012. 5(5): 1277–80.

100. Peng, D.X., et al., Prognostic implications of microRNA-100 and its functional roles in human epithelial ovarian cancer. *Oncol Rep*, 2012. 27(4): 1238–44.

101. Bagnoli, M., et al., Identification of a chrXq27.3 microRNA cluster associated with early relapse in advanced stage ovarian cancer patients. *Oncotarget*, 2011. 2(12): 1265–78.

102. Fu, X., et al., Involvement of microRNA-93, a new regulator of PTEN/Akt signaling pathway, in regulation of chemotherapeutic drug cisplatin chemosensitivity in ovarian cancer cells. *FEBS Lett*, 2012. 586(9): 1279–86.

103. Zhang, Q., et al., [Expression and significance of microRNAs in the p53 pathway in ovarian cancer cells and serous ovarian cancer tissues]. *Zhonghua Zhong Liu Za Zhi*, 2011. 33(12): 885–90.

104. Fiehn, O., Metabolomics—the link between genotypes and phenotypes. *Plant Mol Biol*, 2002. 48(1–2): 155–71.

105. Griffin, J.L. and J.P. Shockcor, Metabolic profiles of cancer cells. *Nat Rev Cancer*, 2004. 4(7): 551–61.

106. Spratlin, J.L., N.J. Serkova, and S.G. Eckhardt, Clinical applications of metabolomics in oncology: a review. *Clin Cancer Res*, 2009. 15(2): 431–40.

107. Odunsi, K., et al., Detection of epithelial ovarian cancer using 1H-NMR-based metabonomics. *Int J Cancer*, 2005. 113(5): 782–88.

108. Ala-Korpela, M., Y. Hiltunen, and J.D. Bell, Quantification of biomedical NMR data using artificial neural network analysis: lipoprotein lipid profiles from 1H NMR data of human plasma. *NMR Biomed*, 1995. 8(6): 235–44.

109. Denkert, C., et al., Mass spectrometry-based metabolic profiling reveals different metabolite patterns in invasive ovarian carcinomas and ovarian borderline tumors. *Cancer Res*, 2006. 66(22): 10795–804.

3.

OVARIAN CANCER IMMUNITY
HOW DOES IMMUNE SUPPRESSION GROW CANCER?

Vincent Lavoué, Patrick Legembre, Jean Levêque,
Fabrice Foucher, Sébastien Henno, and Florian Cabillic

INTRODUCTION

Epithelial ovarian cancer (EOC) is the fifth most common cancer among women and the fourth most common cause of cancer-related death among women in developing countries.[1] The prognosis is poor, with a five-year survival rate of 30%. The majority of patients relapse within 16 to 18 months following the end of treatment and die from the disease despite response to first-line therapy consisting of debulking surgery and chemotherapy.[2,3] Fifteen percent of patients die within the first year. No substantial decrease in the death rate has occurred in the past three decades. Thus, there is an urgent need for basic knowledge of ovarian tumor biology for the development of innovative EOC treatments.

Unlike melanoma or renal and hematologic tumor diseases, EOC is not considered to be immunogenic. However, there is evidence of an immune response against EOC in patients.[4] Experimental data show that the inflammatory microenvironment of EOC prevents the maturation of myeloid cells, favors regulatory cell development, and restrains the cytotoxic activity of effector lymphocytes, leading the tumor to escape from the immune system and triggering cancer progression.[5] Treatments such as chemotherapy with paclitaxel/carboplatin and debulking surgery are traditionally considered to negatively impact the immune system during EOC.[6] However, recent data challenge this concept and highlight the major role of immune response in EOC. Indeed, aforementioned treatments were shown to modulate the host response and to decrease the immunosuppression.[7,8]

EVIDENCE OF AN IMMUNE RESPONSE IN EOC

EOC expresses or overexpresses tumor-associated antigens (TAA), that is, antigens (Ag), acquired by tumor cells in the process of neoplastic transformation that can elicit a specific T-cell immune response by the host. In 1993, EOC ascites was found to contain CD8+ T cells capable of recognizing HER2/neu-positive tumor cells.[9] Five to 66% of EOCs exhibit this epidermal growth factor receptor–related glycoprotein that activates signaling pathways involved in cellular proliferation.[10,11] Many other TAA were described in EOC, such as folate receptor α,[12] epithelial cell adhesion molecule,[13] human epididymis protein 4,[14] p53,[15] mucin-like MUC16 (CA125) and MUC1 (CA15.3),[16] and TAA of the cancer-testis group.[17,18] Tumor-reactive T cells and antibodies (Ab) directed against TAA were detected in the peripheral blood of patients with advanced-stage disease at the time of diagnosis,[15,19] and tumor-reactive T-cells were isolated from tumors or ascites.[20]

Furthermore, there is clinical evidence for the role of immunosurveillance against EOC. The detection of intraepithelial tumor-infiltrating lymphocytes (TIL) correlates with clinical outcome. Zhang et al. detected CD3[+] TIL in 102/186 frozen specimens from patients with stage III/IV EOC.[21] The five-year progression-free survival rates were 31.0% and 8.7% for patients with and without TIL, respectively. The presence of TIL correlated with progression-free survival in multivariate analysis ($p < 0.001$).[21] Recently, other studies confirmed that the CD3[+] TIL count is a significant prognosis factor in EOC (Table 3.1).[22–32] High frequencies and activity levels of immune effector cells such as CD8[+] T-cells, natural killer (NK) cells, and Vγ9Vδ2 T cells are correlated with positive clinical outcomes for EOC patients.[33,34] Thelper (Th) 17 cells, a recently discovered T-lymphocyte subset, were found in proportionally higher number in EOC microenvironments in comparison with other immune cells.[35,36] In EOC patients, Th17 levels in the tumor correlated positively with Th1 cells, cytotoxic CD8[+] T cells, and NK cells, and Th17 levels in ascites correlated positively with patient survival.[35] Intriguingly, Th17 were reported to promote either tumor cell growth or anti-tumor response, and their role in cancer development is currently under debate.[37,38] Finally, in addition to TIL, the number of peripheral blood immune cells (e.g., NK cells) is also correlated with survival in EOC.[33] All of these results support the existence of immunosurveillance in EOC (Table 3.1).

IMMUNE ESCAPE IN EOC

The tumor immunosurveillance concept was postulated in the 1960s by Burnet and Thomas, who proposed that the immune system patrols the body to recognize and destroy host cells that become cancerous and that the immune system is responsible for preventing cancer development.[39] This concept was then replaced by the cancer-immunoediting hypothesis, in which the immune system shapes tumor immunogenicity with three successive phases: elimination, equilibrium, and escape.[40]

Immune escape in EOC involves several mechanisms that implicate tumor, immune, and stromal cells.

OVARIAN TUMOR CELLS BECOME INVISIBLE

Ovarian tumor cells escape immune recognition by downregulating surface molecules involved in Ag presentation, such as β2-microglobulin and major histocompatibility complex (MHC).[28] Similarly, the downregulation of MHC class I-related chain A expression impedes the detection of tumor cells by innate cytotoxic effector cells through the engagement of the NKG2D-activating receptor.[41,42] Additionally, ovarian tumor cells overexpress molecules that counteract the cytotoxic activities of immune cells: CA125 binds the NK cell inhibitory receptor (KIR) siglec-9, thereby protecting themselves from NK-mediated lysis;[43,44] the macrophage migration inhibitory factor (MIF) downregulates NKG2D-activating receptor expression on NK cells.[45] Furthermore, engagement of programmed death-1 (PD-1) on CD8[+] T-cells by programmed death-1 ligand-1 (PD-L1) expressed by ovarian tumor cells impairs the effector functions of these lymphocytes.[24,46] Wide panels of cancers, including EOC, were also shown to express indolamine-2,3-dioxygenase (IDO), an intracellular enzyme that catalyzes the rate-limiting step in the metabolism of the essential amino acid tryptophan.[47,48] IDO is a beneficial host mechanism regulating immune responses in various contexts such as pregnancy, transplantation, or infection. It was proposed to elicit feedback process, therefore preventing deleterious consequences of excessive immune responses. However, this endogenous mechanism is hijacked by tumors to establish immunotolerance to tumor antigens.[49,50]

Authors	Year	Findings
Zhang et al.[21]	2003	Association between intraepithelial T-cell infiltration (TIL CD3+) and patient survival
Raspollini et al.[22]	2005	Association between intraepithelial T-cell infiltration (TIL CD3+) and patient survival (plus chemotherapeutic response)
Sato et al.[23]	2005	Association between intraepithelial T-cell infiltration (TIL CD8+) and patient survival
Hamanishi et al.[24]	2007	Association between intraepithelial T-cell infiltration (TIL CD3+) and patient survival
Clarke et al.[25]	2008	Association between intraepithelial T-cell infiltration (TIL CD8+) and patient survival (only for high grade serous EOC, but not for endometrioïd or mucinous EOC)
Shah et al.[26]	2008	Association between intraepithelial T-cell infiltration (TIL CD8+) and optimal debulking surgery
Tomsova et al.[27]	2008	Association between intraepithelial T-cell infiltration (TIL CD3+) and patient survival
Callahan et al.[38]	2008	Association between intraepithelial T-cell infiltration (TIL CD8+) and patient survival
Han et al.[28]	2008	Association between intraepithelial T-cell infiltration (TIL CD3+ and CD8+) and patient survival
Stumpf et al.[29]	2009	Association between intraepithelial T-cell infiltration (TIL CD3+ and CD8+) and patient survival
Leffers et al.[30,39]	2009	Association between intraepithelial T-cell infiltration (TIL CD8+) and patient survival
Milne et al.[31]	2009	Association between intraepithelial T-cell infiltration (TIL CD3+ and CD8+) and patient survival
Kryczek et al.[35]	2009	Association between intraepithelial T-cell infiltration (TIL CD4+ with IL-17 secretion) and patient survival
Motz et al.[37]	2014	Association between intraepithelial T-cell infiltration (TIL CD4+ with IL-17 secretion) and patient survival

NOTE: EOC = epithelial ovarian cancer.

ROLE OF IMMUNE CELLS IN IMMUNE SUPPRESSION

Immune cells also play a major role in the immune escape in EOC.[51] The EOC-specific recruitment of CD4+CD25+FoxP3+ regulatory T cells (Treg), tolerogenic dendritic cells (DC), B7-H4+ tumor-associated macrophages (TAM), and myeloid-derived suppressor cells (MDSC) fosters immune privilege and predicts reduced survival in EOC (Table 3.1).[23,36,52-56] Accumulation of Treg is now well documented in various tumors including EOC.[23,36] CCR4 chemokine receptor expression confers to Treg higher capacity than effector T cells to infiltrate the tumor in response to CCL22 chemokine produced by either tumor cells or TAM.[36] In addition, Treg could originate from in situ expansion. In that setting, ICOS-ligand co-stimulation provided by plasmacytoid DC (pDC) was recently highlighted as a prominent signal triggering in situ Treg expansion in some tumors, including EOC.[57,58] Lastly, de novo conversion of FoxP3- cells into Treg was shown to occur in the tumor as a consequence of TGF-β stimulation or IDO induction.[59,60] Treg mainly mediate immunosuppression through cell-cell contacts with DC or effector cells or by the secretion of immunosuppressive cytokines, including IL-10, IL-35, and TGF-β. [61] Treg notably contribute to DC tolerization, thereby further reducing the effector T-cell activation and proliferation. Interestingly, association of tumor regulatory T cells with high hazard ratio for death and decreased survival times is currently well documented in EOC.[23,36,62] Besides Treg, DC are instrumental in establishing immunosuppression in cancer. While DC were initially recognized as the primary orchestrators of the immune response, their role in the immunotolerance is now well established.[63] Importantly, both conventional myeloid DC and pDC are characterized by high plasticity.[64] Consequently, their immune properties could be modulated by environmental stimuli, and tumors may benefit from this Achille's heel to induce DC tolerization and to reduce the adaptive immunity to tumor antigens. Accordingly, studies showed that the EOC microenvironment converts DC toward an immunosuppressive phenotype.[65] In a mouse model of EOC, Scarlett et al. showed that the DC phenotype controls EOC progression. Indeed, the switch of infiltrating DC from activating to regulatory phenotype coincides with rapid tumor progression to terminal disease.[56] The role of pDC in EOC immunity was proposed by Zou et al. that evidenced the recruitment of pDC in response to stromal-derived factor-1 (SDF-1/CXCL-12) secretion by EOC.[66] The accumulation of pDC within the EOC was shown to be associated with shorter progression-free survival.[54] Tolerogenic DC may exert profound immunosuppressive effects on effector lymphocytes. Alteration of the IFN-α production by pDC was recently documented in EOC.[54] Moreover, through PD-L1/PD-L2 expression,

DC can engage the PD-1 inhibitory pathway, thus inhibiting lymphocyte proliferation and effector functions,[67,68] inducing tumor-specific T-cell apoptosis,[69] and promoting the differentiation of CD4+ T-cells into Treg.[70] Tolerogenic DC can also turn down the immune response through the induction of IDO activity that inhibits CD8+ T-cell proliferation[71] and decreases NKG2D expression on NK cells.[72] As mentioned for DC, the tumor microenvironment also strongly polarizes the macrophage differentiation and gives rise to TAM.[37] B7-H4+ macrophages, a subset of TAM, was shown to suppress TAA-specific T-cell immunity.[53] An inverse correlation was evidenced between the intensity of B7-H4 expression on macrophages in EOC and patient survival.[62] Moreover, average five-year survival rate was found significantly higher in EOC patients with low densities of TAM than in patients with increased TAM populations.[73] Lastly, MDSC are immature myeloid cells with immunosuppressive properties that were evidenced in both mouse model of EOC and EOC patients.[55,74,75] MDSC exhibit increased level of arginase-1 (ARG-1) and inductible nitric oxide synthase (iNOS) activities. Deprivation of L-arginine in the tumor microenvironment is emerging as a key immunosuppressive mechanism. It leads to CD3-zeta chain downregulation, thereby inhibiting effector T-cell activation.[76] Increased levels of nitric oxide, along with reactive oxygen and nitrogen species, disrupt signaling through the IL-2 receptor[77] and alter Ag recognition by nitrating the TCR.[78] Moreover, MDSC were shown to facilitate effector T-cell conversion into Treg[79] and to inhibit intratumoral migration of CD8+ effectors because of the nitration of CCL2 chemoattractant (Table 3.2).[80]

ROLE OF STROMA CELLS IN IMMUNE SUPPRESSION

The third player in tumor escape is the stromal cell population. Overexpression of the endothelin-B receptor by tumor endothelial cells inhibits concurrent

TABLE 3.2 CLINICAL ARGUMENTS FOR IMMUNE SUPPRESSION IN EPITHELIAL OVARIAN CARCINOMA

Authors	Year	Findings
Curiel et al.[36]	2004	Inverse association between survival and intratumoral regulatory T cells (CD4+CD25+FoxP3+)
Wolf et al.[40]	2005	Inverse association between survival and intratumoral regulatory T cells (FoxP3+)
Dong et al.[41]	2006	Inverse association between survival and intratumoral NK (CD3- CD16+) or B cells (CD19+)
Kryczek et al.[42]	2007	Inverse association between survival and intratumoral B7-H4+ macrophage or regulatory T cells (FoxP3+)
Hamanishi et al.[24]	2007	PD-L1 expression by tumor predicts low T-cell infiltration
Buckanovitch et al.[43]	2008	Endothelin B receptor (ET$_B$R) expression restricts T-cell infiltration and predicts poor survival
Labidi-Galy[44,45]	2011	Inverse association between survival and intratumoral pDC (CD4+, CD123+, BDCA2+)

NOTE: PD-1 = programmed cell death 1; PD-L1 = PD-1 ligand 1; ET$_B$R = endothelin B receptor; pDC = plasmacytoïd dendritic cells.

ICAM-1 expression, thereby impairing the ICAM-1/LFA-1-mediated transmigration of leukocytes.[81] Overexpression of the endothelin-B receptor is associated with the absence of TIL and short survival time in EOC patients.[82] Furthermore, stromal cells may provide chemoattractants for the immune cells (e.g., SDF-1/CXCL12) that recruit Pdc.[66] They are also able to secrete soluble immunosuppressive factors (e.g., prostaglandin-E2 [PGE2], which is produced by mesenchymal stem cells [MSC]). Furthermore, expression of CD95L by tumor endothelial cells selects immune cells intratumor recruitment. Indeed, in EOCs, soluble factors such as vascular endothelial growth factor A, interleukin 10 (IL-10), and PGE2[83] cooperatively induced CD95L expression in endothelial cells, which thereby acquired the ability to kill effector CD8+ T cells but not Treg cells because of higher levels of c-FLIP expression in Treg cells.[84] CD95L belongs to the tumor necrosis factor (TNF) family and is the ligand of the death receptor CD95. While CD95 is ubiquitously expressed, CD95L exhibits a restricted expression pattern, mainly detected at the surface of lymphocytes, where it contributes to the elimination of infected and transformed cells.

IMMUNOSUPPRESSIVE SOLUBLE FACTORS

Finally, the EOC microenvironment is characterized by the presence of numerous immunosuppressive soluble or cellular factors (IL-10, TGF-β, PGE2, MIF, HLA-G, IDO, arginase-1, PD-L1, B7-H4, and Fas-ligand), which can originate from various sources, including tumor, immune, and stromal cells.[85–89] PGE2 can be secreted by both MSC and EOC tumor cells. Of note, overexpression of COX-2, an inducible enzyme that triggers PGE2 synthesis, by ovarian tumor cells correlates with resistance to chemotherapy and poor prognosis.[90] PGE2 inhibits NK and γδ T-cell cytotoxicity[91–93] and induces the differentiation of CD4+ T cells into Treg.[94] Similarly, IDO is expressed in ovarian tumor cells and tumor-infiltrating DC.[47,48,95] IDO expression was reported in 43% of analyzed EOC tissues (83/192).[96] Moreover, its expression was correlated with worse patient survival[47,48] and with enhanced peritoneal tumor dissemination.[48,97] IDO is currently thought to be one of the main factors that contribute to tumor-induced immunosuppression by depleting tryptophan from the microenvironment and producing tryptophan metabolite kynurenine. Depletion of tryptophan is sensed by GCN2 kinase pathway driving effector T-cell anergy and apoptosis.[98] Effects of kynurenine are mediated by the aryl hydrocarbon receptor transcription factor that induces increased survival and motility in cancer cells while favoring Treg expansion and suppressive effects in effector T cells.[99,100]

Thus, regulatory cells, along with soluble and cellular immunosuppressive factors, create a tolerogenic microenvironment in EOC that compromises the anti-tumor immune response. These EOC immunosuppressive networks characterize the "cancer immunoediting" concept, which emphasizes a dynamic process of interaction between cancer and the host immune system (Figure 3.1).[40]

IMMUNOMMODULATORY TOOLS TO COUNTERACT IMMUNE SUPPRESSION IN OVARIAN CANCER

Next we review some immunomodulatory tools already in clinical use or likely to be

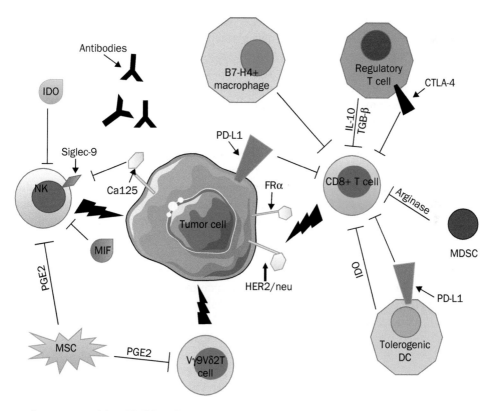

Figure 3.1 Immune network in epithelial ovarian carcinoma. EOC is immunogenic and expresses tumor-associated antigens such as HER2/neu, Ca125, or FRa. Various immune effectors such as the CD8+ T cell, NK cell, or Vg9Vd2 T cell can attack tumor cells, but immunosuppressive crosstalks counteract effector cell attacks. Regulatory T cells, tolerogenic DC, MDSC, B7-H4+ macrophages, or nonimmune cells such as MSC or tumor cells themself halt immune anti-tumor activities through cell-cell contacts or soluble factors (i.e., IL-10, TGF-b, arginase, MIF, IDO, PGE2). For example, immunosuppressive cell-cell contacts involve the Ca125/siglec pathway or programmed death 1/PD-L1 pathway. CTLA-4 is an other example of an immunosuppressive checkpoint in the tumor microenvironment. Reprinted with permission from Lavoue V, et al. Immunity of human epithelial ovarian carcinoma: the paradigm of immune suppression in cancer. *J Transl Med.* 2013 Jun 13;11: 147. doi: 10.1186/1479-5876-11-147

assessed in the near future that interact with the immunosuppressive factors found in the EOC microenvironment.

DEPLETE RECRUITMENT OF REGULATORY CELLS

The first approach may consist of depleting the host of the regulatory cells or limiting their recruitment within the tumor. Treg depletion may be achieved using low-dose cyclophosphamide which prevents, under an incompletely understood mechanism, Treg development and functionality.[101,102] An alternative strategy uses the expression by Treg of the IL-2 receptor alpha (CD25). Recombinant fusion protein of IL-2 and diphtheria toxin (Ontak®, Eisai) was tested in EOC patients and showed effective depletion of circulating Treg.[103] Moreover, in patients with metastatic breast cancer, the anti-CD25 mAb daclizumab (Zenapax®, Roche) demonstrated selective T-lymphocyte killing properties, allowing Treg depletion for several weeks.[104] However, it is unclear if Treg depletion occurs at EOC locations (solid tumor, malignant ascites) and results in tumor regression.[103-105] Moreover, as effector cells also express CD25, anti-CD25 mAb may also induce unwanted depletion of effector cells.[106] In addition, blocking the ICOS pathway could inhibit the pDC-triggered proliferation of Treg within the tumor.[58] However, as the ICOS pathway also favors the differentiation of Th17 cells, which might either promote tumor growth or anti-tumor response,[35,37,107-110] careful preclinical investigations of ICOS inhibitors (314.8 mAb) is needed.[57]

The role of chemoattractants in the recruitment of immune cells also gives a great opportunity to reduce the infiltration of regulatory cells within the tumor.[111] First candidates are under investigation. CCR4 antagonists were shown to block the recruitment of Treg instructed by CCL22 and CCL17 and to favor the induction of antigen-specific CD8+ T cell response after vaccination.[112] Similarly, Bindarit®, which inhibits CCL2

synthesis and therefore restricts the recruitment in the tumor of immature myeloid cells, was shown to induce tumor regression in prostate and breast cancer animal models.[113] Regulatory cell depletion could also be achieved by improving the maturation of immature myeloid cells[114] using all trans retinoic acid[115] or ultra-low non-cytotoxic doses of paclitaxel (chemo-immunomodulation).[116]

USE OF ANTAGONISTS OF IMMUNE-REPRESSOR MOLECULES OR AGONISTS OF IMMUNE-ACTIVATING RECEPTORS

Another attractive approach is the use of either antagonists of immune-repressor molecules or agonists of immune-activating receptors.[117] Checkpoint blockade receptors comprise CTLA-4, PD-1, and KIR that, upon engagement, dampen the immune response. CTLA-4 predominantly regulates T cells at the priming phase of activation by competing with CD28+ for binding of B7-1 and B7-2 on DC. CTLA-4 engagement prevents T cells from achieving full activation. Accordingly, anti-CTLA-4 mAb were shown to activate CD4+ and CD8+ effector T cells both directly by removing inhibitory checkpoints and indirectly via the inhibition of regulatory T-cell activity.[118] Eleven EOC patients, previously vaccinated with GM-CSF and irradiated autologous tumor cells, received anti-CTLA-4 ipilimumab (Yervoy®, Bristol-Myers-Squibb [BMS]). Significant anti-tumor effects were observed in a minority of these patients and were correlated with increased CD8+ T-cells/Treg ratio.[119] In contrast to CTLA-4, PD-1 signaling occurs in the tumor, where PD-L1-expressing tumor cells can signal through PD-1 on TIL to turn down the anti-tumor T-cell response. In EOC, the PD-1/PD-L1 pathway seems to be a dominant immunosuppression mechanism.[68] PD-L1 expression in EOC was demonstrated to be an independent unfavorable prognostic factor and to promote peritoneal dissemination.[24,120] Several PD-1/PD-L1-pathway blocking agents were assessed in various cancer types, and promising results were recently reported. Nivolumab (BMS-936558, Bristol-Myers-Squibb) was tested in 296 patients, most harboring lung cancer, renal cell cancer, and melanoma, with clinical benefits apparent in 20% to 25% of the patients.[121] Impressive durable responses were reported: 25/42 patients with PD-L1-positive tumor experienced an objective response while none of the 17/42 PD-L1-negative patients did. However, lack of prognostic association was reported elsewhere, and the usefulness of PD-L1 as a biomarker needs to be explored in larger prospective studies.[122] In addition, Bramher and colleagues reported that 1/17 EOC patients treated with anti-PD-L1 mAb (BMS-936559) experienced an objective response.[123] New trials enrolling patients with solid tumor of multiple origins are underway and informative data in EOC are expected.[124] Inhibition of the cytotoxic properties of NK cells through KIR engagement may also contribute to the tumor escape. Some anti-KIR antibodies, such as lilirumab (Bristol-Myers-Squibb), recently entered clinical development phases. First data were obtained in hematological diseases, and Phase I studies recruiting patients with solid tumors are ongoing.[125,126] As a corollary, agonistic agents of costimulatory molecules such as glucocorticoid-induced TNFR (GITR), OX40, and CD137 are candidates to boost the anti-tumor immune response. A dose-escalation Phase I clinical trial (NCT01239134) with agonist anti-GITR mAb (TRX518) was recently initiated.

REPRESS ENZYME ACTIVITIES THAT INHIBIT IMMUNE RESPONSE

The third possibility is to repress the activity of enzymes (IDO, ARG-1, iNOS) that were shown to inhibit the immune response. Data from the first clinical trials using IDO inhibitors, notably the isomers of 1-methyl-tryptophan, were disappointing, but these studies may suffer from lack of potent and selective IDO inhibitors. New compounds recently entered clinical trials.[127] A Phase II study of IDO inhibitor INCB024360 is currently recruiting patients with biochemical recurrent only EOC following complete remission with first-line chemotherapy (clinical trial: NCT01685255). In addition, inhibitors of phosphodiesterase (PDE)-5 (e.g., sildenafil) were reported to increase intracellular concentrations of cGPM, resulting in the inhibition of both ARG-1 and iNOS. PDE-5 inhibitors along with nitroaspirin or specific ARG-1/iNOS inhibitors might provide new therapeutic strategy to recover potent anti-tumor immune response.[114]

Lastly, PGE2 was shown to be a crucial immunosuppressive factor in EOC, as it impairs the cytotoxic properties of effector cells such as $V\gamma9V\delta2$ T cells[92] and also induces the differentiation of MDSC from bone marrow stem cells in a mouse model.[128] PGE2 biosynthesis is regulated by the inducible COX-2 enzyme and could be inhibited by the COX-2-specific inhibitor celecoxib (Celebrex®, Pfizer). In a mouse model, celecoxib prevented the local and systemic expansion of MDSC, impaired the suppressive function of these cells, and significantly improved vaccine immunotherapy.[129] Thus, celecoxib, currently used in the prevention of colorectal adenomatous polyps,[130] could be tested in combination with immunotherapy to reduce the immunosuppression by MDSC in EOC. Another possible strategy to counteract the immunosuppressive influence of PGE2 on $V\gamma9V\delta2$ T cells could be to restore the cytotoxic properties of these cells with a zoledronate perfusion.[92] In addition, zoledronate was shown to prevent the immunosuppressive polarization of TAM,[131,132] which is a major component of the leukocyte infiltrate in the tumor microenvironment and plays a dominant role in the production of immune suppressive cytokines in EOC.[53] Thus, zoledronate, which is currently used for the management of osteoporosis and bone metastasis, appears to be an attractive molecule to reinforce the immune response. Altogether, these data warrant further exploration of combinatorial therapies with immunotherapy and bisphosphonates.

CONCLUSION

In conclusion, accumulated evidence supports the immunoediting hypothesis and the idea that EOC is immunogenic. Immunotherapeutic protocols aimed at modulating the immune system to strengthen the spontaneous anti-tumor immune response are under investigation. Targeting the immunosuppressive mechanisms could be the key to fully unleash the potential of immunotherapy. The combination of molecules endowed with immuno-modulatory properties with immunotherapy targeting the tumor cells will hopefully increase the survival of EOC patients. Careful preclinical evaluation will be necessary to screen optimal combinations before clinical trials.

REFERENCES

1. Jemal A, Siegel R, Ward E, Hao Y, Xu J, Thun MJ. Cancer statistics, 2009. *CA Cancer J Clin.* 2009;59:225–49.
2. Pfisterer J, Ledermann JA. Management of platinum-sensitive recurrent ovarian cancer. *Semin Oncol.* 2006;33:S12–16.
3. Hoskins P, Vergote I, Cervantes A, Tu D, Stuart G, Zola P, et al. Advanced ovarian cancer: phase III randomized study of sequential cisplatin-topotecan and carboplatin-paclitaxel vs carboplatin-paclitaxel. *J Natl Cancer Inst.* 2010;102:1547–56.
4. Knutson KL, Curiel TJ, Salazar L, Disis ML. Immunologic principles and immunotherapeutic approaches in ovarian cancer. *Hematol Oncol Clin North Am.* 2003;17:1051–73.
5. Cubillos-Ruiz JR, Rutkowski M, Conejo-Garcia JR. Blocking ovarian cancer progression by targeting tumor microenvironmental leukocytes. *Cell Cycle.* 2010;9:260–68.
6. Brune IB, Wilke W, Hensler T, Holzmann B, Siewert JR. Downregulation of T helper type 1 immune response and altered pro-inflammatory and anti-inflammatory T cell cytokine balance following conventional but not laparoscopic surgery. *Am J Surg.* 1999;177:55–60.
7. Napoletano C, Bellati F, Landi R, Pauselli S, Marchetti C, Visconti V, et al. Ovarian cancer cytoreduction induces changes in T cell population subsets reducing immunosuppression. *J Cell Mol Med.* 2010;14:2748–59.
8. Coleman S, Clayton A, Mason MD, Jasani B, Adams M, Tabi Z. Recovery of CD8+ T-cell function during systemic chemotherapy in advanced ovarian cancer. *Cancer Res.* 2005;65:7000–7006.
9. Ioannides CG, Fisk B, Fan D, Biddison WE, Wharton JT, O'Brian CA. Cytotoxic T cells isolated from ovarian malignant ascites recognize a peptide derived from the HER-2/neu proto-oncogene. *Cell Immunol.* 1993;151:225–34.
10. Bookman MA, Darcy KM, Clarke-Pearson D, Boothby RA, Horowitz IR. Evaluation of monoclonal humanized anti-HER2 antibody, trastuzumab, in patients with recurrent or refractory ovarian or primary peritoneal carcinoma with overexpression of HER2: a phase II trial of the Gynecologic Oncology Group. *J Clin Oncol.* 2003;21:283–90.
11. Camilleri-Broet S, Hardy-Bessard AC, Le Tourneau A, Paraiso D, Levrel O, Leduc B, et al. HER-2 overexpression is an independent marker of poor prognosis of advanced primary ovarian carcinoma: a multicenter study of the GINECO group. *Ann Oncol.* 2004;15:104–12.
12. Peoples GE, Anderson BW, Fisk B, Kudelka AP, Wharton JT, Ioannides CG. Ovarian cancer-associated lymphocyte recognition of folate binding protein peptides. *Ann Surg Oncol.* 1998;5:743–50.
13. Runz S, Keller S, Rupp C, Stoeck A, Issa Y, Koensgen D, et al. Malignant ascites-derived exosomes of ovarian carcinoma patients contain CD24 and EpCAM. *Gynecol Oncol.* 2007;107:563–71.
14. Drapkin R, von Horsten HH, Lin Y, Mok SC, Crum CP, Welch WR, et al. Human epididymis protein 4 (HE4) is a secreted glycoprotein that is overexpressed by serous and endometrioid ovarian carcinomas. *Cancer Res.* 2005;65:2162–69.
15. Goodell V, Salazar LG, Urban N, Drescher CW, Gray H, Swensen RE, et al. Antibody immunity to the p53 oncogenic protein is a prognostic indicator in ovarian cancer. *J Clin Oncol.* 2006;24:762–68.
16. Chauhan SC, Singh AP, Ruiz F, Johansson SL, Jain M, Smith LM, et al. Aberrant expression of MUC4 in ovarian carcinoma: diagnostic significance alone and in combination with MUC1 and MUC16 (CA125). *Mod Pathol.* 2006;19:1386–94.
17. Zhang S, Zhou X, Yu H, Yu Y. Expression of tumor-specific antigen MAGE, GAGE and BAGE in ovarian cancer tissues and cell lines. *BMC Cancer.* 2010;10:163.
18. Chiriva-Internati M, Wang Z, Salati E, Timmins P, Lim SH. Tumor vaccine for ovarian carcinoma targeting sperm protein 17. *Cancer.* 2002;94:2447–53.
19. Schlienger K, Chu CS, Woo EY, Rivers PM, Toll AJ, Hudson B, et al. TRANCE- and CD40 ligand-matured dendritic cells reveal MHC class I-restricted T cells specific for autologous tumor in late-stage ovarian cancer patients. *Clin Cancer Res.* 2003;9:1517–27.
20. Peoples GE, Schoof DD, Andrews JV, Goedegebuure PS, Eberlein TJ. T-cell recognition of ovarian cancer. *Surgery.* 1993;114:227–34.
21. Zhang L, Conejo-Garcia JR, Katsaros D, Gimotty PA, Massobrio M, Regnani G, et al. Intratumoral T

cells, recurrence, and survival in epithelial ovarian cancer. *N Engl J Med.* 2003;348:203–13.

22. Raspollini MR, Castiglione F, Rossi Degl'innocenti D, Amunni G, Villanucci A, Garbini F, et al. Tumour-infiltrating gamma/delta T-lymphocytes are correlated with a brief disease-free interval in advanced ovarian serous carcinoma. *Ann Oncol.* 2005;16:590–96.

23. Sato E, Olson SH, Ahn J, Bundy B, Nishikawa H, Qian F, et al. Intraepithelial CD8+ tumor-infiltrating lymphocytes and a high CD8+/regulatory T cell ratio are associated with favorable prognosis in ovarian cancer. *Proc Natl Acad Sci U S A.* 2005;102:18538–43.

24. Hamanishi J, Mandai M, Iwasaki M, Okazaki T, Tanaka Y, Yamaguchi K, et al. Programmed cell death 1 ligand 1 and tumor-infiltrating CD8+ T lymphocytes are prognostic factors of human ovarian cancer. *Proc Natl Acad Sci U S A.* 2007;104:3360–65.

25. Clarke B, Tinker AV, Lee CH, Subramanian S, van de Rijn M, Turbin D, et al. Intraepithelial T cells and prognosis in ovarian carcinoma: novel associations with stage, tumor type, and BRCA1 loss. *Mod Pathol.* 2009;22:393–402.

26. Shah CA, Allison KH, Garcia RL, Gray HJ, Goff BA, Swisher EM. Intratumoral T cells, tumor-associated macrophages, and regulatory T cells: association with p53 mutations, circulating tumor DNA and survival in women with ovarian cancer. *Gynecol Oncol.* 2008;109:215–19.

27. Tomsova M, Melichar B, Sedlakova I, Steiner I. Prognostic significance of CD3+ tumor-infiltrating lymphocytes in ovarian carcinoma. *Gynecol Oncol.* 2008;108:415–20.

28. Han LY, Fletcher MS, Urbauer DL, Mueller P, Landen CN, Kamat AA, et al. HLA class I antigen processing machinery component expression and intratumoral T-Cell infiltrate as independent prognostic markers in ovarian carcinoma. *Clin Cancer Res.* 2008;14:3372–79.

29. Stumpf M, Hasenburg A, Riener MO, Jutting U, Wang C, Shen Y, et al. Intraepithelial CD8-positive T lymphocytes predict survival for patients with serous stage III ovarian carcinomas: relevance of clonal selection of T lymphocytes. *Br J Cancer.* 2009;101:1513–21.

30. Leffers N, Gooden MJ, de Jong RA, Hoogeboom BN, ten Hoor KA, Hollema H, et al. Prognostic significance of tumor-infiltrating T-lymphocytes in primary and metastatic lesions of advanced stage ovarian cancer. *Cancer Immunol Immunother.* 2009;58:449–59.

31. Milne K, Kobel M, Kalloger SE, Barnes RO, Gao D, Gilks CB, et al. Systematic analysis of immune infiltrates in high-grade serous ovarian cancer reveals CD20, FoxP3 and TIA-1 as positive prognostic factors. *PLoS One.* 2009;4:e6412.

32. Adams SF, Levine DA, Cadungog MG, Hammond R, Facciabene A, Olvera N, et al. Intraepithelial T cells and tumor proliferation: impact on the benefit from surgical cytoreduction in advanced serous ovarian cancer. *Cancer.* 2009;115:2891–902.

33. Garzetti GG, Cignitti M, Ciavattini A, Fabris N, Romanini C. Natural killer cell activity and progression-free survival in ovarian cancer. *Gynecol Obstet Invest.* 1993;35:118–20.

34. Thedrez A, Lavoue V, Dessarthe B, Daniel P, Henno S, Jaffre I, et al. A quantitative deficiency in peripheral blood Vgamma9Vdelta2 cells is a negative prognostic biomarker in ovarian cancer patients. *PLoS One.* 2013;8(5):e63322.

35. Kryczek I, Banerjee M, Cheng P, Vatan L, Szeliga W, Wei S, et al. Phenotype, distribution, generation, and functional and clinical relevance of Th17 cells in the human tumor environments. *Blood.* 2009;114:1141–49.

36. Curiel TJ, Coukos G, Zou L, Alvarez X, Cheng P, Mottram P, et al. Specific recruitment of regulatory T cells in ovarian carcinoma fosters immune privilege and predicts reduced survival. *Nat Med.* 2004;10:942–49.

37. Wilke CM, Kryczek I, Zou W. Antigen-presenting cell (APC) subsets in ovarian cancer. *Int Rev Immunol.* 2011;30:120–26.

38. Motz GT, Santoro SP, Wang LP, Garrabrant T, Lastra RR, Hagemann IS, et al. Tumor endothelium FasL establishes a selective immune barrier promoting tolerance in tumors. *Nat Med.* 2014;20:607–15.

39. Burnet FM. The concept of immunological surveillance. *Prog Exp Tumor Res.* 1970;13:1–27.

40. Schreiber RD, Old LJ, Smyth MJ. Cancer immunoediting: integrating immunity's roles in cancer suppression and promotion. *Science.* 2011;331:1565–70.

41. Lu J, Aggarwal R, Kanji S, Das M, Joseph M, Pompili V, et al. Human ovarian tumor cells escape gammadelta T cell recognition partly by down regulating surface expression of MICA and limiting cell cycle related molecules. *PLoS One.* 2011;6:e23348.

42. Thedrez A, Sabourin C, Gertner J, Devilder MC, Allain-Maillet S, Fournie JJ, et al. Self/non-self discrimination by human gammadelta T cells: simple solutions for a complex issue? *Immunol Rev.* 2007;215:123–35.

43. Gubbels JA, Felder M, Horibata S, Belisle JA, Kapur A, Holden H, et al. MUC16 provides immune protection by inhibiting synapse formation between NK and ovarian tumor cells. *Mol Cancer.* 2010;9:11.

44. Belisle JA, Horibata S, Jennifer GA, Petrie S, Kapur A, Andre S, et al. Identification of Siglec-9 as the receptor for MUC16 on human NK cells, B cells, and monocytes. *Mol Cancer.* 2010;9:118.

45. Krockenberger M, Dombrowski Y, Weidler C, Ossadnik M, Honig A, Hausler S, et al. Macrophage migration inhibitory factor contributes to the immune escape of ovarian cancer by down-regulating NKG2D. *J Immunol.* 2008;180:7338–48.

46. Matsuzaki J, Gnjatic S, Mhawech-Fauceglia P, Beck A, Miller A, Tsuji T, et al. Tumor-infiltrating NY-ESO-1-specific CD8+ T cells are negatively

regulated by LAG-3 and PD-1 in human ovarian cancer. *Proc Natl Acad Sci U S A.* 2010;107:7875–80.

47. Okamoto A, Nikaido T, Ochiai K, Takakura S, Saito M, Aoki Y, et al. Indoleamine 2,3-dioxygenase serves as a marker of poor prognosis in gene expression profiles of serous ovarian cancer cells. *Clin Cancer Res.* 2005;11:6030–39.

48. Inaba T, Ino K, Kajiyama H, Yamamoto E, Shibata K, Nawa A, et al. Role of the immunosuppressive enzyme indoleamine 2,3-dioxygenase in the progression of ovarian carcinoma. *Gynecol Oncol.* 2009;115:185–92.

49. Mellor AL, Munn DH. Creating immune privilege: active local suppression that benefits friends, but protects foes. *Nat Rev Immunol.* 2008;8:74–80.

50. Johnson TS, Munn DH. Host indoleamine 2,3-dioxygenase: contribution to systemic acquired tumor tolerance. *Immunol Invest.* 2012;41:765–97.

51. Ostrand-Rosenberg S, Sinha P, Beury DW, Clements VK. Cross-talk between myeloid-derived suppressor cells (MDSC), macrophages, and dendritic cells enhances tumor-induced immune suppression. *Semin Cancer Biol.* 2012;22:275–81.

52. Curiel TJ, Wei S, Dong H, Alvarez X, Cheng P, Mottram P, et al. Blockade of B7-H1 improves myeloid dendritic cell-mediated antitumor immunity. *Nat Med.* 2003;9:562–67.

53. Kryczek I, Zou L, Rodriguez P, Zhu G, Wei S, Mottram P, et al. B7-H4 expression identifies a novel suppressive macrophage population in human ovarian carcinoma. *J Exp Med.* 2006;203:871–81.

54. Labidi-Galy SI, Sisirak V, Meeus P, Gobert M, Treilleux I, Bajard A, et al. Quantitative and functional alterations of plasmacytoid dendritic cells contribute to immune tolerance in ovarian cancer. *Cancer Res.* 2011;71:5423–34.

55. Yang R, Cai Z, Zhang Y, Yutzy WHt, Roby KF, Roden RB. CD80 in immune suppression by mouse ovarian carcinoma-associated Gr-1+CD11b+ myeloid cells. *Cancer Res.* 2006;66:6807–15.

56. Scarlett UK, Rutkowski MR, Rauwerdink AM, Fields J, Escovar-Fadul X, Baird J, et al. Ovarian cancer progression is controlled by phenotypic changes in dendritic cells. *J Exp Med.* 2012;209:495–506.

57. Faget J, Bendriss-Vermare N, Gobert M, Durand I, Olive D, Biota C, et al. ICOS-ligand expression on plasmacytoid dendritic cells supports breast cancer progression by promoting the accumulation of immunosuppressive CD4+ T cells. *Cancer Res.* 2012;72:6130–41.

58. Conrad C, Gregorio J, Wang YH, Ito T, Meller S, Hanabuchi S, et al. Plasmacytoid dendritic cells promote immunosuppression in ovarian cancer via ICOS costimulation of Foxp3(+) T-regulatory cells. *Cancer Res.* 2012;72:5240–49.

59. Liu VC, Wong LY, Jang T, Shah AH, Park I, Yang X, et al. Tumor evasion of the immune system by converting CD4+CD25- T cells into CD4+CD25+ T regulatory cells: role of tumor-derived TGF-beta. *J Immunol.* 2007;178:2883–92.

60. Curti A, Pandolfi S, Valzasina B, Aluigi M, Isidori A, Ferri E, et al. Modulation of tryptophan catabolism by human leukemic cells results in the conversion of CD25- into CD25+ T regulatory cells. *Blood.* 2007;109:2871–77.

61. Oleinika K, Nibbs RJ, Graham GJ, Fraser AR. Suppression, subversion and escape: the role of regulatory T cells in cancer progression. *Clin Exp Immunol.* 2013;171:36–45.

62. Kryczek I, Wei S, Zhu G, Myers L, Mottram P, Cheng P, et al. Relationship between B7-H4, regulatory T cells, and patient outcome in human ovarian carcinoma. *Cancer Res.* 2007;67:8900–905.

63. Steinman RM, Hawiger D, Nussenzweig MC. Tolerogenic dendritic cells. *Annu Rev Immunol.* 2003;21:685–711.

64. Ito T, Liu YJ, Kadowaki N. Functional diversity and plasticity of human dendritic cell subsets. *Int J Hematol.* 2005;81:188–96.

65. Scarlett UK, Cubillos-Ruiz JR, Nesbeth YC, Martinez DG, Engle X, Gewirtz AT, et al. In situ stimulation of CD40 and Toll-like receptor 3 transforms ovarian cancer-infiltrating dendritic cells from immunosuppressive to immunostimulatory cells. *Cancer Res.* 2009;69:7329–37.

66. Zou W, Machelon V, Coulomb-L'Hermin A, Borvak J, Nome F, Isaeva T, et al. Stromal-derived factor-1 in human tumors recruits and alters the function of plasmacytoid precursor dendritic cells. *Nat Med.* 2001;7:1339–46.

67. Tseng SY, Otsuji M, Gorski K, Huang X, Slansky JE, Pai SI, et al. B7-DC, a new dendritic cell molecule with potent costimulatory properties for T cells. *J Exp Med.* 2001;193:839–46.

68. Krempski J, Karyampudi L, Behrens MD, Erskine CL, Hartmann L, Dong H, et al. Tumor-infiltrating programmed death receptor-1+ dendritic cells mediate immune suppression in ovarian cancer. *J Immunol.* 2011;186:6905–13.

69. Dong H, Strome SE, Salomao DR, Tamura H, Hirano F, Flies DB, et al. Tumor-associated B7-H1 promotes T-cell apoptosis: a potential mechanism of immune evasion. *Nat Med.* 2002;8:793–800.

70. Wang L, Pino-Lagos K, de Vries VC, Guleria I, Sayegh MH, Noelle RJ. Programmed death 1 ligand signaling regulates the generation of adaptive Foxp3+CD4+ regulatory T cells. *Proc Natl Acad Sci U S A.* 2008;105:9331–36.

71. Munn DH, Sharma MD, Hou D, Baban B, Lee JR, Antonia SJ, et al. Expression of indoleamine 2,3-dioxygenase by plasmacytoid dendritic cells in tumor-draining lymph nodes. *J Clin Invest.* 2004;114:280–90.

72. Della Chiesa M, Carlomagno S, Frumento G, Balsamo M, Cantoni C, Conte R, et al. The tryptophan catabolite L-kynurenine inhibits the surface expression of NKp46- and NKG2D-activating receptors and regulates NK-cell function. *Blood.* 2006;108:4118–25.

73. Wan T, Liu JH, Zheng LM, Cai MY, Ding T. Prognostic significance of tumor-associated

macrophage infiltration in advanced epithelial ovarian carcinoma. *Ai Zheng*. 2009;28:323–27.

74. Bak SP, Alonso A, Turk MJ, Berwin B. Murine ovarian cancer vascular leukocytes require arginase-1 activity for T cell suppression. *Mol Immunol*. 2008;46:258–68.

75. Obermajer N, Muthuswamy R, Odunsi K, Edwards RP, Kalinski P. PGE(2)-induced CXCL12 production and CXCR4 expression controls the accumulation of human MDSCs in ovarian cancer environment. *Cancer Res*. 2011;71:7463–70.

76. Ezernitchi AV, Vaknin I, Cohen-Daniel L, Levy O, Manaster E, Halabi A, et al. TCR zeta downregulation under chronic inflammation is mediated by myeloid suppressor cells differentially distributed between various lymphatic organs. *J Immunol*. 2006;177:4763–72.

77. Mazzoni A, Bronte V, Visintin A, Spitzer JH, Apolloni E, Serafini P, et al. Myeloid suppressor lines inhibit T cell responses by an NO-dependent mechanism. *J Immunol*. 2002;168:689–95.

78. Nagaraj S, Gupta K, Pisarev V, Kinarsky L, Sherman S, Kang L, et al. Altered recognition of antigen is a mechanism of CD8+ T cell tolerance in cancer. *Nat Med*. 2007;13:828–35.

79. Huang B, Pan PY, Li Q, Sato AI, Levy DE, Bromberg J, et al. Gr-1+CD115+ immature myeloid suppressor cells mediate the development of tumor-induced T regulatory cells and T-cell anergy in tumor-bearing host. *Cancer Res*. 2006;66:1123–31.

80. Molon B, Ugel S, Del Pozzo F, Soldani C, Zilio S, Avella D, et al. Chemokine nitration prevents intratumoral infiltration of antigen-specific T cells. *J Exp Med*. 2011;208:1949–62.

81. Yang L, Froio RM, Sciuto TE, Dvorak AM, Alon R, Luscinskas FW. ICAM-1 regulates neutrophil adhesion and transcellular migration of TNF-alpha-activated vascular endothelium under flow. *Blood*. 2005;106:584–92.

82. Buckanovich RJ, Facciabene A, Kim S, Benencia F, Sasaroli D, Balint K, et al. Endothelin B receptor mediates the endothelial barrier to T cell homing to tumors and disables immune therapy. *Nat Med*. 2008;14:28–36.

83. Lavoue V, Cabillic F, Toutirais O, Thedrez A, Dessarthe B, de La Pintiere CT, et al. Sensitization of ovarian carcinoma cells with zoledronate restores the cytotoxic capacity of Vgamma9Vdelta2 T cells impaired by the prostaglandin E2 immunosuppressive factor: implications for immunotherapy. *Int J Cancer*. 2012;131:E449–62.

84. Motz GT, Santoro SP, Wang LP, Garrabrant T, Lastra RR, Hagemann IS, et al. Tumor endothelium FasL establishes a selective immune barrier promoting tolerance in tumors. *Nat Med*. 2014;20(6):607–15.

85. Sebti Y, Le Friec G, Pangault C, Gros F, Drenou B, Guilloux V, et al. Soluble HLA-G molecules are increased in lymphoproliferative disorders. *Hum Immunol*. 2003;64:1093–101.

86. Freedman RS, Deavers M, Liu J, Wang E. Peritoneal inflammation—A microenvironment for epithelial ovarian cancer (EOC). *J Transl Med*. 2004;2:23.

87. Nelson BH. The impact of T-cell immunity on ovarian cancer outcomes. *Immunol Rev*. 2008;222:101–16.

88. Lin A, Zhang X, Zhou WJ, Ruan YY, Xu DP, Wang Q, et al. Human leukocyte antigen-G expression is associated with a poor prognosis in patients with esophageal squamous cell carcinoma. *Int J Cancer*. 2011;129:1382–90.

89. Rodriguez GC, Haisley C, Hurteau J, Moser TL, Whitaker R, Bast RC Jr, et al. Regulation of invasion of epithelial ovarian cancer by transforming growth factor-beta. *Gynecol Oncol*. 2001;80:245–53.

90. Ferrandina G, Lauriola L, Zannoni GF, Fagotti A, Fanfani F, Legge F, et al. Increased cyclooxygenase-2 (COX-2) expression is associated with chemotherapy resistance and outcome in ovarian cancer patients. *Ann Oncol*. 2002;13:1205–11.

91. Martinet L, Jean C, Dietrich G, Fournie JJ, Poupot R. PGE2 inhibits natural killer and gamma delta T cell cytotoxicity triggered by NKR and TCR through a cAMP-mediated PKA type I-dependent signaling. *Biochem Pharmacol*. 2010;80:838–45.

92. Lavoue V, Cabillic F, Toutirais O, Thedrez A, Dessarthe B, Thomas de La Pintiere C, et al. Sensitization of ovarian carcinoma cells with zoledronate restores the cytotoxic capacity of Vgamma9Vdelta2 T cells impaired by the prostaglandin E2 immunosuppressive factor: Implications for immunotherapy. *Int J Cancer*. 2011;131(4):E449–62.

93. Komarova S, Kawakami Y, Stoff-Khalili MA, Curiel DT, Pereboeva L. Mesenchymal progenitor cells as cellular vehicles for delivery of oncolytic adenoviruses. *Mol Cancer Ther*. 2006;5:755–66.

94. Baratelli F, Lin Y, Zhu L, Yang SC, Heuze-Vourc'h N, Zeng G, et al. Prostaglandin E2 induces FOXP3 gene expression and T regulatory cell function in human CD4+ T cells. *J Immunol*. 2005;175:1483–90.

95. Harden JL, Egilmez NK. Indoleamine 2,3-dioxygenase and dendritic cell tolerogenicity. *Immunol Invest*. 2012;41:738–64.

96. Qian F, Villella J, Wallace PK, Mhawech-Fauceglia P, Tario JD Jr, Andrews C, et al. Efficacy of levo-1-methyl tryptophan and dextro-1-methyl tryptophan in reversing indoleamine-2,3-dioxygenase-mediated arrest of T-cell proliferation in human epithelial ovarian cancer. *Cancer Res*. 2009;69:5498–504.

97. Nonaka H, Saga Y, Fujiwara H, Akimoto H, Yamada A, Kagawa S, et al. Indoleamine 2,3-dioxygenase promotes peritoneal dissemination of ovarian cancer through inhibition of natural killercell function and angiogenesis promotion. *Int J Oncol*. 2011;38:113–20.

98. Munn DH, Sharma MD, Baban B, Harding HP, Zhang Y, Ron D, et al. GCN2 kinase in T cells mediates proliferative arrest and anergy induction in response to indoleamine 2,3-dioxygenase. *Immunity*. 2005;22:633–42.

99. Fallarino F, Grohmann U, You S, McGrath BC, Cavener DR, Vacca C, et al. The combined effects of tryptophan starvation and tryptophan catabolites down-regulate T cell receptor zeta-chain and induce a regulatory phenotype in naive T cells. *J Immunol.* 2006;176:6752–61.

100. Platten M, Wick W, Van den Eynde BJ. Tryptophan catabolism in cancer: beyond IDO and tryptophan depletion. *Cancer Res.* 2011;72:5435–40.

101. Berd D, Maguire HC, Jr., Mastrangelo MJ. Induction of cell-mediated immunity to autologous melanoma cells and regression of metastases after treatment with a melanoma cell vaccine preceded by cyclophosphamide. *Cancer Res.* 1986;46:2572–77.

102. Ghiringhelli F, Menard C, Puig PE, Ladoire S, Roux S, Martin F, et al. Metronomic cyclophosphamide regimen selectively depletes CD4+CD25+ regulatory T cells and restores T and NK effector functions in end stage cancer patients. *Cancer Immunol Immunother.* 2007;56:641–48.

103. Attia P, Maker AV, Haworth LR, Rogers-Freezer L, Rosenberg SA. Inability of a fusion protein of IL-2 and diphtheria toxin (Denileukin Diftitox, DAB389IL-2, ONTAK) to eliminate regulatory T lymphocytes in patients with melanoma. *J Immunother.* 2005;28:582–92.

104. Rech AJ, Mick R, Martin S, Recio A, Aqui NA, Powell DJ Jr, et al. CD25 blockade depletes and selectively reprograms regulatory T cells in concert with immunotherapy in cancer patients. *Sci Transl Med.* 2012;4:134ra62.

105. Barnett B, Kryczek I, Cheng P, Zou W, Curiel TJ. Regulatory T cells in ovarian cancer: biology and therapeutic potential. *Am J Reprod Immunol.* 2005;54:369–77.

106. Sutmuller RP, van Duivenvoorde LM, van Elsas A, Schumacher TN, Wildenberg ME, Allison JP, et al. Synergism of cytotoxic T lymphocyte-associated antigen 4 blockade and depletion of CD25(+) regulatory T cells in antitumor therapy reveals alternative pathways for suppression of autoreactive cytotoxic T lymphocyte responses. *J Exp Med.* 2001;194:823–32.

107. Wilke CM, Kryczek I, Wei S, Zhao E, Wu K, Wang G, et al. Th17 cells in cancer: help or hindrance? *Carcinogenesis.* 2011;32:643–49.

108. Greten TF, Zhao F, Gamrekelashvili J, Korangy F. Human Th17 cells in patients with cancer: Friends or foe? *Oncoimmunology.* 2012;1:1438–39.

109. Martin-Orozco N, Muranski P, Chung Y, Yang XO, Yamazaki T, Lu S, et al. T helper 17 cells promote cytotoxic T cell activation in tumor immunity. *Immunity.* 2009;31:787–98.

110. Charles KA, Kulbe H, Soper R, Escorcio-Correia M, Lawrence T, Schultheis A, et al. The tumor-promoting actions of TNF-alpha involve TNFR1 and IL-17 in ovarian cancer in mice and humans. *J Clin Invest.* 2009;119:3011–23.

111. Wu X, Lee VC, Chevalier E, Hwang ST. Chemokine receptors as targets for cancer therapy. *Curr Pharm Des.* 2009;15:742–57.

112. Pere H, Montier Y, Bayry J, Quintin-Colonna F, Merillon N, Dransart E, et al. A CCR4 antagonist combined with vaccines induces antigen-specific CD8+ T cells and tumor immunity against self antigens. *Blood.* 2011;118:4853–62.

113. Zollo M, Di Dato V, Spano D, De Martino D, Liguori L, Marino N, et al. Targeting monocyte chemotactic protein-1 synthesis with bindarit induces tumor regression in prostate and breast cancer animal models. *Clin Exp Metastasis.* 2012;29:585–601.

114. Sevko A, Umansky V. Myeloid-derived suppressor cells interact with tumors in terms of myelopoiesis, tumorigenesis and immunosuppression: thick as thieves. *J Cancer.* 2013;4:3–11.

115. Mirza N, Fishman M, Fricke I, Dunn M, Neuger AM, Frost TJ, et al. All-trans-retinoic acid improves differentiation of myeloid cells and immune response in cancer patients. *Cancer Res.* 2006;66:9299–307.

116. Shurin MR, Naiditch H, Gutkin DW, Umansky V, Shurin GV. ChemoImmuno Modulation: immune regulation by the antineoplastic chemotherapeutic agents. *Curr Med Chem.* 2012;19:1792–803.

117. Melero I, Grimaldi AM, Perez-Gracia JL, Ascierto PA. Clinical development of immunostimulatory monoclonal antibodies and opportunities for combination. *Clin Cancer Res.* 2013;19:997–1008.

118. Peggs KS, Quezada SA, Chambers CA, Korman AJ, Allison JP. Blockade of CTLA-4 on both effector and regulatory T cell compartments contributes to the antitumor activity of anti-CTLA-4 antibodies. *J Exp Med.* 2009;206:1717–25.

119. Hodi FS, Butler M, Oble DA, Seiden MV, Haluska FG, Kruse A, et al. Immunologic and clinical effects of antibody blockade of cytotoxic T lymphocyte-associated antigen 4 in previously vaccinated cancer patients. *Proc Natl Acad Sci U S A.* 2008;105:3005–10.

120. Abiko K, Mandai M, Hamanishi J, Yoshioka Y, Matsumura N, Baba T, et al. PD-L1 on tumor cells is induced in ascites and promotes peritoneal dissemination of ovarian cancer through CTL dysfunction. *Clin Cancer Res.* 2013;19:1363–74.

121. Topalian SL, Hodi FS, Brahmer JR, Gettinger SN, Smith DC, McDermott DF, et al. Safety, activity, and immune correlates of anti-PD-1 antibody in cancer. *N Engl J Med.* 2012;366(26):2443–54.

122. Karim R, Jordanova ES, Piersma SJ, Kenter GG, Chen L, Boer JM, et al. Tumor-expressed B7-H1 and B7-DC in relation to PD-1+ T-cell infiltration and survival of patients with cervical carcinoma. *Clin Cancer Res.* 2009;15:6341–47.

123. Brahmer JR, Tykodi SS, Chow LQ, Hwu WJ, Topalian SL, Hwu P, et al. Safety and activity of anti-PD-L1 antibody in patients with advanced cancer. *N Engl J Med.* 2012;366:2455–65.

124. Hamid O, Carvajal RD. Anti-programmed death-1 and anti-programmed death-ligand 1 antibodies

in cancer therapy. *Expert Opin Biol Ther.* 2013;13(6):847–61.

125. Benson DM, Jr., Hofmeister CC, Padmanabhan S, Suvannasankha A, Jagannath S, Abonour R, et al. A phase I trial of the anti-KIR antibody IPH2101 in patients with relapsed/refractory multiple myeloma. *Blood.* 2012;120:4324–33.

126. Vey N, Bourhis JH, Boissel N, Bordessoule D, Prebet T, Charbonnier A, et al. A phase 1 trial of the anti-inhibitory KIR mAb IPH2101 for AML in complete remission. *Blood.* 2012;120:4317–23.

127. Liu X, Shin N, Koblish HK, Yang G, Wang Q, Wang K, et al. Selective inhibition of IDO1 effectively regulates mediators of antitumor immunity. *Blood.* 2010;115:3520–30.

128. Sinha P, Clements VK, Fulton AM, Ostrand-Rosenberg S. Prostaglandin E2 promotes tumor progression by inducing myeloid-derived suppressor cells. *Cancer Res.* 2007;67:4507–13.

129. Veltman JD, Lambers ME, van Nimwegen M, Hendriks RW, Hoogsteden HC, Aerts JG, et al. COX-2 inhibition improves immunotherapy and is associated with decreased numbers of myeloid-derived suppressor cells in mesothelioma. Celecoxib influences MDSC function. *BMC Cancer.* 2010;10:464.

130. Arber N, Eagle CJ, Spicak J, Racz I, Dite P, Hajer J, et al. Celecoxib for the prevention of colorectal adenomatous polyps. *N Engl J Med.* 2006;355:885–95.

131. Rogers TL, Holen I. Tumour macrophages as potential targets of bisphosphonates. *J Transl Med.* 2011;9:177.

132. Veltman JD, Lambers ME, van Nimwegen M, Hendriks RW, Hoogsteden HC, Hegmans JP, et al. Zoledronic acid impairs myeloid differentiation to tumour-associated macrophages in mesothelioma. *Br J Cancer.* 2010;103:629–41.

4.

OVARIAN TUMOR MICROENVIRONMENT AND INNATE IMMUNE RECOGNITION

Jocelyn Reader, Sarah Lynam, Amy Harper, Gautam Rao, Maya Matheny, and Dana M. Roque

INTRODUCTION

Ovarian adenocarcinoma is typified by detection at late stages with dissemination of cancer cells into the peritoneal cavity and frequent acquisition of chemoresistance. These characteristics can be explained in part by the intrinsic properties of ovarian cancer cells. A number of studies show the importance of the tumor microenvironment in tumor progression. Ovarian cancer cells can regulate the composition of their stroma to promote the formation of ascitic fluid rich in cytokines and bioactive lipids and to stimulate the differentiation of stromal cells into a pro-tumoral phenotype. In response, cancer-associated fibroblasts, cancer-associated mesenchymal stem cells, tumor-associated macrophages, and other peritoneal cells such as adipocytes and mesothelial cells, can regulate tumor growth, angiogenesis, dissemination, and chemoresistance. This chapter deciphers the current knowledge about the role of stromal cells, associated secreted factors, and the immune system on tumor progression. This provides a foundation to suggest that targeting the microenvironment holds great potential to improve the prognosis of patients with ovarian adenocarcinoma.

INNATE IMMUNE SYSTEM: DEFINITIONS AND COMPONENTS

Immune surveillance plays an important role in tumor kinetics. Distinct populations of immune cells are recruited to the tumor site with the potential to play a tumor-promoting or tumor-inhibiting role. The innate immune system (natural killer [NK] cells, monocytes/macrophages, neutrophils) is linked via antigen-presenting cells (dendritic cells [DC]) to the adaptive immune system (B cells, helper T cells [CD4+T_h], cytotoxic T cells [CD8+T_c]). Resultant cytokine responses may be classified as Th1 (proinflammatory: interferon [IFN]-γ/interleukin [IL]-2/IL-12) or Th2 (inactivating: IL-4/IL-5/IL-13 [important to eosinophilic responses]; IL-10 [important to anti-inflammatory responses]).[1] As such, tumors generally induce Th2 immunity to allow escape from tumor surveillance.

NATURAL KILLER CELLS

NK cells are lymphoid cells void of antigen-specific receptors. They attack cells which lack class I major histocompatibility complex (MHC) through release of cytokines and cell lysis. NK cells are governed by toll-like receptors (TLRs) under the influence of IL-15 and IL-18. Natural killers are converted into lymphokine-activated killers by the Th1 response[2] and lyse cells bearing non-self antigens without prior sensitization.[3] Using cells from malignant ovarian ascites, Wong and colleagues illustrated that primed NK cells promote DC and type-1 immune responses against cancer.[4] Treatment of ovarian cancer cells with oxaliplatin but not cisplatin also increases NK cytolysis through enhancement of the Th1 response,[5] making NK therapy in concert with cytotoxic chemotherapy an attractive doublet. Others have suggested a role for intraperitoneal delivery of allogenic NK cells based on efficacy in mouse models.[6] Administration of donor NK cells with aldesleukin (IL-2) to ovarian cancer patients treated with cyclophosphamide, fludarabine, and total-body irradiation has been explored, but the study was terminated due to toxicity.[7]

Tumors may evade detection through secretion of indolamine 2,3-dioxygenase (IDO)[8] and transforming growth factor (TGF)-β[9] to decrease NK response, and shedding of lipids later presented on CD1 molecules in ascites to abrogate NK cell activation.[10] Chemoresistant ovarian cancers often have defective tumor necrosis factor (TNF)-related apoptosis-inducing ligand (TRAIL) signaling, and NK cells that express TRAIL resensitize ovarian cancer cells to apoptosis *in vitro* and *in vivo*.[11] Small molecule inhibitors of IDO[12] and TGF-β[13] and soluble recombinant TRAIL and TRAIL agonist antibodies[14] therefore remain under active investigation.

MYELOID-DERIVED SUPPRESSOR CELLS: MONOCYTES/MACROPHAGES AND NEUTROPHILS

Myeloid-derived suppressor cells (MDSCs) are immature precursors to monocytes/macrophages, granulocytes, and DCs. Macrophages are classified by phenotype, though many patients may reveal mixed patterns not amenable to such assignment. M1 cells remain cytotoxic under the influence of IFN-γ, granulocyte monocyte colony stimulating factor, lipopolysaccharide, and TNF. M2 cells exert tumor-promoting effects, driven by IL-4, -6, -10, -13, monocyte colony stimulating factor (M-CSF), CD163, TLR, and TGF-β.[15-18]

Tumor-associated macrophages (TAMs) can represent up to 50% of the tumor mass and constitute a heterogeneous population with the potential to differentiate into distinct macrophage types,[19] based on a bidirectional exchange of local microenvironment soluble mediators which influence phenotype. Cancer cells often secrete IL-10, C-C chemokine ligands (CCL) -2, -3, -4, -5, -7, -8, C-X-C chemokine ligand (CXCL)-12, vascular endothelial growth factor (VEGF), and platelet-derived growth factor (PDGF) to recruit monocytes/macrophages. Tumor extracellular matrix and associated fibroblasts secrete M-CSF,[20] which has been shown to modulate vascular leakage; blockade of M-CSF using receptor kinases reverses vascular leakage.[21] M1 TAMs release inflammatory cytokines (e.g., IL-1b, IL-6, IL-12, IL-23, and TNF) and reactive oxygen species (ROS) that kill cancer cells; M2 TAMs—once "educated" by the tumor release growth factors (e.g., EGF, fibroblast growth factor [FGF], VEGF) associated with vascularization and expansion of the cancer mass.[22] Ovarian TAM expression of hypoxia-inducible factor 1-α (HIF-1α), programmed death ligand 1 (PD-L1; B7-H1), PD-1 (CD279),[23] and B7H4 co-inhibitory molecule (CD80)[24] suppresses T-cell responses.[25] TAMs herald poor outcome in epithelial ovarian cancer.[26] In a study of 112 ovarian cancer patients, TAMs most frequently infiltrated serous histology, followed by mucinous, undifferentiated, endometrioid, and clear cell subtypes ($p = 0.049$). Intratumoral TAM density significantly increased with stage ($p = 0.023$) and grade ($p = 0.006$); however, the overall M1/M2 TAM ratio decreased with advancing stage ($p = 0.012$).[22]

Neutrophils represent the most abundant circulating leukocyte population. Analogous to macrophage phenotypes, neutrophils dichotomize into N1 (anti-tumoral) and N2 (pro-tumoral) paradigms under the influence of IFN-β and TGF-β, respectively. N1 neutrophils promote CD8+ T cell recruitment through TNF-α, CCL3, CXCL9, and CXCL10 and may exert a direct cytotoxic effect on tumor cells through ROS.[27] TGF-β blockade increases the number of tumor-associated neutrophils. Neutrophils accomplish transendothelial migration through the integrin mac-1, L-selectin, and leukocyte function associated antigen-1. Bednarska and colleagues demonstrated that neutrophil expression of mac-1 is higher in patients with ovarian cancer compared to controls and highest in undifferentiated compared to other histologic subtypes of ovarian carcinoma.[28] Among 519 women with ovarian cancer, high neutrophil-to-lymphocyte ratio correlated with CA-125 and poor prognosis in a multivariate analysis.[29]

TUMOR-ASSOCIATED LYMPHOCYTES

Tumor-infiltrating CD3+ T-lymphocytes are tumor-specific cells with prognostic and therapeutic implications. In a cohort of 174 ovarian cancer patients treated with surgical cytoreduction and chemotherapy, detection of intratumoral T cells was associated with improved progression-free (3.9-fold) and overall survival (2.8-fold).[30] CD4+CD25+FOXp3+ regulatory T cells (T_{reg}) are a major factor in preventing the immune response from destroying ovarian cancers.[31] A thorough discussion of the role of the adaptive immune response is beyond the scope of this chapter.

Natural killer T cells (NKT) also bridge the innate and adaptive immune responses. When functional, they allow the host to mount an effective immune response against disease.[32-34] NKT cells represent a unique population of T lymphocytes that share features of both T cells and NK cells. Unlike classic T cells that recognize protein-derived antigens presented on MHC class I and class II molecules, the T-cell receptors on NKT cells recognize both exogenous and endogenous lipids presented on non-polymorphic, MHC class I-like CD1d molecules. There are two main NKT-cell subsets, invariant or type I NKT cells and diverse or type II NKT cells.[34] NKT cells respond to glycolipid antigens and bridge the innate/adaptive immune responses by influencing effector functions of macrophages, DCs, NK cells, as well as T and B cells.[33] Alteration of the tumor microenvironment allows NKT immune evasion by ovarian cancer. Ganglioside GD3, a major factor in ovarian cancer ascites, can inhibit NKT cell activation by blocking the natural stimulatory ligands of NKT cells.[35] A high concentration of circulating gangliosides is associated with poor prognosis.

BASOPHILS AND EOSINOPHILS

Basophils contain cytoplasmic granules that stain with basophilic dyes. These cells were discovered by Paul Ehrlich in 1879 and account for less than 1% of blood leukocytes. Historically, basophil function was felt to be aligned with allergic or parasitic disease, but more recently, human basophils have been found to support Th2 polarization through their synthesis of IL-4 and IL-13; they also secrete IL-3, VEGF, and other pro-angiogenic molecules and constitutively express CD40 ligand that binds CD40 on antigen-presenting cells.[36,37] There is growing excitement regarding the exploitation of basophils to promote tumor rejection.[38]

Eosinophils harbor large secretory granules within the cytoplasm and incorporate acidophilic stains. Inflammation and tissue damage prompt their activation. Eosinophils express MHC class II and co-stimulatory molecules (CD40, CD80/86, cytotoxic T lymphocyte associated protein-4) that regulate T-cell activation. Eosinophils can either promote Th1 polarization through IDO or Th2 responses through the secreted granule protein eosinophil-derived, which induces the migration and maturation of DCs.[39] Eosinophils remain under-studied in oncologic populations, but recently their infiltration of tumor stroma has been shown to correlate with improved outcome in certain solid tumors.[40]

COMPLEMENT

Classical, Alternative, and Lectin Pathways

Complement activation is a vital part of innate immunity in which foreign or damaged cells are targeted and destroyed by specialized proteins. Circulating complement proteins are primarily synthesized by hepatocytes but are also produced by white blood cells, endothelial cells, and epithelial cells. Complement activation occurs via one of three pathways: the classical, alternative, or lectin pathway (Figure 4.1). All of these pathways converge at the formation of C3 convertase, which cleaves C3 and triggers a proteolytic cascade that ends in the formation of a membrane attack complex (MAC), leading to a pore in the cell wall with resultant cell lysis. Proteolytic cleavage of C3 and C5 creates anaphylatoxins C3a and C5a

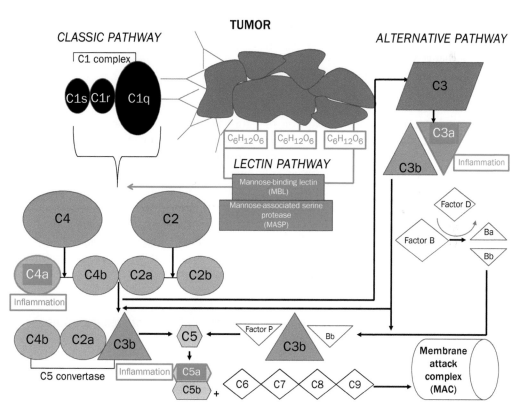

Figure 4.1 The complement cascade consists of classic, alternative, and mannose-binding lectin pathways. In the classical pathway, immunoglobulins bind tumor antigen; the Fc portion activates the C1 complex (C1q, C1r, C1s), which catalyzes the creation complex of C4a and C4b from C4 and C2a and C2b from C2. The complex of C2a4b activates cleavage of C3 into C3a and C3b. C3b combines with C2a4b to create C5 convertase (C2a4b3b). C5 convertase cleaves C5 into C5a and C5b, the latter of which combines with C6, C7, C8, and C9 to form the membrane attack complex (MAC), which leads to pore formation and cell lysis. Byproducts C3a, C4a, and C5a play key roles in inflammation. Neoplastic cells may also activate the alternative pathway, whereby constitutive C3 cleavage occurs. C3b combines with factor B breakdown products and is stabilized by factor P; together this complex also converts C5 into C5a and C5b. In the lectin pathway, carbohydrate modifications of tumor-associated antigens allow mannose-associated serine proteases to activate C4 and C2 in a manner similar to the C1 complex.

that draw the cellular components of the immune system to the site, thus promoting a state of chronic inflammation.[41] Complement also plays a role in cellular communication, migration, angiogenesis, and tissue proliferation. Ovarian tumor cells have the ability to produce large amounts of complement, through which autocrine stimulation occurs.

Membrane Complement Regulatory Proteins

Initially, the innate immune system recognizes and destroys the glycosylated cell surface proteins and phospholipids of malignant cells through activation of the complement cascade.[42,43] Unfortunately, tumors can develop resistance to these cytotoxic effects via several escape mechanisms. One evasion strategy is the overexpression of membrane complement regulatory proteins (mCRPs). These proteins block complement-mediated killing of the neoplastic cells by inhibiting or causing degradation of the complement cascade, thus preventing the deposition of the membrane attack complex (MAC) components and subsequent cell lysis.[44–48] mCRPs include complement receptor 1 (CR1; CD35) and membrane cofactor protein (MCP; CD46), which promote the degradation of C3b via factor I. CR1 and decay accelerating factor (CD55) degrade C3/C5 convertases. Protectin (CD59) prevents the formation of the MAC, thus preventing cell lysis. Both uterine and ovarian carcinomas have been shown to upregulate mCRPs.[49,50] Another evasion strategy occurs through efficient internalization of MAC formed on the tumor cell surface.[44–48]

Secreted Inhibitory Proteins

In addition to these membrane-bound modulators, soluble secreted inhibitory proteins may play a role in blunting the complement response. Factor H and its alternative splice variant factor H-like protein 1 may be found in high concentrations in malignant ascites; these proteins contain three C3b binding sites that prevent activation of C3b convertase.[45,46] C1 inhibitor (C1INH) inactivates C1s and C1r and has been found in conjunction with Factor I (a heterodimer that inactivates C4b and C3b in the presence of cofactors C4 binding protein and Factor H), to be upregulated in drug-selected P-glycoprotein multidrug resistant ovarian carcinoma cells.[51] Elevated levels of soluble CD59 and CD46 have also been isolated in ovarian cancer ascites, suggesting that ovarian tumor cells selectively upregulate secretion of these factors as a protective mechanism.[46] Thus, while some of the tumor cells will succumb to complement-mediated killing, others may go undetected, leading to more immune-resistant tumor cells and eventual development of metastatic disease.

Inflammation

C3a, C4a, and C5a cause an inflammatory response to tumor cells by attracting eosinophils, monocytes, and T cells, and promoting release of granzymes, ROS, and cytokines upon binding to immune cells. In the acute phase, this inflammation can be particularly cytotoxic. Chronic inflammation, however, encourages neoplastic transformation through the activation of oncogenes, further promoting the development of immune-resistant tumor cells.[1,43]

Autocrine Effects and Neoangiogenesis

Within the tumor microenvironment, C3a and C5a have been found to have anti-apoptotic effects on ovarian cancer. Binding of the MAC is thought to cause a cascade of oncogenic cell processes, and binding of anaphylatoxins C3a and C5a to their receptors can upregulate the expression of growth factor genes within the cancer cells and activate the cell cycle via mitogenic signaling pathways including phosphatidylinositol-3-phosphate kinase (PI3K)/AKT, among others (Table 4.1). This leads to proliferation and

TABLE 4.1 **COMPLEMENT PROTEIN INTERACTIONS WITH THE TUMOR MICROENVIRONMENT**

Protein	Effect	Reference
C1q	Cell adhesion; ligand for $\alpha2\beta1$ integrin	1, 2
C1r/s	Matrix degradation of type I/II collagen; co-localizes with matrix metalloproteinase-9	34
	Ligand for TGF-β; induction of SMAD2/3; promotion of the epithelial-mesenchymal transition	5
C3	Interacts with laminin of the basement membrane	6
	De-differentiation	7, 8
C3a	Chemoattractant for mesenchymal stem cells, activation of ERK 1/2 and AKT	9
	Stimulation of IL-6 mRNA	10
	Neovascularization; stimulation of vascular endothelial growth factor	11
C5a	Promotion of cell migration via p38MAPK	9
	Stimulation of IL-6 mRNA	11
	Neovascularization; stimulation of vascular endothelial growth factor	9
	Stimulation of cyclin E / D1 mRNA	12
	Stimulation of CD8+ T_{reg}	13
MAC	Increase release of fibroblast growth factor and platelet-derived growth factor	14
	Stimulation of cell cycle progression through cdk2/4 and ERK 1/2 activation	15
Bb	regulation/possible induction of apoptosis during differentiation	16

1. Feng X, Tonnesen MG, Peerschke EIB, Ghebrehiwet B. Cooperation of C1q receptors and integrins in C1q-mediated endothelial cell adhesion and spreading. J Immunol Baltim Md 1950. 2002;168(5):2441–2448.

2. Kim K-B, Yi J-S, Nguyen N, et al. Cell-surface receptor for complement component C1q (gC1qR) is a key regulator for lamellipodia formation and cancer metastasis. J Biol Chem. 2011;286(26):23093–23101. doi:10.1074/jbc.M111.233304.

3. Sakiyama H, Inaba N, Toyoguchi T, et al. Immunolocalization of complement C1s and matrix metalloproteinase 9 (92kDa gelatinase/type IV collagenase) in the primary ossification center of the human femur. Cell Tissue Res. 1994;277(2):239–245.

4. Wu Y-Y, Peck K, Chang Y-L, et al. SCUBE3 is an endogenous TGF-β receptor ligand and regulates the epithelial-mesenchymal transition in lung cancer. Oncogene. 2011;30(34):3682–3693. doi:10.1038/onc.2011.85.

5. Leivo I, Engvall E. C3d fragment of complement interacts with laminin and binds to basement membranes of glomerulus and trophoblast. J Cell Biol. 1986;103(3):1091–1100.

6. Del Rio-Tsonis K, Tsonis PA, Zarkadis IK, Tsagas AG, Lambris JD. Expression of the third component of complement, C3, in regenerating limb blastema cells of urodeles. J Immunol Baltim Md 1950. 1998;161(12):6819–6824.

7. Schraufstatter IU, Discipio RG, Zhao M, Khaldoyanidi SK. C3a and C5a are chemotactic factors for human mesenchymal stem cells, which cause prolonged ERK1/2 phosphorylation. J Immunol Baltim Md 1950. 2009;182(6):3827–3836. doi:10.4049/jimmunol.0803055.

8. Venkatesha RT, Berla Thangam E, Zaidi AK, Ali H. Distinct regulation of C3a-induced MCP-1/CCL2 and RANTES/CCL5 production in human mast cells by extracellular signal regulated kinase and PI3 kinase. Mol Immunol. 2005;42(5):581–587. doi:10.1016/j.molimm.2004.09.009.

9. Sayah S, Ischenko AM, Zhakhov A, Bonnard AS, Fontaine M. Expression of cytokines by human astrocytomas following stimulation by C3a and C5a anaphylatoxins: specific increase in interleukin-6 mRNA expression. J Neurochem. 1999;72(6):2426–2436.

10. Nozaki M, Raisler BJ, Sakurai E, et al. Drusen complement components C3a and C5a promote choroidal neovascularization. Proc Natl Acad Sci U S A. 2006;103(7):2328–2333. doi:10.1073/pnas.0408835103.

11. Rousseau S, Dolado I, Beardmore V, et al. CXCL12 and C5a trigger cell migration via a PAK1/2-p38alpha MAPK-MAPKAP-K2-HSP27 pathway. Cell Signal. 2006;18(11):1897–1905. doi:10.1016/j.cellsig.2006.02.006.

12. Daveau M, Benard M, Scotte M, et al. Expression of a functional C5a receptor in regenerating hepatocytes and its involvement in a proliferative signaling pathway in rat. J Immunol Baltim Md 1950. 2004;173(5):3418–3424.

13. Vadrevu SK, Chintala NK, Sharma SK, et al. Complement c5a receptor facilitates cancer metastasis by altering T-cell responses in the metastatic niche. Cancer Res. 2014;74(13):3454–3465. doi:10.1158/0008-5472.CAN-14-0157.

14. Benzaquen LR, Nicholson-Weller A, Halperin JA. Terminal complement proteins C5b-9 release basic fibroblast growth factor and platelet-derived growth factor from endothelial cells. J Exp Med. 1994;179(3):985–992.

15. Niculescu F, Badea T, Rus H. Sublytic C5b-9 induces proliferation of human aortic smooth muscle cells: role of mitogen activated protein kinase and phosphatidylinositol 3-kinase. Atherosclerosis. 1999;142(1):47–56.

16. Uwai M, Terui Y, Mishima Y, et al. A new apoptotic pathway for the complement factor B-derived fragment Bb. J Cell Physiol. 2000;185(2):280–292. doi:10.1002/1097-4652(200011)185:2<280::AID-JCP13>3.0.CO;2-L.

triggers the production of tumor-promoting cytokines such as IL-6, TNF-α, and TGF.[52]

C5a in particular promotes neovascularization by upregulating VEGF.[52–54]

Accordingly, many studies have shown that inhibition of C5a prevents tumor angiogenesis.[53,54] Similarly, C3-deficient tumors display decreased proliferation and angiogenesis.[52–54] Lung and ovarian cancer patients with overexpression of C3 or its proteolytic byproducts have worse overall survival, reinforcing the important role of complement in the tumor microenvironment on oncogenesis.[52]

TUMOR MICROENVIRONMENT: DEFINITIONS AND COMPONENTS

The tumor microenvironment consists of any biologic component that interacts with tumor cells which can include but is not limited to stromal cells, extracellular matrix molecules, and cytokines.[55] Cancer progression, once thought to be an autonomous process, is now recognized as one that engages extensive crosstalk between tumor cells with the surrounding microenvironment.[55,56]

STROMA

Extracellular matrix (ECM) and nonmalignant cells of the tumor define the tumor stroma.[57] The tumor stroma plays a disparate role in cancer development: it can impede cancer growth in normal tissues but can ironically also spurn migration and tumor progression as part of a co-opted desmoplastic response.[58] This duality arises from the ability of malignancy to alter cell behavior or even generate stroma important to proliferation and invasion.[55,59] A variety of stromal cells have been implicated in ovarian tumor progression including adipocytes, endothelial cells, fibroblasts, mesenchymal stem cells, macrophages, other immune cells, and the ECM, among others. Stromal cells produce growth factors, chemokines, collagens, and matrix-degrading enzymes that together provide a three-dimensional tumor scaffold and govern proliferation of cancer cells, tumor invasion, and metastasis.[60,61]

EXTRACELLULAR MATRIX

ECM is the noncellular component surrounding cells that provides physical scaffolding as well as biochemical and biomechanical cues required for morphogenesis, differentiation, and homeostasis.[62] Like cancers originating at other sites, ovarian cancer cells have the ability to alter the expression of surface receptors for ECM, as well as produce ECM molecules themselves.[55,59,63,64]

Collagen

Collagen is one of the most abundant ECM fibrous proteins.[65,66] The collagen family consists of at least 16 members which play a fundamental role in conferring elasticity to tissues but also have functional and structural properties. Using the OV2008 cell line, collagen I has been shown to catalyze migration;[67] in the same study, fibronectin—a high molecular weight glycoprotein that can bind collagen—led to a decrease in directional migration and has been shown to enhance proliferation and adhesion.[68] Expression of α1 chain of collagen XI (colXIα1), whose main physiologic function is to regulate the diameter of major collagen fibrils, correlates with advanced stages of disease;[69,70] as such, colXIα1 was the most highly overexpressed gene in a microarray comparing metastatic versus primary ovarian serous carcinomas.[69,71] Alterations in collagen IV and laminin have been associated with premalignant transformation and metastasis in ovarian cancer. Capo-Chichi and colleagues showed that the majority of primary ovarian tumors lack local collagen IV and laminin in their extracellular matrix in order to facilitate spread through the basement membrane; however, metastatic implants appear to restore expression, perhaps thereby anchoring the metastasis.[72] Consistent with this hypothesis, a study by Cheon and colleagues demonstrated enrichment of a collagen-remodeling gene signature in metastatic compared to primary ovarian serous carcinomas.[66]

Alterations in collagen and other ECM proteins may coincide with acquisition of chemoresistance. In a series of studies,

Januchowski and colleagues generated drug-resistant ovarian cancer cell lines and analyzed them for changes in gene expression relative to the parent line. A2780 cell line variants resistant to cisplatin, doxorubicin, topotecan, and paclitaxel overexpressed collagens, laminin, integrin β1, as well as matrix metalloproteinases;[73] ovarian cancer cell line W1 rendered resistant to methotrexate, cisplatin, doxorubicin, vincristine, topotecan, and paclitaxel overexpressed several types of collagen and periostin, which has been shown to support the epithelial to mesenchymal transition.[73] Ovarian cancer ascites contains high concentrations of procollagen I and III and M-CSF.[73] Together, these studies highlight the important role that collagen plays in ovarian cancer pathogenesis, metastasis, and drug resistance. Therapeutic strategies involving monoclonal antibodies against C-terminal telopeptide of type I collagen to inhibit fibril formation[73] and collagen IV-based chemotherapy delivery paradigms,[74] among others, are underway.

Hyaluronic Acid and Versican

ECM polysaccharides and glycoasminoglycans also influence adhesion, motility, and differentiation.[64] High levels of hyaluronic acid (HA), a large polymer synthesized at the cell surface, correlate with tumor progression, aggressiveness, and poor prognosis in ovarian cancer.[75-77] Versican is a secreted proteoglycan with multiple functions that can promote motility and invasion.[78] Overexpression of versican in malignant ovarian stroma is associated with increased invasive potential and unfavorable prognosis,[79,80] likely strengthening adhesion of epithelial ovarian carcinoma cells to mesothelial cells.[63,64] Versican and HA interact to form a pericellular matrix around ovarian cancer cells which may protect them against mechanical forces within the peritoneal cavity and allow seeding.[78] Treatment of peritoneal macrophages with low molecular weight HA stimulates production of IL-12,

RANTES (regulated on activation, normal T cell expressed and secreted; also known as CCL5), and macrophage inflammatory proteins 1α/1β.[81] MicroRNA-based translational repression of versican represents an intriguing construct for anti-cancer therapy that exploits tumor microenvironment properties.[82]

Integrins

Integrins are cellular surface glycoprotein receptors which are noncovalent heterodimers between one of 18 α and 8 β subunits.[83] The integrin heterodimer can bind to a unique set of ligands including components of the ECM and regulate ovarian cancer migration, invasion, proliferation, and survival.[68,83] The most highly expressed integrin subunits in ovarian cancer cells and stromal cells are αV and $β_1$.[84]

Among integrins, β1 is among the most well-studied. Interactions between α5β1-integrin and fibronectin mediate formation of ovarian carcinoma spheroids in NIH:OVCAR5 cells; blockade of the β1-integrin subunit inhibits adhesion of spheroids to fibronectin, laminin, and type IV collagen.[85] In a confirmatory study by Casey and Skubitz using NIH:OVCAR5 and SKOV3 cells, β1 integrin-matrix interactions including α5β1 with fibronectin, α2β1 with type IV collagen, and α6β1 with laminin regulated cell migration.[86] Ahmed and colleagues showed that αVβ1, α6β1, α3β1 are highly expressed in ovarian cancer cell lines Hey, Ovcar3, and Peo36;[68] proliferation was stimulated by collagen 1, laminin, and fibronectin, and adhesion by collagen and laminin. Accordingly, integrin function-blocking antibodies against α4β1 integrin augment sensitivity to carboplatin both *in vitro* and in murine models.[87]

Other β integrins have been implicated in aggressive phenotypes of ovarian cancer. αVβ3, which binds vitronectin, stimulates proliferation, drug resistance, and escape from anoikis—the programmed cell death of anchorage-dependent cells that normally occurs at the time of detachment from surrounding ECM.[88–90] Stromal cell-derived factor-1 enhances ovarian cancer cell invasion through $\alpha V \beta 6$-mediated signaling.[91] $\beta 5$ integrin may serve as a biomarker for serous ovarian carcinoma cells that possess active focal adhesion kinase signaling.[92–94] $\alpha V \beta 3$ integrin-targeted drug delivery systems are being explored.[95]

CD157

CD157 is an adenosine diphosphate (ADP)-ribosyl cyclase-related cell surface molecule on mesothelial cells that is involved in humoral immune response and transendoethelial leukocyte trafficking.[90] Forced expression induces morphological and phenotypic changes characterized by disruption of intercellular junctions and an epithelial-to-mesenchymal transition, which reduces sensitivity to anoikis and increases anchorage-independent growth, cell motility, and mesothelial invasion. Knockdown of CD157 in OV-90 and OC314 cells induces reversion to a mesenchymal phenotype and reduces migratory potential.

Tetraspanin

Tetraspanins are a family of transmembrane proteins present on plasma membrane and within intracellular organelles and granules in nearly all cell and tissue types. They organize laterally with integrins, membrane-anchored growth factors, and other tetraspanin family proteins.[96,97] Tetraspanin-1 (Tspan-1) is overexpressed in endometrioid and mucinous subtypes of ovarian carcinoma,[98] while tetraspanin-29 (CD9) is upregulated in borderline and serous-type ovarian carcinomas. There have been contradictory results surrounding the role of the latter in ovarian cancer progression.[97,99,100] Overexpression of CD9 in SKOV3 cells that typically have low CD9 expression led to an increase in cell growth

and expression of TNF-α, IL-6, IL-8, and NF-kB activation;[97] however, in another study malignant progression of epithelial ovarian carcinomas was associated with downregulation and altered cellular location of CD9, in which a shift occurred from localization within the membrane in grade 1 tumors to the cytoplasm in grade 3 tumors.[101] These changing patterns of expression from the membrane to the cytoplasm may be a mechanism by which tumor cells lose their adhesive properties during transformation. Furuya provided evidence that such downregulation in CD9 may be an acquired event in the process of tumor dissemination to the peritoneum.[102] CD151 (Tspan-24) is expressed in both epithelial ovarian carcinoma and normal surface epithelial cells. CD151 expression reduces migration of SKOV3 and OVCAR5 and invasion in SKOV3 ovarian cancer cell lines.[103] Interestingly, Baldwin and colleagues demonstrated that knockdown of CD151 or $\alpha 3$ integrin enhances tumor cell proliferation, growth, and formation of ascites in nude mice, suggesting a tumor suppressor role for CD151 and its associated $\alpha 3 \beta 1$ integrin in ovarian cancer.[104] Interestingly, MDSCs derived from Tspan-28 (CD81) knockout mice implanted with orthotopic cancer cell lines demonstrated reduced function relative to MDSCs from CD81 wild-type models.[105]

Tissue Transglutaminase

Tissue transglutaminase (TG2) is an enzyme involved in cross-linking proteins and in integrin-fibronectin networks.[55,106] TG2 mRNA expression is upregulated in ovarian tumor and ascites compared to normal ovarian surface epithelial cells.[107,108] Diminished TG2 expression decreases $\beta 1$ integrin in the plasma membrane of SKOV3 cells[108] and inhibits tumor spread to the peritoneal surface. Blocking transpeptidase activity though use of small molecule inhibitors like ITP-79 inhibits cancer cell adhesion by at least 50%.[106,108]

Matrix Metalloproteinases

Cancer cells participate in ECM remodeling[109] through a family of proteolytic enzymes known as matrix metalloproteinases (MMPs) and their inhibitors, tissue inhibitors of metalloproteinases. Increased expression of MMP9 confers a higher hazard ratio for death in high-grade serous ovarian carcinoma.[110,111] MMP14 (also known as membrane type 1 matrix metalloproteinase) induces the release of CA-125 from the cell surface; high expression of MMP14 leads to a decrease in adhesion of ovarian cancer cells to meso-mimetic culture, yet these cells become more invasive in the setting of collagen matrix which suggests that proteolytic clearing of CA-125 may expose integrins for high-affinity cell binding.[112] MMP overexpression has been associated with increased metastatic potential of ovarian tumors, but the expression pattern of each MMP is highly variable and dependent upon tumor type, stage, and means of MMP identification.[109] An extensive review covering the topic of MMPs in ovarian cancer was recently published by Al-Alem and Curry.[109] Unfortunately, a Phase III trial of the MMP-2, -3, -9 inhibitor tanomastat (BAY 12-9566) as maintenance therapy in ovarian cancer patients failed to provide benefit progression-free or overall survival, albeit well-tolerated.[113]

CA-125

MUC16, or CA-125, is a 22,152-amino acid glycoprotein that can interact with a variety of microenvironment constituents. In postmenopausal women, an elevated CA 125 >35 U/mL has sensitivity and specificity for ovarian cancer of 69% to 87% and 81% to 93%, respectively.[114] CA-125 influences tumor cell implantation through its ability to bind mesothelin expressed by meso-thelial cells and selectins,[115,116] decreases immunosurveillance through siglec-9 receptors on the surface of NK cells and monocytes, enhances proliferation through interactions with cytoplasmic tyrosine kinase JAK2, and upregulates *LMO2* and *NANOG* resulting in a cancer stem cell phenotype.[117] Accordingly, CA-125 has long been a target of antigen-specific immunotherapy.[118] Patients who are immunologically tolerant to CA-125 who respond to the anti-idiotypic antibody ACA125 demonstrate progression-free survival of 11.0 ± 5.6 months, in contrast to 8.0 ± 4.2 months in nonresponders.[119] Similarly, responders to abagovomab, an anti-idiotypic antibody produced by a mouse hybridoma and generated against OC125 epitope of CA 125, have significantly longer overall survival (23.4 months) compared to nonresponders (4 months) (*p* < 0.0001). Unfortunately, as maintenance therapy for patients with ovarian cancer in first remission, abagovomab does not prolong recurrence-free or overall survival.[120] Oregovomab is a high-affinity murine monoclonal antibody specific for CA-125 that leads to immune processing of antibody and antigen. In a trial involving 184 patients with ovarian cancer stages I to IV,[121] those who mounted an immune response had a longer survival compared with non-responders (22.9 vs. 13.5 months; *p* = 0.009).

CANCER-ASSOCIATED FIBROBLASTS

Cancer-associated fibroblasts (CAFs) are another major constituent of tumor stroma. Fibroblasts are essential components of connective tissue and are recruited and activated during wound repair.[55,58] During wound healing, fibroblasts become specialized into myofibroblasts, capable of contractility and increased extracellular matrix synthesis.[122] Compared to normal fibroblasts and myofibroblasts, CAFs are perpetually activated, neither reverting back to a normal phenotype nor undergoing apoptosis.[123] Absent in normal ovary, CAFs are present in benign ovarian tumors and borderline ovarian cancers and are abundant in epithelial ovarian carcinoma.[76] CAFs play an active role in immune tolerance, support of stem-like cancer cells, and cancer initiation through the secretion of various signaling factors.[57,123–127]

CAFs have unique traits that distinguish them from normal fibroblasts. Several immunohistochemical CAF markers have been identified including α smooth muscle actin, fibroblast activation protein (FAP), Thy-1, desmin, and S100A4 protein.[123] In two recent studies conducted by Mhawech-Fauceglia and colleagues,[128,129] FAP immunoexpression in stroma of epithelial ovarian cancer was identified as a significant predictive factor for platinum resistance and shorter time to progression compared to those with FAP-negative stroma. Recently, natriuretic peptide B (NPPB) was identified as a novel CAF-specific biomarker for ovarian cancer.[130] NPPB was expressed in 60% of primary ovarian cancer stroma tissues but not normal ovarian stroma and was found to be elevated in the blood of 50% of women with ovarian cancer.

Multiple origins have been proposed as the source for activated fibroblasts in tumor stroma, including both mesenchymal stem cell (MSC) and non-stem cell progenitors. Resting fibroblasts that surround the tumor can be recruited and activated. Additionally, smooth muscle cells, pericytes, adipocytes, and inflammatory cells may transdifferentiate into active fibroblasts.[59,131] Another source for activated fibroblasts occurs via epithelial-to-mesenchymal or endothelial-to-mesenchymal transition (EMT or EndMT).[131] Several cytokines activate fibroblasts such as hepatocyte growth factor, FGF-2, TGF-β, CXCL12, and PDGF.[59]

CAFs and cancer cells engage in cross-talk that has an effect on the physiology of both. Tumor-derived chemoattractants lead to recruitment of fibroblasts and to their phenotypic changes.[131] Fu and colleagues demonstrated that conditioned media obtained from co-culturing CAFs with epithelial ovarian cancer cell lines OVCAR-3 and SKOV-3 stimulated tumor cell proliferation, migration, and invasion.[124] CAFs may also induce epigenetic alterations leading to increased migratory ability in tumor cells. Co-culture of ovarian cancer cell lines A2780, SKOV-3, and ES-2 increases migration compared to cells cultured alone or with normal fibroblasts, in conjunction with enhanced expression of the histone methyltransferase enhancer of zeste homologue 2.[132] CAFs also induce stem-like properties of ovarian cancer cells through upregulation of FGF-4.[125] Recently, Shen and colleagues demonstrated that anti-tumor treatments applied to ovarian CAFs results in the production of wingless-type MMTV integration site (WNT) 16B, a newly discovered member of the WNT family that regulates DCs and T_{reg}, leading to alterations in tumor immune tolerance.[127] A multikinase inhibitor against FGF receptors 1 to 4 in solid tumors with aberrant FGF signaling is currently underway.[133]

ENDOTHELIAL CELLS

Endothelial cells that form the tumor vasculature represent another important component of the tumor microenvironment. Neovascularization is essential for tumor growth, and high tumor microvessel density portends poor outcome in ovarian cancer patients.[115,134–136] Neoangiogenesis is a dynamic process involving interplay of pro- and anti-angiogenic factors.[115]

The impact of endothelial cells on cancer cells has not been fully explored. Franses and colleagues demonstrated that culturing MDA-MB-231 breast or A549 lung carcinoma cells in endothelial cell-conditioned media resulted in a decrease in proliferation and migration via multiple pathways;[137] whether similar results would be observed in ovarian cancer remains to be determined.

MESOTHELIAL CELLS

Mesothelial cells form a protective monolayer that lines peritoneal, pleural, and pericardial surfaces.[115] Mesothelium is the first point-of-contact for floating ovarian cancer cells. It acts as a mechanical and paracrine barrier to inhibit the spread of ovarian cancer by blocking access to the stroma beneath the mesothelium.[138] Accordingly, a dysfunctional mesothelium becomes permissive of metastases due to secretion of paracrine factors.[115] Iwanicki and colleagues observed that mesothelial cells are generally absent beneath tumor implants; they illustrated that ovarian cancer spheroids that are successful in implantation use integrin- and talin-dependent activation of myosin and traction force to promote mesothelial cell displacement.[139] Co-culture of peritoneal mesothelial cells with ovarian cancer cells enhances the production of CCL (also known as MCP-1), prostaglandin E_2 (PGE_2), isoprostane-8, and urokinase-type plasminogen activator (uPA).[76,140] Mesothelial cells within the omentum, a frequent site of ovarian cancer metastasis, secrete cytokines and fibronectin in the presence of ovarian cancer cells, to enable attachment, invasion, and proliferation.[115,139,141,142] Via mesothelial crosstalk, ovarian cancer cells that invade omentum downregulate miR193b, a regulator of uPA, in *ex vivo* and mouse xenograft models.[143]

ADIPOCYTES

Adipocytes are the predominant component of fatty tissue. They specialize in energy storage and secretion of growth factors. Ovarian cancer cells exhibit trophism for adipocytes of the omentum, mesentery, and gonadal tissues.[115,144] Adipocytes promote tumorigenesis through production of adipokines, hormones, and growth factors.[55] Leptin, a hormone produced by adipocytes which is involved in regulation of body weight and sexual maturation, can stimulate ovarian cancer cell growth.[115,145] In a study performed by Nieman and colleagues, omentum served as a potent chemoattractant for ovarian cancer cells, which were then further stimulated by adipocytes via direct transfer of lipids to tumor cells.[146] Recently,

using a mouse model of ovarian cancer, metformin successfully reversed the proliferative and migratory effects of adipocyte-conditioned media on mouse ovarian cancer cell line ID8, suggesting its potential as a therapeutic modality through modulation of the cancer milieu.[147]

MESENCHYMAL STEM CELLS

Mesenchymal stem cells (MSCs) are adult stem cells that can be recruited to the tumor microenvironment and differentiate into a multitude of different cell types including osteogenic, myogenic, chondrogenic, and adipogenic lineages, or CAFs.[55,115] MSCs contribute to ovarian cancer pathogenesis through cell-cell interactions as well as secreted factors, such as IL-6.[21,76,148,149] MSCs may render ovarian cancer cells resistant to hyperthermia.[76,150] Touboul and colleagues have recently provided an in-depth review of the role of MSCs in ovarian cancer.[148]

BIOACTIVE LIPIDS

Lysophosphatidic Acid

Lysophosphatidic acid (LPA) is a water-soluble bioactive lipid that regulates diverse cellular functions through binding of G-protein-coupled receptors.[151] LPA can be found in ascites and sera of patients with ovarian cancer; its presence correlates with poor prognosis and chemoresistance, and it has been explored as a marker of ovarian cancer, with sensitivity as high as 94% and a specificity of 88% for the diagnosis of ovarian cancer in a pooled meta-analysis.[76,151,152] LPA promotes production of PGE_2, a bioactive lipid linked to ovarian cancer progression,[140] as well as C-X-C chemokine receptor 4 and its ligand CXCL-12, IL-8, and IL-6.[153–157] It also fosters long-term survival of ovarian cancer cells through the upregulation of telomerase, a deoxyribonucleic acid (DNA) polymerase that adds telomere repeat segments to the ends of DNA to prevent replicative sensescence[158,159] and proliferation in ovarian cancer cells via HIF-1α and PI3K. LPA inhibits NK activity.[160]

Sphingosine-1-Phosphate

Sphingosine-1-phosphate (S1P) has also been identified at micrometric concentrations in ascites.[161] Chemotherapy appears to upregulate S1P, which stimulates migration and invasion in epithelial ovarian cancer cells but not in human ovarian surface epithelial cells.[162,163] S1P induces an M2 phenotype and inhibits NK-mediated cell lysis of immature DCs.[164]

Cyclooxygenase Pathway and Prostaglandin E$_2$

The cyclooxygenase (COX) enzymes catalyze the rate-limiting step in the conversion of arachidonic acid to prostaglandins (Figure 4.2) and are involved in solid tumor progression.[164] Three isoforms exist for COX enzymes: constitutively expressed COX-1, inducible COX-2, and COX-3, a slice variant of COX-1. COX-2, absent from most cells, can be induced by cytokines and growth factors and is involved in the regulation of inflammatory responses.[164] Synthesis of PGE$_2$, the most abundant prostanoid in the body, is driven by COX enzymes.[164] Both COX-1 and COX-2 are expressed in ovarian epithelial ovarian cancer with varying intensities across different histological types and correlate with tumor proliferation.[165] COX-1 is expressed in both primary and metastatic cancers, ovarian cancer cell lines, the epithelium of inclusion cysts, and surface epithelium of normal ovaries;[165] COX-2 is highly expressed in metastatic compared to primary ovarian cancers and correlates with tumor proliferation.[165,166] COX-1 is thought to be the primary source of PGE$_2$ production in ovarian cancer; however, several studies have shown increased COX-2 expression and PGE$_2$ secretion in ovarian cancer cell lines.[167–170] Interestingly, silencing of COX-2 expression leads to a decrease in proliferation, migration,

and invasion in ovarian cancer cells.[171] Pharmacological antagonism of COX-1—and to a lesser extent COX-2—in an *in vivo* model decreases PGE$_2$, angiogenesis, and tumor growth.[171,172] While preclinical data suggested that COX inhibitors, such as indomethacin, may augment the effectiveness of platinum-based chemotherapy,[173] unfortunately, in the Phase II setting for ovarian cancer, the addition of COX-2 inhibition in the first-line setting has been disappointing,[174] possibly due to compensatory upregulation of COX-1 and abolition of the protective effects of EP1 (described later). COX inhibition may remain a viable option for heavily pretreated recurrent disease, despite side effects.[175,176] PGE$_2$ induces chemokines that attract MDSCs, T$_{regs}$, and suppressive DCs and suppresses local influx of Th1 and NK cells.[177]

PGE$_2$ interacts with four subtypes of G-protein-coupled receptors, EP1 to EP4, which lead to downstream intracellular signaling pathways.[164] Increased PGE$_2$ levels have been detected in the serum of women with ovarian cancer.[171,178,179] PGE$_2$ stimulates cell invasion and MMP-2/MMP-9 activity in SKOV-3 cells.[179] PGE$_2$ acting through the EP4 receptor stimulates cell invasion and production of VEGF in the HEY serous ovarian carcinoma cell line.[170] PGE$_2$ stimulates M2 macrophage polarization through cyclic AMP pathways.[180] While EP1 functions as a metastasis suppressor and its loss portends poorer overall survival, EP4 may occupy an opposite role. We have shown by immunohistochemistry that ovarian cancer tissues express EP4 and that pharmacologic antagonism of EP4 in ovarian cancer cell lines results in a decrease in proliferation and migration.[181] EP4 receptor inhibition may thus emerge as a bona fide treatment for ovarian cancer that circumvents the pitfalls of global COX inhibition.

CYTOKINES AND GROWTH FACTORS

"Cytokines," derived from the Greek words referring to "cell" and "movement," are small proteins that modulate cell signaling.

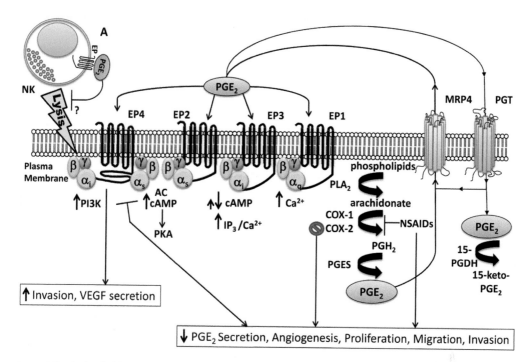

Figure 4.2 Prostaglandin biosynthesis and signaling. Phospholipase A2 (PLA$_2$) converts mobilized phospholipids from the plasma membrane to arachidonate. Cyclooxygenase enzymes, COX-1 or COX-2, in a rate-limiting step catalyze arachidonate to the precursor molecule prostaglandin H2 (PGH$_2$). PGH$_2$ is then converted to prostaglandin E2 (PGE$_2$) by PGES synthase. PGE$_2$ is then exported to the extracellular environment via the multidrug resistance-associated protein four (MRP4) where PGE$_2$ can exert its effects via autocrine/ paracrine signaling. PGE$_2$ can bind to four subtypes of G-protein-coupled receptors, EP1–EP4, which are coupled to different intracellular signaling pathways. EP2 and EP4 receptors are linked to cyclic AMP (cAMP) and protein kinase A (PKA) signaling through sequential activation of Ga(alpha)s and adenylate cyclase (AC). EP4 can also activate phosphoinositide-3-kinase (PI3K) through Ga(alpha)i. Elevation of intracellular calcium results from the activation of EP1 though Ga(alpha)q. Multiple isoforms exist for the EP3 receptor that can result in different responses, but the majority of isoforms act to inhibit cAMP generation through Ga(alpha)i. Ligand binding to EP3 can also result in an increase in IP$_3$/intracellular calcium as well as an increase in cAMP. In ovarian cancer, signaling through the EP4 receptor leads to an increase in invasion and VEGF secretion. Conversely, blocking the production of PGE$_2$ by genetic silencing of the COX-2 enzyme leads to a decrease in proliferation, migration, and invasion. Pharmacologic antagonism of COX-1 and COX-2 by nonsteroidal anti-inflammatories, which also results in a reduction in PGE$_2$ synthesis, has been shown to decrease angiogenesis. At the receptor level, pharmacological antagonism of the EP4 receptor results in a decrease in ovarian cancer proliferation and migration. Once signaling is complete, PGE$_2$ can be imported inside of the cell via prostaglandin transporter (PGT) where it can be converted to an inactive form 15-keto-PGE$_2$ by 15-hydroxyprostaglandin dehydrogenase (15-PGDH). In breast cancer, PGE$_2$ exerts immunosuppressive effects by blocking NK cell mediated tumor lysis. The potential for a similar immunosuppressive effect in ovarian cancer could exist but has yet to be explored.

Interleukin-6 and Interleukin-8

IL-6 is a cytokine central to inflammation.[182] It is constitutively secreted from ovarian cancer cells, mesothelial cells, fibroblasts, and macrophages, or through secondary inflammation.[183] In epithelial ovarian cancer, high levels of IL-6 and TNF-α together correlate with worse overall and progression-free survival.[184,185] IL-6 is capable of promoting proliferation, adhesion, invasion, angiogenesis, and immune suppression (as reviewed in Macchio et al. 2013), as well as prevention of apoptosis.[186,187,188] Increased expression of IL-6 receptor has been observed in epithelial ovarian cancer; the soluble form affects tumor cells as well as adjacent stromal or peritoneal cells.[183]

IL-8 was initially described as a neutrophil and monocyte chemoattractant of the

CXC family and is frequently overexpressed in malignancies and by monocytes and mesothelial cells.[189,190] IL-8 levels are elevated in ovarian cyst fluid, ascites, serum, and ovarian carcinoma.[191–193] Like IL-6, IL-8 is associated with poor prognosis in epithelial ovarian cancer patients.[185,194] IL-8 expression by ovarian cancer cells correlates with *in vivo* and *in vitro* cell proliferation.[195] Concentration of IL-8 found in ascites correlates with increased angiogenesis index as measured by a murine model.[196] IL-8 increases ovarian cancer cell migration through the induction of the EMT program and can also increase anchorage-independent growth, adhesion, and invasion through the activation of multiple signaling pathways including cyclins and MMPs.[189,197]

Both IL-6 and IL-8 have been found in significantly higher levels in peritoneal fluid of ovarian cancer patients compared with peritoneal fluid from patients with other gynecological diagnoses, and these proteins may serve as important diagnostic biomarkers for ovarian cancer.[198] Functional inhibition of these cytokines is a potential therapeutic target in the treatment of ovarian cancer;[173,199,200] Dijkgraaf and colleagues suggest that IL-6 receptor antibodies, such as the monoclonal antibody tocilizumab, may enhance platinum-based chemotherapy.[173] Secreted protein acidic and rich in cysteine is another secreted extracellular matrix protein that inhibits proliferation induced by IL-6, as well as the LPA-induced secretion of proliferative cytokines IL-6 and IL-8.[201]

Vascular Endothelial Growth Factor

VEGF is a proangiogenic cytokine that enhances proliferation, invasion, and migration of endothelial cells, as well as vascular permeability.[76] VEGF promotes stabilization and survival of endothelial progenitor cells from bone marrow.[202–204] Tumor vasculature possesses VEGF-mediated ultrastructural abnormalities including exceptional permeability and vascular wall infiltration by tumor cells,[202] which both contribute to metastasis

and malignant ascites formation.[202] In some models, VEGF inhibits DC migration.[204]

Tumor Necrosis Factor-α

TNF-α is a major mediator of inflammation.[205–208] Local administration of TNF-α is anti-angiogenic and has a powerful antitumor effect, yet endogenous TNF-α in the tumor microenvironment enhances growth and invasion by inducing other cytokines/chemokines such as IL-6, IL-8, and VEGF.[207,209–211] TNF-α heralds an increased risk of ovarian cancer; in a study analyzing serum levels of various inflammatory mediators, elevated TNF-α conferred an increased risk of developing ovarian cancer between 2 and 14 years later.[212] Patients with epithelial ovarian cancer have increased plasma levels of TNF-α and several other inflammatory mediators compared to those with benign conditions,[213] and high pretreatment levels of TNF-α correlate with poor prognosis.[184] Immunohistochemical analysis of paraffin-embedded tissues also demonstrates a correlation between TNF-α (and IL-1 and COX-2) immunoreactivity with stage in both serous and mucinous tumors.[214,215]

Biologically, TNF-α has pleiotropic effects in various ovarian cancer cells, dependent on their ability to activate c-Jun NH2-terminal kinase (JNK). An increase in CD44 expression, a marker of stemness, along with enhanced migration and invasion is observed only in cells capable of activating JNK; opposite effects are observed in patients incapable of activating JNK.[216]

Transforming Growth Factor-β

TGF-β is a superfamily of peptide growth factors.[217] In normal ovarian and some cancer cells, TGF-β induces growth arrest; however, in other cancer cells—particularly those with mutant or null p53—this ability is lost and TGF-β can instead promote cellular invasion.[217,218] In NIH-OVCAR3 ovarian cancer cells, TGF-β isoforms inhibit proliferation and promote migration accompanied by incomplete EMT transformation.[219] Enhanced migration may relate to TGF-β-related upregulation of versican expression by stromal cells, leading to activation of CD44 and MMP expression.[220]

MICROENVIRONMENT CROSSTALK IN EPITHELIAL OVARIAN CANCER

INFLAMMATION AND THE PATHOGENESIS OF OVARIAN CANCER

Types of Ovarian Cancer

The characteristic changes of ovarian surface epithelium and subsequent pathways leading to ovarian carcinogenesis continue to challenge the medical community. Historically, pathophysiologic models assumed malignant conversion of mesothelium into distinct histologic subtypes with spread to surrounding adnexal structures; newer paradigms suggest extraovarian or fallopian tube origins of epithelial ovarian cancer.[221-223] Clinical presentation at advanced stages of disease further limits identification of a precursor lesion for ovarian cancer. Regardless of the location of inciting events that trigger epithelial ovarian tumorigenesis, these lesions vary in patterns of genetic alterations and disease progression.[224]

Mounting molecular evidence in conjunction with histopathologic findings suggests that two distinct epithelial ovarian cancer phenotypes exist. Classification as Type I or II disease is related to histology, grade, stage, and patterns of DNA mutations (Table 4.2). Type I tumors, including low-grade serous, endometrioid, mucinous, and clear cell histologies, are characterized by a more indolent disease course. Precursor lesions acquire mutations in *KRAS, PTEN, ERBB2,* and other cell signaling pathways and progress in a stepwise fashion to larger tumors that generally remain confined to the ovary.[225-227]

TABLE 4.2 **DIFFERENCES BETWEEN TYPE I AND II OVARIAN CANCERS**

	Type I	Type II
Histology	Clear cell Endometrioid Low-grade serous Mucinous	Carcinosarcoma High-grade serous Undifferentiated carcinoma
Suspected precursor	Endometriomas Benign cystadenomas	Likely *de novo* Fallopian tube epithelial cells (serous tubal *in situ* carcinomas)
Associated mutations	**Clear cell:** *ARID1A* (50%), *PIK3CA* (50%), *PTEN* (20%) **Endometrioid:** β-catenin/*CTNNB1* (40%), *PIK3CA* (20%) **Low-grade serous:** *BRAF* (30%) **Mucinous:** *KRAS* (75%)	**High-grade serous:** *TP53* (95%) Inactivation of *BRCA1/2* (20%)
Stage	I (confined to ovary)[a]	III/IV[a]
Survival	Favorable	Poor

[a] Based on International Federation of Gynecology and Obstetrics (FIGO) 2014 ovarian cancer staging guidelines.

Type II tumors, including high-grade serous carcinoma, carcinosarcoma, and undifferentiated carcinomas, are more aggressive with a predilection for distant metastasis at the time of diagnosis. Current evidence suggests that these lesions, which more closely resemble to fallopian tube epithelium, develop de novo after mutations in tumor suppressor *TP53* and cell cycle regulating pathways and are marked by genetic instability.[166,222,223] Several theories suggest that physiologic processes including ovulation and menstruation may generate an inflammatory microenvironment that contributes to subsequent mutagenesis.

Theory of Incessant Ovulation

First described by Fathalla in 1971, the theory of incessant ovulation suggests the process of ovulation repetitively inflicts trauma to ovarian surface epithelium and predisposes tissue to aberrant repair mechanisms eventually resulting in malignancy.[166] Animal models have demonstrated oxidative DNA damage and a concomitant increase in p53 expression in ovarian surface epithelial cells located immediately adjacent to the site of follicle rupture at the time of ovulation.[228] This process is thought to be a result of neutrophil and macrophage infiltration of the ovary following the luteinizing hormone surge and complex interactions between cytokines (e.g., IL-1, TNF-α), prostaglandins, plasminogen activators, and nitric oxide that characterize ovulation. In support of this theory is the predominance of epithelial ovarian cancers in humans and hens, another "extravagantly" ovulating animal, compared to non-human primates whose ovulatory patterns are confined to breeding seasons.[229]

Decades of epidemiologic evidence suggest that factors associated with a decreased number of lifetime ovulatory cycles are highly protective against development of ovarian cancer. A meta-analysis of 23,257 women with ovarian cancer and over 87,000 controls reveals combined oral contraceptive use is associated with an overall relative risk reduction

in ovarian cancer of 20% for each five years of use.[230] This benefit persists for over 30 years after cessation but progressively declines over time. Pregnancy has also been demonstrated to consistently reduce the risk of ovarian cancer, with increasing parity and pregnancy over age 35 years conferring greater protective benefit.[231] Case-control studies conducted by Purdie and colleagues among Australian women estimate a 6% increase in risk of ovarian cancer per single year of ovulation.[232]

Molecular data further suggest a role of ovulation in ovarian pathogenesis. Patterns of *TP53* mutation seen in patients with more ovulatory cycles are associated with development of epithelial ovarian cancer, particularly in Type II disease. Accumulation of p53, increased IL-8 expression, and higher incidence of double stand breaks in DNA were noted in fallopian tube epithelial cells exposed to follicular fluid *in vitro*,[233] invoking a role for the ovulatory milieu in early mutagenesis associated with high-grade serous ovarian cancer. When examining patient reproductive history, an analysis of 197 women with invasive ovarian cancer revealed that women with overexpression in p53 ($n = 105$) were approximately seven times more likely to have had moderate to high numbers of lifetime ovulatory cycles when compared to controls. Similar findings were demonstrated among *BRCA*-mutated women undergoing prophylactic salpingectomy: strong nuclear localization of p53 in morphologically benign tissue (so-called p53 signatures) inversely correlates with parity.[234,235] Notably, this correlation is not consistently demonstrated in patients with p53-negative tumors.[236]

Several limitations to this theory exist. Marked histologic differences between ovarian surface epithelium and müllerian subtypes (serous, clear cell, endometrioid, and clear cell) suggest alternative origins of ovarian cancer. Additionally, the protective benefit conferred by the use of oral contraceptives and pregnancy in the development of ovarian cancer far exceeds the anticipated risk reduction based on the number of prevented ovulatory cycles alone.[232,237]

Theory of Incessant Menstruation and Iron-induced Oxidative Stress

Dissemination of endometrial tissue within the peritoneal cavity via retrotubal flow during menses is a concept only recently described in ovarian pathogenesis. Historic studies investigating endometriosis identify blood in peritoneal fluid of over 90% of women undergoing diagnostic laparoscopy during menses, suggesting retrograde menstruation through the fallopian tube is a common physiologic phenomenon.[238] Salvador et al. suggest this retrotubal flow during menstruation exposes the fallopian tube and ovary to inflammatory mediators and ultimately leads to carcinogenesis.[223] Disruption of retrograde menstruation via bilateral tubal ligation confers a 34% relative risk reduction for ovarian cancer, with a similar effect among patients undergoing hysterectomy, supporting the hypothesis that such procedures prevent a cascade of events leading to development of ovarian epithelial tumors.[239]

The presence of refluxed blood in the peritoneum as a consequence of menstruation provides a major source of oxidative stress associated with genetic instability.[240] Hemolysis of refluxed erythrocytes in the pelvis containing stored iron in the form of hemoglobin leads to proteolytic digestion of hemoglobin giving rise to heme. Catabolism by heme oxygenase produces reactive iron leading to ROS formation via the Fenton reaction. Excess superoxide anions and hydroxyl radicals overwhelm cellular antioxidant defense mechanisms resulting in oxidative stress (Figure 4.3). The carcinogenic properties of iron and subsequent ROS have been well-elucidated, including oxidation of DNA bases leading to single nucleotide substitutions, epigenetic modifications, and activation of β-catenin pathways *in vivo*. Interestingly, oxidative DNA damage patterns occur nonrandomly.[241] DNA-histone protein complexes likely account for increased vulnerability to oxidative damage for specific sequences coding for telomeres and selected oncogenes.

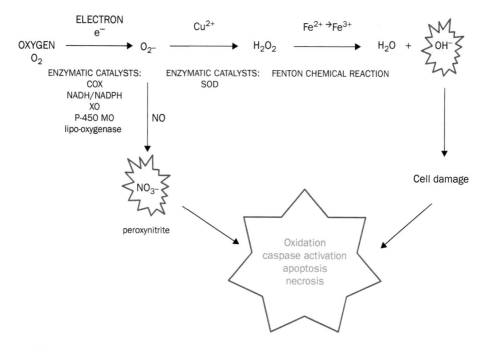

Figure 4.3. Oxidative stress in the tumor microenvironment.

Recent investigations into the role of iron in ovarian cancer have closely examined involvement of the fallopian tube and fimbriae in the disease process. Histologic evidence of iron deposition as reflected by tubal hemosiderin deposits or hemosiderin-laden macrophages are found in over 20% of patients with high-grade serous carcinoma, particularly in fimbrial mucosa when compared to controls with and without endometriosis.[242] These findings indirectly support the theory of incessant retrograde menstruation with localization of deposition in tubal fimbriae. It is unclear, however, if this reflects tumor invasion rather than chronic iron deposition. *In vitro* models of fimbrial secretory epithelial cells exposed to varying physiologic concentrations of catalytic iron demonstrated a marked increase in p53, Ki67, and nitric oxide production as well as cell viability.[243] These characteristic neoplastic changes reflect patterns consistent with serous ovarian cancer and occur in a dose-dependent fashion, suggesting women with greater iron exposure as a result of incessant menstruation may be at increased risk.

Iron overload in the peritoneal cavity as a result of excessive retrograde menstruation additionally affects the function of pelvic macrophages, which sequester iron by phagocytosis. Iron release by M2 macrophages may stimulate tumor cells growth.[244] Increased levels of peritoneal macrophage ferritin levels and iron overload have been well documented in patients with endometriosis.[245] The presence of excessive intracellular unbound iron and ROS in macrophages is associated with constitutive NF-κB activation, a transcription factor associated with cell immortality, proliferation, proinflammatory cytokine expression, and neovascularization that characterizes ovarian carcinogenesis.[246,247] Complex interactions between iron homeostasis and ROS formation with subsequent inflammation as a result of excessive retrograde menstruation thus may contribute to a mutagenic environment favoring ovarian malignancy.

Endometriosis-Related Ovarian Cancers

Not surprisingly, findings from case-control and large cohort studies demonstrate a three-fold increase in the risk of endometrioid and clear cell subtypes of ovarian cancer among women with endometriosis.[248] Although malignant conversion of endometriotic lesions has not been fully characterized, atypical endometrial gland cytology or architecture is identified in 61% of patients with endometriosis-associated ovarian tumors.[249,250] Histopathologic analysis of a subset of these patients with clear cell and endometrioid ovarian cancer shows direct transition from atypical endometriosis to carcinoma, suggesting a bonafide precancerous disease state.

Genetic instability within endometriosis has also been well documented. Loss of heterozygosity resulting in tumor suppressor gene inactivation (particularly at *PTEN* on 10q23.3) has been described in a significant proportion of endometriotic implants and suggests a role of these lesions in ovarian neoplasia.[251] Yamaguchi et al. found endometriotic cysts are rich in catalytic iron with a high concentration of oxidized purine nucleotides, reflecting an inherently higher rate of DNA mutation within these lesions.[252] Unlike high-grade serous lesions, data remain conflicting regarding the role of *TP53* malignant conversion of endometriosis to clear cell and endometrioid subtypes. Instead, loss of *ARID1A*, a regulating factor central to chromatin remodeling, appears to be crucial to pathogenesis of these subtypes. *ARID1A* mutations are seen in 30% of endometrioid carcinomas and 46% of clear-cell carcinomas, with shared patterns of truncated mutations seen in contiguous endometriotic lesions.[253]

WARBURG AND REVERSE WARBURG EFFECTS

Tumor microenvironment appears to regulate metabolism of established tumors. The Warburg effect is named for Otto Warburg who first reported in 1924 that cancer cells metabolize glucose differently than cells in normal tissue. Normal cells use mitochondrial oxidative phosphorylation, while cancer cells rely instead on aerobic glycolysis, a relatively inefficient way to generate 5'-triphospate (ATP). This is not felt to be due to a defect in mitochondrial function in cancer cells. Rather, it may be that signaling pathways that promote cell proliferation may also regulate metabolic pathways such as aerobic glycolysis. Alternatively, cancer cells may have mutations which favor nutrient metabolism for proliferation at the expense of efficient ATP production.[254]

The reverse Warburg effect was described by Lisanti and colleagues to describe tumor-stroma interactions. This model describes the net energy transfer from catabolic tumor stroma to anabolic tumor cells. Oxidative stress promotes autophagy in cancer-associated fibroblasts and other stromal cells which provides nutrients to fuel growth and proliferation of cancer cells.[255] Stromatogenesis—stroma formation during neoplasia—results in unusually edematous and loose stroma, which may actually serve as a buffer through the absorption of lactic acid from cancer cells.[256] Exploiting the altered metabolic properties of tumor cells may augment anti-cancer therapies.

RESISTANCE MECHANISMS

Hypoxia and Class III β-Tubulin

Hypoxia, the lack of sufficient oxygen, is a common feature of solid tumors and may contribute to cancer immune suppression.[257] Hypoxia stimulates the release of angiogenic factors, and promotes EMT and metastasis.[257] HIFs govern cellular responses to low oxygen tension, though some (e.g., HIF-1α) can also be stimulated through factor signaling under normoxic conditions. HIFs prompt the maturation of MDSCs and the recruitment of TAMs, leading to augmentation of an immunosuppressive environment via TGF-β and IL-10, and bind hypoxia-response elements resulting in the transcription of target genes.[257,258]

Hypoxia confers poor prognosis in ovarian carcinoma.[259] One mechanism underlying this phenomenon involves dysregulation of cytoskeletal proteins. Microtubules are dynamic structures that form part of the cytoskeleton with many important intracellular roles including separation of chromosomes during mitosis, transport, locomotion, and maintenance of cell structure.[260] Microtubules consist of eight α- and seven β-tubulin isotypes that form heterodimers and can rapidly lengthen and contract.[261] This dynamic instability is critical to its function within the cell. The β-tubulin subtypes differ in amino acid positions at the carboxy terminus[262] and possess specific tissue and developmental distributions. Class I represents the constitutively expressed subtype of β-tubulin.[263] Several chemotherapeutic agents such as paclitaxel exert their toxic effects by stabilizing or destabilizing microtubules through binding of the β-tubulin subunit. Overexpression of class III β-tubulin may contribute to chemoresistance through alterations in paclitaxel drug affinity as well as cytoskeletal activation of prosurvival kinases. Upregulation of class III β-tubulin (TUBB3) has been implicated in paclitaxel resistance and poor survival in a variety of human tumors, including lung,[264] breast,[265] and colon.[266] We have previously shown that aggressive or chemoresistant subtypes of gynecologic cancer including ovarian clear cell,[267] carcinosarcomas,[269] leiomyosarcoma,[270] uterine serous carcinoma,[271] and ovarian cancer patients treated with neoadjuvant chemotherapy[268] overexpress class III β-tubulin Hypoxia is a strong inducer of TUBB3 in A2780 ovarian cancer cell line.[272] Under hypoxic conditions and as influenced by extent of promoter methylation, HIF-1α/2α may bind the 3' region of TUBB3 to induce transcription.[273] PGE_2 may also control expression of HIF-1α in intracrine fashion,[274] suggesting a role for modulation to contribute to paclitaxel sensitization.

Stemness, Intrinsic Resistance, and Acquired Resistance

Cancer stem cells represent a minute fraction of the tumor mass (0.001%–0.1%) and exhibit self-renewal, heterogeneous differentiation capacity, and exceptional resistance to chemo/radiotherapy. CD44 is a glycoprotein marker of stemness. CD44 may mediate Th2 polarization of naïve T cells with increased IL-4 production.[275] The clinical significance of CD44 is controversial; in some studies but not others expression has been associated with poor prognosis and survival,[275-280] and knockdown of CD44 results in decreased proliferation, migration/invasion, and spheroid formation, as well as enhancement of drug sensititvity.[86,275,281] In a study of 26 patients, Gao and colleagues found that metastatic and recurrent ovarian cancers expressed higher levels of CD44 compared to matched primary tumor.[275] Given its important role in ovarian cancer pathogenesis CD44 has been identified as a potential target against cancer.[64]

In the ovarian tumor microenvironment, carcinoma-associated mesenchymal stem cells (CA-MSCs) play a role in resistance to apoptosis. Castells and colleagues[282] showed that CA-MSC induced activation of the PI3K/Akt pathway and X-linked inhibitor of apoptosis protein, which is in inhibitor of caspases -3 and -7.[282] CA-MSCs play an active role in trogocytosis, the transfer of surface molecules from antigen-presenting cells to lymphocytes. Trogocytosis not only influences the phenotype and function of lymphocytes but can result in negative immunologic feedback whereby NK cells that have adopted antigens of the neighbor cells are rapidly destroyed by naïve NK cells. Trogocytosis may promote the development of chemoresistance via direct exchange of membrane fragments containing multidrug-resistance pumps *MDR1* and *ABCB1*.[283] Oncologic trogocytosis is just one example of acquired resistance to tumor therapy. Additional mechanisms of acquired chemoresistance include alteration of the lipid membrane modifying drug penetrance, increased capacity in DNA repair, modification of drug targets, drug inactivation mediated by metallothionein- or glutathione-dependent mechanisms, and loss of drug surface transporter.[283,284]

Environment-mediated drug resistance arises from signaling interactions between tumor cells and the mesenchymal stroma via either soluble factors (e.g., cytokines, chemokines, growth factors secreted by fibroblast-like tumor stroma) or cell adhesion (e.g., tumor cell integrins to stromal fibroblasts or to components of the ECM such as collagen, fibronectin, and laminin).[285] As a result of these interactions, the microenvironment temporarily protects the ovarian cancer cells while they acquire the genetic changes that make them permanently chemoresistant; any minimal residual disease that persists then becomes responsible for subsequent relapse.

CONCLUSIONS

It is insurmountable in any one chapter to capture fully the tremendous efforts invested by the medical and scientific community toward understanding the complex interactions between the innate immune system and tumor microenvironment. Herein, however, one can see that from decades of inquiry, often met previously with frustration and disillusionment, has emerged a time ripe to harness the diagnostic and therapeutic implications of these endeavors and provide for our patients the opportunity for early detection and cure, toward which all aspire.

REFERENCES

1. Berger A. Th1 and Th2 responses: what are they? *BMJ.* 2000;321(7258):424.
2. Sinkovics JG, Horvath JC. Human natural killer cells: a comprehensive review. *Int J Oncol.* 2005;27(1):5–47.
3. Dana M Roque, Alessandro D Santin. Antigen-specific immunotherapy for ovarian cancer. In: *Advances in Ovarian Cancer Management.*

London: Future Medicine Ltd; 2012:136–54. http://www.futuremedicine.com/doi/abs/10.2217/ebo.11.180. Accessed December 8, 2015.

4. Wong JL, Berk E, Edwards RP, Kalinski P. IL-18-primed helper NK cells collaborate with dendritic cells to promote recruitment of effector CD8+ T cells to the tumor microenvironment. *Cancer Res.* 2013;73(15):4653–62. doi:10.1158/0008-5472. CAN-12-4366.

5. Siew Y-Y, Neo S-Y, Yew H-C, et al. Oxaliplatin regulates expression of stress ligands in ovarian cancer cells and modulates their susceptibility to natural killer cell-mediated cytotoxicity. *Int Immunol.* 2015;27(12): 621–32. doi:10.1093/intimm/dxv041.

6. Geller MA, Knorr DA, Hermanson DA, et al. Intraperitoneal delivery of human natural killer cells for treatment of ovarian cancer in a mouse xenograft model. *Cytotherapy.* 2013;15(10):1297–306. doi:10.1016/j.jcyt.2013.05.022.

7. Geller MA. NCT00652899. Allogeneic Natural Killer Cells in Patients with Recurrent Ovarian Cancer, Fallopian Tube, and Primary Peritoneal Cancer. 2008. http://www.clinicaltrials.gov.

8. Tanizaki Y, Kobayashi A, Toujima S, et al. Indoleamine 2,3-dioxygenase promotes peritoneal metastasis of ovarian cancer by inducing an immunosuppressive environment. *Cancer Sci.* 2014;105(8):966–73. doi:10.1111/cas.12445.

9. Wilson EB, El-Jawhari JJ, Neilson AL, et al. Human tumour immune evasion via TGF-β blocks NK cell activation but not survival allowing therapeutic restoration of anti-tumour activity. *Plos One.* 2011;6(9):e22842. doi:10.1371/journal.pone.0022842.

10. Webb TJ, Giuntoli RL, Rogers O, Schneck J, Oelke M. Ascites specific inhibition of CD1d-mediated activation of natural killer T cells. *Clin Cancer Res.* 2008;14(23):7652–58. doi:10.1158/1078-0432. CCR-08-1468.

11. El-Gazzar A, Perco P, Eckelhart E, et al. Natural immunity enhances the activity of a DR5 agonistic antibody and carboplatin in the treatment of ovarian cancer. *Mol Cancer Ther.* 2010;9(4):1007–18. doi:10.1158/1535-7163.MCT-09-0933.

12. Dolušić E, Frédérick R. Indoleamine 2,3-dioxygenase inhibitors: a patent review (2008–2012). *Expert Opin Ther Pat.* 2013;23(10):1367–81. doi:10.1517/13543776.2013.827662.

13. Herbertz S, Sawyer JS, Stauber AJ, et al. Clinical development of galunisertib (LY2157299 monohydrate), a small molecule inhibitor of transforming growth factor-beta signaling pathway. *Drug Des Devel Ther.* 2015;9:4479–99. doi:10.2147/DDDT.S86621.

14. Abdulghani J, El-Deiry WS. TRAIL receptor signaling and therapeutics. *Expert Opin Ther Targets.* 2010;14(10):1091–108. doi:10.1517/14728222.2010.519701.

15. Cannon MJ, Ghosh D, Gujja S. Signaling circuits and regulation of immune suppression by ovarian tumor-associated macrophages. *Vaccines.* 2015;3(2):448–66. doi:10.3390/vaccines3020448.

16. Gajewski TF, Schreiber H, Fu Y-X. Innate and adaptive immune cells in the tumor microenvironment. *Nat Immunol.* 2013;14(10):1014–22. doi:10.1038/ni.2703.

17. Bellora F, Castriconi R, Dondero A, et al. TLR activation of tumor-associated macrophages from ovarian cancer patients triggers cytolytic activity of NK cells. *Eur J Immunol.* 2014;44(6):1814–22. doi:10.1002/eji.201344130.

18. Khan Z, Marshall JF. The role of integrins in TGFβ activation in the tumour stroma. *Cell Tissue Res.* 2016;365(3):657–73. doi:10.1007/s00441-016-2474-y.

19. Solinas G, Germano G, Mantovani A, Allavena P. Tumor-associated macrophages (TAM) as major players of the cancer-related inflammation. *J Leukoc Biol.* 2009;86(5):1065–73. doi:10.1189/jlb.0609385.

20. Reinartz S, Schumann T, Finkernagel F, et al. Mixed-polarization phenotype of ascites-associated macrophages in human ovarian carcinoma: correlation of CD163 expression, cytokine levels and early relapse. *Int J Cancer.* 2014;134(1):32–42. doi:10.1002/ijc.28335.

21. Moughon DL, He H, Schokrpur S, et al. Macrophage blockade using CSF1R inhibitors reverses the vascular leakage underlying malignant ascites in late-stage epithelial ovarian cancer. *Cancer Res.* 2015;75(22):4742–52. doi:10.1158/0008-5472. CAN-14-3373.

22. Zhang M, He Y, Sun X, et al. A high M1/M2 ratio of tumor-associated macrophages is associated with extended survival in ovarian cancer patients. *J Ovarian Res.* 2014;7:19. doi:10.1186/1757-2215-7-19.

23. Krempski J, Karyampudi L, Behrens MD, et al. Tumor-infiltrating programmed death receptor-1+ dendritic cells mediate immune suppression in ovarian cancer. *J Immunol.* 2011;186(12):6905–13. doi:10.4049/jimmunol.1100274.

24. Kryczek I, Wei S, Zhu G, et al. Relationship between B7-H4, regulatory T cells, and patient outcome in human ovarian carcinoma. *Cancer Res.* 2007;67(18):8900–905. doi:10.1158/0008-5472. CAN-07-1866.

25. Doedens AL, Stockmann C, Rubinstein MP, et al. Macrophage expression of hypoxia-inducible factor-1 alpha suppresses T-cell function and promotes tumor progression. *Cancer Res.* 2010;70(19):7465–75. doi:10.1158/0008-5472. CAN-10-1439.

26. Shah CA, Allison KH, Garcia RL, Gray HJ, Goff BA, Swisher EM. Intratumoral T cells, tumor-associated macrophages, and regulatory T cells: association with p53 mutations, circulating tumor DNA and survival in women with ovarian cancer. *Gynecol Oncol.* 2008;109(2):215–19. doi:10.1016/j.ygyno.2008.01.010.

27. Mishalian I, Bayuh R, Levy L, Zolotarov L, Michaeli J, Fridlender ZG. Tumor-associated neutrophils

(TAN) develop pro-tumorigenic properties during tumor progression. *Cancer Immunol Immunother.* 2013;62(11):1745–56. doi:10.1007/s00262-013-1476-9.

28. Bednarska K, Klink M, Wilczyński JR, et al. Heterogeneity of the Mac-1 expression on peripheral blood neutrophils in patients with different types of epithelial ovarian cancer. *Immunobiology.* 2016;221(2):323–32. doi:10.1016/j.imbio.2015.10.003

29. Williams KA, Labidi-Galy SI, Terry KL, et al. Prognostic significance and predictors of the neutrophil-to-lymphocyte ratio in ovarian cancer. *Gynecol Oncol.* 2014;132(3):542–50. doi:10.1016/j.ygyno.2014.01.026.

30. Zhang L, Conejo-Garcia JR, Katsaros D, et al. Intratumoral T cells, recurrence, and survival in epithelial ovarian cancer. *N Engl J Med.* 2003;348(3):203–13. doi:10.1056/NEJMoa020177.

31. Knutson KL, Maurer MJ, Preston CC, et al. Regulatory T cells, inherited variation, and clinical outcome in epithelial ovarian cancer. *Cancer Immunol Immunother.* 2015;64(12):1495–504. doi:10.1007/s00262-015-1753-x.

32. Taniguchi M, Seino K-I, Nakayama T. The NKT cell system: bridging innate and acquired immunity. *Nat Immunol.* 2003;4(12):1164–65. doi:10.1038/ni1203-1164.

33. Subleski J, Weiss JM, Wiltrout RH. NK and NKT cells: the innate-adaptive interface including humoral responses. In: *Natural Killer Cells: Basic Science and Clinical Application*, MT Lotze, AW Thomsom, eds. San Diego, CA: Academic Press; 2010.

34. McEwen-Smith RM, Salio M, Cerundolo V. The regulatory role of invariant NKT cells in tumor immunity. *Cancer Immunol Res.* 2015;3(5):425–35. doi:10.1158/2326-6066.CIR-15-0062.

35. Webb TJ, Li X, Giuntoli RL, et al. Molecular identification of GD3 as a suppressor of the innate immune response in ovarian cancer. *Cancer Res.* 2012;72(15):3744–52. doi:10.1158/0008-5472.CAN-11-2695.

36. Marone G, Borriello F, Varricchi G, Genovese A, Granata F. Basophils: historical reflections and perspectives. *Chem Immunol Allergy.* 2014;100:172–92. doi:10.1159/000358734.

37. Falcone FH, Haas H, Gibbs BF. The human basophil: a new appreciation of its role in immune responses. *Blood.* 2000;96(13):4028–38.

38. Sektioglu IM, Carretero R, Bulbuc N, et al. Basophils promote tumor rejection via chemotaxis and infiltration of CD8+ T cells. *Cancer Res.* 2017;77(2):291–302. doi:10.1158/0008-5472.CAN-16-0993.

39. Davis BP, Rothenberg ME. Eosinophils and cancer. *Cancer Immunol Res.* 2014;2(1):1–8. doi:10.1158/2326-6066.CIR-13-0196.

40. Prizment AE, Vierkant RA, Smyrk TC, et al. Tumor eosinophil infiltration and improved survival of colorectal cancer patients: Iowa Women's Health

Study. *Mod Pathol.* 2016;29(5):516–27. doi:10.1038/modpathol.2016.42.

41. Ricklin D, Hajishengallis G, Yang K, Lambris JD. Complement: a key system for immune surveillance and homeostasis. *Nat Immunol.* 2010;11(9):785–97. doi:10.1038/ni.1923.

42. Pio R, Ajona D, Lambris JD. Complement inhibition in cancer therapy. *Semin Immunol.* 2013;25(1):54–64. doi:10.1016/j.smim.2013.04.001.

43. Schreiber RD, Old LJ, Smyth MJ. Cancer immunoediting: integrating immunity's roles in cancer suppression and promotion. *Science.* 2011;331(6024):1565–70. doi:10.1126/science.1203486.

44. Gorter A, Meri S. Immune evasion of tumor cells using membrane-bound complement regulatory proteins. *Immunol Today.* 1999;20(12):576–82.

45. Junnikkala S, Hakulinen J, Jarva H, et al. Secretion of soluble complement inhibitors factor H and factor H-like protein (FHL-1) by ovarian tumour cells. *Br J Cancer.* 2002;87(10):1119-1127. doi:10.1038/sj.bjc.6600614.

46. Bjørge L, Hakulinen J, Vintermyr OK, et al. Ascitic complement system in ovarian cancer. *Br J Cancer.* 2005;92(5):895–905. doi:10.1038/sj.bjc.6602334.

47. Bjørge L, Hakulinen J, Wahlström T, Matre R, Meri S. Complement-regulatory proteins in ovarian malignancies. *Int J Cancer.* 1997;70(1):14–25.

48. Bjørge L, Junnikkala S, Kristoffersen EK, Hakulinen J, Matre R, Meri S. Resistance of ovarian teratocarcinoma cell spheroids to complement-mediated lysis. *Br J Cancer.* 1997;75(9):1247–55.

49. Bellone S, Roque D, Cocco E, et al. Downregulation of membrane complement inhibitors CD55 and CD59 by siRNA sensitises uterine serous carcinoma overexpressing Her2/neu to complement and antibody-dependent cell cytotoxicity in vitro: implications for trastuzumab-based immunotherapy. *Br J Cancer.* 2012;106(9):1543–50. doi:10.1038/bjc.2012.132.

50. Shi XX, Zhang B, Zang JL, Wang GY, Gao MH. CD59 silencing via retrovirus-mediated RNA interference enhanced complement-mediated cell damage in ovary cancer. *Cell Mol Immunol.* 2009;6(1):61–66. doi:10.1038/cmi.2009.8.

51. Odening KE, Li W, Rutz R, et al. Enhanced complement resistance in drug-selected P-glycoprotein expressing multi-drug-resistant ovarian carcinoma cells. *Clin Exp Immunol.* 2009;155(2):239–48. doi:10.1111/j.1365-2249.2008.03817.x.

52. Cho MS, Vasquez HG, Rupaimoole R, et al. Autocrine effects of tumor-derived complement. *Cell Rep.* 2014;6(6):1085–95. doi:10.1016/j.celrep.2014.02.014.

53. Kurihara R, Yamaoka K, Sawamukai N, et al. C5a promotes migration, proliferation, and vessel formation in endothelial cells. *Inflamm Res.* 2010;59(8):659–66. doi:10.1007/s00011-010-0178-4.

54. Markiewski MM, DeAngelis RA, Benencia F, et al. Modulation of the antitumor immune response by

complement. *Nat Immunol.* 2008;9(11):1225–35. doi:10.1038/ni.1655.

55. Musrap N, Diamandis EP. Revisiting the complexity of the ovarian cancer microenvironment—clinical implications for treatment strategies. *Mol Cancer Res.* 2012;10(10):1254–64. doi:10.1158/1541-7786. MCR-12-0353.

56. Hanahan D, Weinberg RA. Hallmarks of cancer: the next generation. *Cell.* 2011;144(5):646–74. doi:10.1016/j.cell.2011.02.013.

57. Sund M, Kalluri R. Tumor stroma derived biomarkers in cancer. *Cancer Metastasis Rev.* 2009;28(1–2):177–83. doi:10.1007/s10555-008-9175-2.

58. Schauer IG, Sood AK, Mok S, Liu J. Cancer-associated fibroblasts and their putative role in potentiating the initiation and development of epithelial ovarian cancer. *Neoplasia.* 2011;13(5):393–405.

59. Furuya M. Ovarian cancer stroma: pathophysiology and the roles in cancer development. *Cancers.* 2012;4(3):701–24. doi:10.3390/cancers4030701.

60. Labiche A, Heutte N, Herlin P, Chasle J, Gauduchon P, Elie N. Stromal compartment as a survival prognostic factor in advanced ovarian carcinoma. *Int J Gynecol Cancer.* 2010;20(1):28–33. doi:10.1111/IGC.0b013e3181bda1cb.

61. Ganss R. Tumor stroma fosters neovascularization by recruitment of progenitor cells into the tumor bed. *J Cell Mol Med.* 2006;10(4):857–65.

62. Frantz C, Stewart KM, Weaver VM. The extracellular matrix at a glance. *J Cell Sci.* 2010;123(24):4195–4200. doi:10.1242/jcs.023820.

63. Desjardins M, Xie J, Gurler H, et al. Versican regulates metastasis of epithelial ovarian carcinoma cells and spheroids. *J Ovarian Res.* 2014;7:70. doi:10.1186/1757-2215-7-70.

64. Ween MP, Oehler MK, Ricciardelli C. Role of versican, hyaluronan and CD44 in ovarian cancer metastasis. *Int J Mol Sci.* 2011;12(2):1009–29. doi:10.3390/ijms12021009.

65. Frantz C, Stewart KM, Weaver VM. The extracellular matrix at a glance. *J Cell Sci.* 2010;123(24):4195–4200. doi:10.1242/jcs.023820.

66. Cheon D-J, Tong Y, Sim M-S, et al. A collagen-remodeling gene signature regulated by TGF-β signaling is associated with metastasis and poor survival in serous ovarian cancer. *Clin Cancer Res.* 2014;20(3):711–23. doi:10.1158/1078-0432. CCR-13-1256.

67. Flate E, Stalvey JRD. Motility of select ovarian cancer cell lines: effect of extra-cellular matrix proteins and the involvement of PAK2. *Int J Oncol.* 2014;45(4):1401–11. doi:10.3892/ijo.2014.2553.

68. Ahmed N, Riley C, Rice G, Quinn M. Role of integrin receptors for fibronectin, collagen and laminin in the regulation of ovarian carcinoma functions in response to a matrix microenvironment. *Clin Exp Metastasis.* 2005;22(5):391–402. doi:10.1007/s10585-005-1262-y.

69. Raglow Z, Thomas SM. Tumor matrix protein collagen XIα1 in cancer. *Cancer Lett.* 2015;357(2):448–53. doi:10.1016/j.canlet.2014.12.011.

70. Wu Y-H, Chang T-H, Huang Y-F, Huang H-D, Chou C-Y. COL11A1 promotes tumor progression and predicts poor clinical outcome in ovarian cancer. *Oncogene.* 2014;33(26):3432–40. doi:10.1038/onc.2013.307.

71. Tothill RW, Tinker AV, George J, et al. Novel molecular subtypes of serous and endometrioid ovarian cancer linked to clinical outcome. *Clin Cancer Res.* 2008;14(16):5198–208. doi:10.1158/1078-0432. CCR-08-0196.

72. Capo-Chichi CD, Smith ER, Yang D-H, et al. Dynamic alterations of the extracellular environment of ovarian surface epithelial cells in premalignant transformation, tumorigenicity, and metastasis. *Cancer.* 2002;95(8):1802–15. doi:10.1002/cncr.10870.

73. Januchowski R, Zawierucha P, Ruciński M, Nowicki M, Zabel M. Extracellular matrix proteins expression profiling in chemoresistant variants of the A2780 ovarian cancer cell line. *BioMed Res Int.* 2014;2014:365867. doi:10.1155/2014/365867.

74. Ndinguri MW, Zheleznyak A, Lauer JL, Anderson CJ, Fields GB. Application of collagen-model triple-helical peptide-amphiphiles for CD44-targeted drug delivery systems. *J Drug Deliv.* 2012;2012:592602. doi:10.1155/2012/592602.

75. Anttila MA, Tammi RH, Tammi MI, Syrjänen KJ, Saarikoski SV, Kosma VM. High levels of stromal hyaluronan predict poor disease outcome in epithelial ovarian cancer. *Cancer Res.* 2000;60(1):150–55.

76. Thibault B, Castells M, Delord J-P, Couderc B. Ovarian cancer microenvironment: implications for cancer dissemination and chemoresistance acquisition. *Cancer Metastasis Rev.* 2014;33(1):17–39. doi:10.1007/s10555-013-9456-2.

77. Hiltunen ELJ, Anttila M, Kultti A, et al. Elevated hyaluronan concentration without hyaluronidase activation in malignant epithelial ovarian tumors. *Cancer Res.* 2002;62(22):6410–13.

78. Ween MP, Hummitzsch K, Rodgers RJ, Oehler MK, Ricciardelli C. Versican induces a pro-metastatic ovarian cancer cell behavior which can be inhibited by small hyaluronan oligosaccharides. *Clin Exp Metastasis.* 2011;28(2):113–25. doi:10.1007/s10585-010-9363-7.

79. Ghosh S, Albitar L, LeBaron R, et al. Up-regulation of stromal versican expression in advanced stage serous ovarian cancer. *Gynecol Oncol.* 2010;119(1):114–20. doi:10.1016/j.ygyno.2010.05.029.

80. Voutilainen K, Anttila M, Sillanpää S, et al. Versican in epithelial ovarian cancer: relation to hyaluronan, clinicopathologic factors and prognosis. *Int J Cancer.* 2003;107(3):359–64. doi:10.1002/ijc.11423.

81. Hodge-Dufour J, Noble PW, Horton MR, et al. Induction of IL-12 and chemokines by hyaluronan requires adhesion-dependent priming of resident but not elicited macrophages. *J Immunol.* 1997;159(5):2492–500.

82. Seto AG. The road toward microRNA therapeutics. *Int J Biochem Cell Biol.* 2010;42(8):1298–305. doi:10.1016/j.biocel.2010.03.003.

83. Sawada K, Ohyagi-Hara C, Kimura T, Morishige K-I. Integrin inhibitors as a therapeutic agent for ovarian cancer. *J Oncol.* 2012;2012:915140. doi:10.1155/2012/915140.

84. Davidson B, Goldberg I, Gotlieb WH, et al. Coordinated expression of integrin subunits, matrix metalloproteinases (MMP), angiogenic genes and Ets transcription factors in advanced-stage ovarian carcinoma: a possible activation pathway? *Cancer Metastasis Rev.* 2003;22(1):103–15.

85. Casey RC, Burleson KM, Skubitz KM, et al. Beta 1-integrins regulate the formation and adhesion of ovarian carcinoma multicellular spheroids. *Am J Pathol.* 2001;159(6):2071–80.

86. Casey RC, Skubitz AP. CD44 and beta1 integrins mediate ovarian carcinoma cell migration toward extracellular matrix proteins. *Clin Exp Metastasis.* 2000;18(1):67–75.

87. Scalici JM, Harrer C, Allen A, et al. Inhibition of α4β1 integrin increases ovarian cancer response to carboplatin. *Gynecol Oncol.* 2014;132(2):455–61. doi:10.1016/j.ygyno.2013.12.031.

88. Hapke S, Kessler H, Luber B, et al. Ovarian cancer cell proliferation and motility is induced by engagement of integrin alpha(v)beta3/Vitronectin interaction. *Biol Chem.* 2003;384(7):1073–83. doi:10.1515/BC.2003.120.

89. Gao J, Hu Z, Liu D, et al. Expression of Lewis y antigen and integrin αv, β3 in ovarian cancer and their relationship with chemotherapeutic drug resistance. *J Exp Clin Cancer Res.* 2013;32:36. doi:10.1186/1756-9966-32-36.

90. Carduner L, Picot CR, Leroy-Dudal J, Blay L, Kellouche S, Carreiras F. Cell cycle arrest or survival signaling through αv integrins, activation of PKC and ERK1/2 lead to anoikis resistance of ovarian cancer spheroids. *Exp Cell Res.* 2014;320(2):329–42. doi:10.1016/j.yexcr.2013.11.011.

91. Xue B, Wu W, Huang K, et al. Stromal cell-derived factor-1 (SDF-1) enhances cells invasion by αvβ6 integrin-mediated signaling in ovarian cancer. *Mol Cell Biochem.* 2013;380(1–2):177–84. doi:10.1007/s11010-013-1671-1.

92. Tancioni I, Uryu S, Sulzmaier FJ, et al. FAK Inhibition disrupts a β5 integrin signaling axis controlling anchorage-independent ovarian carcinoma growth. *Mol Cancer Ther.* 2014;13(8):2050–61. doi:10.1158/1535-7163.MCT-13-1063.

93. Ortolan E, Arisio R, Morone S, et al. Functional role and prognostic significance of CD157 in ovarian carcinoma. *J Natl Cancer Inst.* 2010;102(15):1160–77. doi:10.1093/jnci/djq256.

94. Morone S, Lo-Buono N, Parrotta R, et al. Overexpression of CD157 contributes to epithelial ovarian cancer progression by promoting mesenchymal differentiation. *Plos One.* 2012;7(8):e43649. doi:10.1371/journal.pone.0043649.

95. Zhong P, Meng H, Qiu J, et al. αvβ3 Integrin-targeted reduction-sensitive micellar mertansine prodrug: superb drug loading, enhanced stability, and effective inhibition of melanoma growth in vivo. *J Control Release.* 2017;259:176–86. doi:10.1016/j.jconrel.2016.12.011.

96. Hemler ME. Tetraspanin proteins promote multiple cancer stages. *Nat Rev Cancer.* 2014;14(1):49–60. doi:10.1038/nrc3640.

97. Hwang JR, Jo K, Lee Y, Sung B-J, Park YW, Lee J-H. Upregulation of CD9 in ovarian cancer is related to the induction of TNF-α gene expression and constitutive NF-κB activation. *Carcinogenesis.* 2012;33(1):77–83. doi:10.1093/carcin/bgr257.

98. Scholz C-J, Kurzeder C, Koretz K, et al. Tspan-1 is a tetraspanin preferentially expressed by mucinous and endometrioid subtypes of human ovarian carcinomas. *Cancer Lett.* 2009;275(2):198–203. doi:10.1016/j.canlet.2008.10.014.

99. Santin AD, Zhan F, Bellone S, et al. Gene expression profiles in primary ovarian serous papillary tumors and normal ovarian epithelium: identification of candidate molecular markers for ovarian cancer diagnosis and therapy. *Int J Cancer.* 2004;112(1):14–25. doi:10.1002/ijc.20408.

100. Drapkin R, Crum CP, Hecht JL. Expression of candidate tumor markers in ovarian carcinoma and benign ovary: evidence for a link between epithelial phenotype and neoplasia. *Hum Pathol.* 2004;35(8):1014–21.

101. Houle CD, Ding X-Y, Foley JF, Afshari CA, Barrett JC, Davis BJ. Loss of expression and altered localization of KAI1 and CD9 protein are associated with epithelial ovarian cancer progression. *Gynecol Oncol.* 2002;86(1):69–78.

102. Furuya M, Kato H, Nishimura N, et al. Down-regulation of CD9 in human ovarian carcinoma cell might contribute to peritoneal dissemination: morphologic alteration and reduced expression of beta1 integrin subsets. *Cancer Res.* 2005;65(7):2617–25. doi:10.1158/0008-5472.CAN-04-3123.

103. Mosig RA, Lin L, Senturk E, et al. Application of RNA-Seq transcriptome analysis: CD151 is an invasion/migration target in all stages of epithelial ovarian cancer. *J Ovarian Res.* 2012;5:4. doi:10.1186/1757-2215-5-4.

104. Baldwin LA, Hoff JT, Lefringhouse J, et al. CD151-α3β1 integrin complexes suppress ovarian tumor growth by repressing slug-mediated EMT and canonical Wnt signaling. *Oncotarget.* 2014;5(23):12203–17.

105. Vences-Catalán F, Rajapaksa R, Srivastava MK, et al. Tetraspanin CD81 promotes tumor growth and metastasis by modulating the functions of T regulatory and myeloid-derived suppressor cells. *Cancer Res.* 2015;75(21):4517–26. doi:10.1158/0008-5472.CAN-15-1021.

106. Khanna M, Chelladurai B, Gavini A, et al. Targeting ovarian tumor cell adhesion mediated by tissue transglutaminase. *Mol Cancer Ther.* 2011;10(4):626–36. doi:10.1158/1535-7163.MCT-10-0912.

107. Matei D, Graeber TG, Baldwin RL, Karlan BY, Rao J, Chang DD. Gene expression in epithelial

ovarian carcinoma. *Oncogene.* 2002;21(41):6289–98. doi:10.1038/sj.onc.1205785.

108. Satpathy M, Cao L, Pincheira R, et al. Enhanced peritoneal ovarian tumor dissemination by tissue transglutaminase. *Cancer Res.* 2007;67(15):7194–202. doi:10.1158/0008-5472.CAN-07-0307.

109. Al-Alem L, Curry T. Ovarian cancer: involvement of the matrix metalloproteinases. *Reproduction.* 2015;150(2): R55–64. doi:10.1530/REP-14-0546

110. Desmeules P, Trudel D, Turcotte S, et al. Prognostic significance of TIMP-2, MMP-2, and MMP-9 on high-grade serous ovarian carcinoma using digital image analysis. *Hum Pathol.* 2015;46(5):739–45. doi:10.1016/j.humpath.2015.01.014.

111. Fu Z, Xu S, Xu Y, Ma J, Li J, Xu P. The expression of tumor-derived and stromal-derived matrix metalloproteinase 2 predicted prognosis of ovarian cancer. *Int J Gynecol Cancer.* 2015;25(3):356–62. doi:10.1097/IGC.0000000000000386.

112. Bruney L, Conley KC, Moss NM, Liu Y, Stack MS. Membrane-type I matrix metalloproteinase-dependent ectodomain shedding of mucin16/CA-125 on ovarian cancer cells modulates adhesion and invasion of peritoneal mesothelium. *Biol Chem.* 2014;395(10):1221–31. doi:10.1515/hsz-2014-0155.

113. Hirte H, Vergote IB, Jeffrey JR, et al. A phase III randomized trial of BAY 12-9566 (tanomastat) as maintenance therapy in patients with advanced ovarian cancer responsive to primary surgery and paclitaxel/platinum containing chemotherapy: a National Cancer Institute of Canada Clinical Trials Group Study. *Gynecol Oncol.* 2006;102(2):300–308. doi:10.1016/j.ygyno.2005.12.020.

114. Myers ER, Bastian LA, Havrilesky LJ, et al. Management of adnexal mass. *Evid Report Technology Assess.* 2006;130:1–145.

115. Naora H. Heterotypic cellular interactions in the ovarian tumor microenvironment: biological significance and therapeutic implications. *Front Oncol.* 2014;4:18. doi:10.3389/fonc.2014.00018.

116. Kaneko O, Gong L, Zhang J, et al. A binding domain on mesothelin for CA125/MUC16. *J Biol Chem.* 2009;284(6):3739–49. doi:10.1074/jbc.M806776200.

117. Das S, Batra SK. Understanding the unique attributes of MUC16 (CA125): potential implications in targeted therapy. *Cancer Res.* 2015;75(22):4669–74. doi:10.1158/0008-5472.CAN-15-1050.

118. Schwab CL, English DP, Roque DM, Pasternak M, Santin AD. Past, present and future targets for immunotherapy in ovarian cancer. *Immunotherapy.* 2014;6(12):1279–93. doi:10.2217/imt.14.90.

119. Wagner U, Schlebusch H, Köhler S, Schmolling J, Grünn U, Krebs D. Immunological responses to the tumor-associated antigen CA125 in patients with advanced ovarian cancer induced by the murine monoclonal anti-idiotype vaccine ACA125. *Hybridoma.* 1997;16(1):33–40.

120. Sabbatini P, Harter P, Scambia G, et al. Abagovomab as maintenance therapy in patients with epithelial ovarian cancer: a phase III trial of the AGO OVAR, COGI, GINECO, and GEICO--the MIMOSA study. *J Clin Oncol.* 2013;31(12):1554–61. doi:10.1200/JCO.2012.46.4057.

121. Noujaim AA, Schultes BC, Baum RP, Madiyalakan R. Induction of CA125-specific B and T cell responses in patients injected with MAb-B43.13—evidence for antibody-mediated antigen-processing and presentation of CA125 in vivo. *Cancer Biother Radiopharm.* 2001;16(3):187–203. doi:10.1089/10849780152389384.

122. Tomasek JJ, Gabbiani G, Hinz B, Chaponnier C, Brown RA. Myofibroblasts and mechano-regulation of connective tissue remodelling. *Nat Rev Mol Cell Biol.* 2002;3(5):349–363. doi:10.1038/nrm809.

123. Xing F, Saidou J, Watabe K. Cancer associated fibroblasts (CAFs) in tumor microenvironment. *Front Biosci.* 2010;15:166–79.

124. Fu S, Dong L, Sun W, Xu Y, Gao L, Miao Y. Stromal-epithelial crosstalk provides a suitable microenvironment for the progression of ovarian cancer cells in vitro. *Cancer Invest.* 2013;31(9):616–24. doi:10.3109/07357907.2013.849723.

125. Yasuda K, Torigoe T, Mariya T, et al. Fibroblasts induce expression of FGF4 in ovarian cancer stem-like cells/cancer-initiating cells and upregulate their tumor initiation capacity. *Lab Investig J Tech Methods Pathol.* 2014;94(12):1355–69. doi:10.1038/labinvest.2014.122.

126. Xu LN, Xu BN, Cai J, Yang JB, Lin N. Tumor-associated fibroblast-conditioned medium promotes tumor cell proliferation and angiogenesis. *Genet Mol Res.* 2013;12(4):5863–71. doi:10.4238/2013.November.22.14.

127. Shen C-C, Kang Y-H, Zhao M, et al. WNT16B from ovarian fibroblasts induces differentiation of regulatory T cells through β-catenin signal in dendritic cells. *Int J Mol Sci.* 2014;15(7):12928–39. doi:10.3390/ijms150712928.

128. Mhawech-Fauceglia P, Yan L, Sharifian M, et al. Stromal expression of fibroblast activation protein alpha (FAP) predicts platinum resistance and shorter recurrence in patients with epithelial ovarian cancer. *Cancer Microenviron.* 2015;8(1):23–31. doi:10.1007/s12307-014-0153-7

129. Mhawech-Fauceglia P, Wang D, Samrao D, et al. Clinical implications of marker expression of carcinoma-associated fibroblasts (CAFs) in patients with epithelial ovarian carcinoma after treatment with neoadjuvant chemotherapy. *Cancer Microenviron.* 2014;7(1–2):33–39. doi:10.1007/s12307-013-0140-4.

130. Lawrenson K, Grun B, Lee N, et al. NPPB is a novel candidate biomarker expressed by cancer-associated fibroblasts in epithelial ovarian cancer. *Int J Cancer.* 2015;136(6):1390–401. doi:10.1002/ijc.29092.

131. Xouri G, Christian S. Origin and function of tumor stroma fibroblasts. *Semin Cell Dev Biol.* 2010;21(1):40–46. doi:10.1016/j.semcdb.2009.11.017.

132. Xu L, Deng Q, Pan Y, et al. Cancer-associated fibroblasts enhance the migration ability of ovarian cancer cells by increasing EZH2 expression. *Int J Mol Med.* 2014;33(1):91–96. doi:10.3892/ijmm.2013.1549.

133. Helsten T. NCT00652899. Study of Lenvatinib in Patients with Advanced Cancer and Aberrations in FGF/FGFR Signaling. 2016. http://www.clinicaltrials.gov.

134. Hollingsworth HC, Kohn EC, Steinberg SM, Rothenberg ML, Merino MJ. Tumor angiogenesis in advanced stage ovarian carcinoma. *Am J Pathol.* 1995;147(1):33–41.

135. Alvarez AA, Krigman HR, Whitaker RS, Dodge RK, Rodriguez GC. The prognostic significance of angiogenesis in epithelial ovarian carcinoma. *Clin Cancer Res.* 1999;5(3):587–91.

136. Stone PJB, Goodheart MJ, Rose SL, Smith BJ, DeYoung BR, Buller RE. The influence of microvessel density on ovarian carcinogenesis. *Gynecol Oncol.* 2003;90(3):566–71.

137. Franses JW, Baker AB, Chitalia VC, Edelman ER. Stromal endothelial cells directly influence cancer progression. *Sci Transl Med.* 2011;3(66):66ra5. doi:10.1126/scitranslmed.3001542.

138. Stadlmann S, Feichtinger H, Mikuz G, et al. Interactions of human peritoneal mesothelial cells with serous ovarian cancer cell spheroids—evidence for a mechanical and paracrine barrier function of the peritoneal mesothelium. *Int J Gynecol Cancer.* 2014;24(2):192–200. doi:10.1097/IGC.0000000000000036.

139. Iwanicki MP, Davidowitz RA, Ng MR, et al. Ovarian cancer spheroids use myosin-generated force to clear the mesothelium. *Cancer Discov.* 2011;1(2):144–57. doi:10.1158/2159-8274.CD-11-0010.

140. Said NA, Elmarakby AA, Imig JD, Fulton DJ, Motamed K. SPARC ameliorates ovarian cancer-associated inflammation. *Neoplasia.* 2008;10(10):1092–104.

141. Kenny HA, Chiang C-Y, White EA, et al. Mesothelial cells promote early ovarian cancer metastasis through fibronectin secretion. *J Clin Invest.* 2014;124(10):4614–28. doi:10.1172/JCI74778.

142. Mikuła-Pietrasik J, Sosińska P, Kucińska M, et al. Peritoneal mesothelium promotes the progression of ovarian cancer cells in vitro and in a mice xenograft model in vivo. *Cancer Lett.* 2014;355(2):310–15. doi:10.1016/j.canlet.2014.09.041.

143. Mitra AK, Chiang CY, Tiwari P, et al. Microenvironment-induced downregulation of miR-193b drives ovarian cancer metastasis. *Oncogene.* 2015;34(48):5923–32. doi:10.1038/onc.2015.43

144. Lengyel E. Ovarian cancer development and metastasis. *Am J Pathol.* 2010;177(3):1053–64. doi:10.2353/ajpath.2010.100105.

145. Chen C, Chang Y-C, Lan MS, Breslin M. Leptin stimulates ovarian cancer cell growth and inhibits apoptosis by increasing cyclin D1 and Mcl-1 expression via the activation of the MEK/ERK1/2 and PI3K/Akt signaling pathways. *Int J Oncol.* 2013;42(3):1113–19. doi:10.3892/ijo.2013.1789.

146. Nieman KM, Kenny HA, Penicka CV, et al. Adipocytes promote ovarian cancer metastasis and provide energy for rapid tumor growth. *Nat Med.* 2011;17(11):1498–503. doi:10.1038/nm.2492.

147. Tebbe C, Chhina J, Dar SA, et al. Metformin limits the adipocyte tumor-promoting effect on ovarian cancer. *Oncotarget.* 2014;5(13):4746–64.

148. Touboul C, Vidal F, Pasquier J, Lis R, Rafii A. Role of mesenchymal cells in the natural history of ovarian cancer: a review. *J Transl Med.* 2014;12(1):271. doi:10.1186/s12967-014-0271-5.

149. Touboul C, Lis R, Al Farsi H, et al. Mesenchymal stem cells enhance ovarian cancer cell infiltration through IL6 secretion in an amniochorionic membrane based 3D model. *J Transl Med.* 2013;11:28. doi:10.1186/1479-5876-11-28.

150. McLean K, Gong Y, Choi Y, et al. Human ovarian carcinoma–associated mesenchymal stem cells regulate cancer stem cells and tumorigenesis via altered BMP production. *J Clin Invest.* 2011;121(8):3206–19. doi:10.1172/JCI45273.

151. Lu Z, Chen Y, Hu Z, Hu C. Diagnostic value of total plasma lysophosphatidic acid in ovarian cancer: a meta-analysis. *Int J Gynecol Cancer.* 2015;25(1):18–23. doi:10.1097/IGC.0000000000000319.

152. Xu Y, Shen Z, Wiper DW, et al. Lysophosphatidic acid as a potential biomarker for ovarian and other gynecologic cancers. *JAMA.* 1998;280(8):719–23.

153. So J, Navari J, Wang F-Q, Fishman DA. Lysophosphatidic acid enhances epithelial ovarian carcinoma invasion through the increased expression of interleukin-8. *Gynecol Oncol.* 2004;95(2):314–22. doi:10.1016/j.ygyno.2004.08.001.

154. Schwartz BM, Hong G, Morrison BH, et al. Lysophospholipids increase interleukin-8 expression in ovarian cancer cells. *Gynecol Oncol.* 2001;81(2):291–300. doi:10.1006/gyno.2001.6124.

155. Fang X, Schummer M, Mao M, et al. Lysophosphatidic acid is a bioactive mediator in ovarian cancer. *Biochim Biophys Acta.* 2002;1582(1–3):257–64.

156. Fang X, Yu S, Bast RC, et al. Mechanisms for lysophosphatidic acid-induced cytokine production in ovarian cancer cells. *J Biol Chem.* 2004;279(10):9653–61. doi:10.1074/jbc.M306662200.

157. Wang H, Liu W, Wei D, Hu K, Wu X, Yao Y. Effect of the LPA-mediated CXCL12-CXCR4 axis in the tumor proliferation, migration and invasion of ovarian cancer cell lines. *Oncol Lett.* 2014;7(5):1581–85. doi:10.3892/ol.2014.1926.

158. Hanahan D, Weinberg RA. Hallmarks of cancer: the next generation. *Cell.* 2011;144(5):646–74. doi:10.1016/j.cell.2011.02.013.

159. Yang K, Zheng D, Deng X, Bai L, Xu Y, Cong Y-S. Lysophosphatidic acid activates telomerase in ovarian cancer cells through hypoxia-inducible factor-1alpha and the PI3K pathway. *J Cell Biochem.* 2008;105(5):1194–201. doi:10.1002/jcb.21919.

160. Lagadari M, Truta-Feles K, Lehmann K, et al. Lysophosphatidic acid inhibits the cytotoxic activity of NK cells: involvement of Gs protein-mediated signaling. *Int Immunol.* 2009;21(6):667–77. doi:10.1093/intimm/dxp035.

161. Hong G, Baudhuin LM, Xu Y. Sphingosine-1-phosphate modulates growth and adhesion of ovarian cancer cells. *FEBS Lett.* 1999;460(3):513–18.

162. Wang D, Zhao Z, Caperell-Grant A, et al. S1P differentially regulates migration of human ovarian cancer and human ovarian surface epithelial cells. *Mol Cancer Ther.* 2008;7(7):1993–2002. doi:10.1158/1535-7163.MCT-08-0088.

163. Ratajczak MZ, Jadczyk T, Schneider G, Kakar SS, Kucia M. Induction of a tumor-metastasis-receptive microenvironment as an unwanted and underestimated side effect of treatment by chemotherapy or radiotherapy. *J Ovarian Res.* 2013;6(1):95. doi:10.1186/1757-2215-6-95.

164. Reader J, Holt D, Fulton A. Prostaglandin E2 EP receptors as therapeutic targets in breast cancer. *Cancer Metastasis Rev.* 2011;30(3-4):449–63. doi:10.1007/s10555-011-9303-2.

165. Li S, Miner K, Fannin R, Carl Barrett J, Davis BJ. Cyclooxygenase-1 and 2 in normal and malignant human ovarian epithelium. *Gynecol Oncol.* 2004;92(2):622–27. doi:10.1016/j.ygyno.2003.10.053.

166. Ali-Fehmi R, Morris RT, Bandyopadhyay S, et al. Expression of cyclooxygenase-2 in advanced stage ovarian serous carcinoma: correlation with tumor cell proliferation, apoptosis, angiogenesis, and survival. *Am J Obstet Gynecol.* 2005;192(3):819–25. doi:10.1016/j.ajog.2004.10.587.

167. Rask K, Zhu Y, Wang W, Hedin L, Sundfeldt K. Ovarian epithelial cancer: a role for PGE2-synthesis and signalling in malignant transformation and progression. *Mol Cancer.* 2006;5:62. doi:10.1186/1476-4598-5-62.

168. Gupta RA, Tejada LV, Tong BJ, et al. Cyclooxygenase-1 is overexpressed and promotes angiogenic growth factor production in ovarian cancer. *Cancer Res.* 2003;63(5):906–11.

169. Kino Y, Kojima F, Kiguchi K, Igarashi R, Ishizuka B, Kawai S. Prostaglandin E2 production in ovarian cancer cell lines is regulated by cyclooxygenase-1, not cyclooxygenase-2. *Prostaglandins Leukot Essent Fatty Acids.* 2005;73(2):103–11. doi:10.1016/j.plefa.2005.04.014.

170. Spinella F, Rosanò L, Di Castro V, Natali PG, Bagnato A. Endothelin-1-induced prostaglandin E2-EP2, EP4 signaling regulates vascular endothelial growth factor production and ovarian carcinoma cell invasion. *J Biol Chem.* 2004;279(45):46700–705. doi:10.1074/jbc.M408584200.

171. Lin Y, Cui M, Xu T, Yu W, Zhang L. Silencing of cyclooxygenase-2 inhibits the growth, invasion and migration of ovarian cancer cells. *Mol Med Rep.* 2014;9(6):2499–504. doi:10.3892/mmr.2014.2131.

172. Li W, Zhang H, Xu R, Zhuo G, Hu Y, Li J. Effects of a selective cyclooxygenase-2 inhibitor, nimesulide, on the growth of ovarian carcinoma in vivo. *Med Oncol.* 2008;25(2):172–77. doi:10.1007/s12032-007-9016-0.

173. Dijkgraaf EM, Heusinkveld M, Tummers B, et al. Chemotherapy alters monocyte differentiation to favor generation of cancer-supporting M2 macrophages in the tumor microenvironment. *Cancer Res.* 2013;73(8):2480–92. doi:10.1158/0008-5472.CAN-12-3542.

174. Reyners AKL, de Munck L, Erdkamp FLG, et al. A randomized phase II study investigating the addition of the specific COX-2 inhibitor celecoxib to docetaxel plus carboplatin as first-line chemotherapy for stage IC to IV epithelial ovarian cancer, fallopian tube or primary peritoneal carcinomas: the DoCaCel study. *Ann Oncol.* 2012;23(11):2896–902. doi:10.1093/annonc/mds107.

175. Funk CD, FitzGerald GA. COX-2 inhibitors and cardiovascular risk. *J Cardiovasc Pharmacol.* 2007;50(5):470–79. doi:10.1097/FJC.0b013e318157f72d.

176. Legge F, Paglia A, D'Asta M, Fuoco G, Scambia G, Ferrandina G. Phase II study of the combination carboplatin plus celecoxib in heavily pre-treated recurrent ovarian cancer patients. *BMC Cancer.* 2011;11:214. doi:10.1186/1471-2407-11-214.

177. Obermajer N, Muthuswamy R, Odunsi K, Edwards RP, Kalinski P. PGE2-induced CXCL12 production and CXCR4 expression controls the accumulation of human MDSCs in ovarian cancer environment. *Cancer Res.* 2011;71(24):7463. doi:10.1158/0008-5472.CAN-11-2449.

178. Cordes T, Hoellen F, Dittmer C, et al. Correlation of prostaglandin metabolizing enzymes and serum PGE2 levels with vitamin D receptor and serum 25(OH)2D3 levels in breast and ovarian cancer. *Anticancer Res.* 2012;32(1):351–57.

179. Lau M-T, Wong AST, Leung PCK. Gonadotropins induce tumor cell migration and invasion by increasing cyclooxygenases expression and prostaglandin E(2) production in human ovarian cancer cells. *Endocrinology.* 2010;151(7):2985–93. doi:10.1210/en.2009-1318.

180. Luan B, Yoon Y-S, Le Lay J, Kaestner KH, Hedrick S, Montminy M. CREB pathway links PGE2 signaling with macrophage polarization. *Proc Natl Acad Sci U S A.* 2015;112(51):15642–47. doi:10.1073/pnas.1519644112.

181. Reader JC, Staats P, Goloubeva O, et al. Functional studies of EP4 in ovarian cancer. *Cancer Res 2016.* 76((14 Supplement)):5169–5169.

182. Scheller J, Garbers C, Rose-John S. Interleukin-6: from basic biology to selective blockade of pro-inflammatory activities. *Semin Immunol.* 2014;26(1):2–12. doi:10.1016/j.smim.2013.11.002.

183. Kumar J, Ward AC. Role of the interleukin 6 receptor family in epithelial ovarian cancer and its clinical implications. *Biochim Biophys Acta.* 2014;1845(2):117–25. doi:10.1016/j.bbcan.2013.12.003.

184. Kolomeyevskaya N, Eng KH, Khan ANH, et al. Cytokine profiling of ascites at primary surgery identifies an interaction of tumor necrosis factor-α and interleukin-6 in predicting reduced progression-free survival in epithelial ovarian cancer. *Gynecol Oncol.* 2015;138(2):352–57. doi:10.1016/j.ygyno.2015.05.009.

185. Dobrzycka B, Mackowiak-Matejczyk B, Terlikowska KM, Kulesza-Bronczyk B, Kinalski M, Terlikowski SJ. Serum levels of IL-6, IL-8 and CRP as prognostic factors in epithelial ovarian cancer. *Eur Cytokine Netw.* 2013;24(3):106–13. doi:10.1684/ecn.2013.0340.

186. Macciò A, Madeddu C. The role of interleukin-6 in the evolution of ovarian cancer: clinical and prognostic implications--a review. *J Mol Med.* 2013;91(12):1355–68. doi:10.1007/s00109-013-1080-7.

187. Syed V, Ulinski G, Mok SC, Ho S-M. Reproductive hormone-induced, STAT3-mediated interleukin 6 action in normal and malignant human ovarian surface epithelial cells. *J Natl Cancer Inst.* 2002;94(8):617–29.

188. Obata NH, Tamakoshi K, Shibata K, Kikkawa F, Tomoda Y. Effects of interleukin-6 on in vitro cell attachment, migration and invasion of human ovarian carcinoma. *Anticancer Res.* 1997;17(1A):337–42.

189. Yin J, Zeng F, Wu N, Kang K, Yang Z, Yang H. Interleukin-8 promotes human ovarian cancer cell migration by epithelial-mesenchymal transition induction in vitro. *Clin Transl Oncol.* 2015;17(5):365–70. doi:10.1007/s12094-014-1240-4.

190. Waugh DJJ, Wilson C. The interleukin-8 pathway in cancer. *Clin Cancer Res.* 2008;14(21):6735–41. doi:10.1158/1078-0432.CCR-07-4843.

191. Kristjánsdóttir B, Partheen K, Fung ET, Yip C, Levan K, Sundfeldt K. Early inflammatory response in epithelial ovarian tumor cyst fluids. *Cancer Med.* 2014;3(5):1302–12. doi:10.1002/cam4.282.

192. Ivarsson K, Runesson E, Sundfeldt K, et al. The chemotactic cytokine interleukin-8—a cyst fluid marker for malignant epithelial ovarian cancer? *Gynecol Oncol.* 1998;71(3):420–23. doi:10.1006/gyno.1998.5198.

193. Lokshin AE, Winans M, Landsittel D, et al. Circulating IL-8 and anti-IL-8 autoantibody in patients with ovarian cancer. *Gynecol Oncol.* 2006;102(2):244–51. doi:10.1016/j.ygyno.2005.12.011.

194. Kassim SK, El-Salahy EM, Fayed ST, et al. Vascular endothelial growth factor and interleukin-8 are associated with poor prognosis in epithelial ovarian cancer patients. *Clin Biochem.* 2004;37(5):363–69. doi:10.1016/j.clinbiochem.2004.01.014.

195. Xu L, Fidler IJ. Interleukin 8: an autocrine growth factor for human ovarian cancer. *Oncol Res.* 2000;12(2):97–106.

196. Gawrychowski K, Szewczyk G, Skopińska-Różewska E, et al. The angiogenic activity of ascites in the course of ovarian cancer as a marker of disease progression. *Dis Markers.* 2014;2014:683757. doi:10.1155/2014/683757.

197. Wang Y, Xu RC, Zhang XL, et al. Interleukin-8 secretion by ovarian cancer cells increases anchorage-independent growth, proliferation, angiogenic potential, adhesion and invasion. *Cytokine.* 2012;59(1):145–55. doi:10.1016/j.cyto.2012.04.013.

198. Chudecka-Głaz AM, Cymbaluk-Płoska AA, Menkiszak JL, et al. Assessment of selected cytokines, proteins, and growth factors in the peritoneal fluid of patients with ovarian cancer and benign gynecological conditions. *OncoTargets Ther.* 2015;8:471–85. doi:10.2147/OTT.S73438.

199. Guo Y, Xu F, Lu T, Duan Z, Zhang Z. Interleukin-6 signaling pathway in targeted therapy for cancer. *Cancer Treat Rev.* 2012;38(7):904–10. doi:10.1016/j.ctrv.2012.04.007.

200. Cohen S, Bruchim I, Graiver D, et al. Platinum-resistance in ovarian cancer cells is mediated by IL-6 secretion via the increased expression of its target cIAP-2. *J Mol Med.* 2013;91(3):357–68. doi:10.1007/s00109-012-0946-4.

201. Said NA, Najwer I, Socha MJ, Fulton DJ, Mok SC, Motamed K. SPARC inhibits LPA-mediated mesothelial-ovarian cancer cell crosstalk. *Neoplasia.* 2007;9(1):23–35.

202. Amini A, Masoumi Moghaddam S, Morris DL, Pourgholami MH. Utility of vascular endothelial growth factor inhibitors in the treatment of ovarian cancer: from concept to application. *J Oncol.* 2011;2012:e540791. doi:10.1155/2012/540791.

203. Frumovitz M, Sood AK. Vascular endothelial growth factor (VEGF) pathway as a therapeutic target in gynecologic malignancies. *Gynecol Oncol.* 2007;104(3):768–78. doi:10.1016/j.ygyno.2006.10.062.

204. Duhoux FP, Machiels J-P. Antivascular therapy for epithelial ovarian cancer. *J Oncol.* 2010;2010:372547. doi:10.1155/2010/372547.

205. Beutler BA. The role of tumor necrosis factor in health and disease. *J Rheumatol Suppl.* 1999;57:16–21.

206. Hussain SP, Hofseth LJ, Harris CC. Radical causes of cancer. *Nat Rev Cancer.* 2003;3(4):276–85. doi:10.1038/nrc1046.

207. Balkwill F, Joffroy C. TNF: a tumor-suppressing factor or a tumor-promoting factor? *Future Oncol.* 2010;6(12):1833–36. doi:10.2217/fon.10.155.

208. Wang X, Lin Y. Tumor necrosis factor and cancer, buddies or foes? *Acta Pharmacol Sin.* 2008;29(11):1275–88. doi:10.1111/j.1745-7254.2008.00889.x.

209. Madhusudan S, Muthuramalingam SR, Braybrooke JP, et al. Study of etanercept, a tumor necrosis factor-alpha inhibitor, in recurrent ovarian cancer. *J Clin Oncol.* 2005;23(25):5950–59. doi:10.1200/JCO.2005.04.127.

210. Yoshida S, Ono M, Shono T, et al. Involvement of interleukin-8, vascular endothelial growth factor, and basic fibroblast growth factor in tumor necrosis factor alpha-dependent angiogenesis. *Mol Cell Biol.* 1997;17(7):4015–23.

211. Szlosarek PW, Grimshaw MJ, Kulbe H, et al. Expression and regulation of tumor necrosis factor alpha in normal and malignant ovarian epithelium. *Mol Cancer Ther.* 2006;5(2):382–90. doi:10.1158/1535-7163.MCT-05-0303.

212. Trabert B, Pinto L, Hartge P, et al. Pre-diagnostic serum levels of inflammation markers and risk of ovarian cancer in the prostate, lung, colorectal and ovarian cancer (PLCO) screening trial. *Gynecol Oncol.* 2014;135(2):297–304. doi:10.1016/j.ygyno.2014.08.025.

213. Block MS, Maurer MJ, Goergen K, et al. Plasma immune analytes in patients with epithelial ovarian cancer. *Cytokine.* 2015;73(1):108–13. doi:10.1016/j.cyto.2015.01.035.

214. Plewka D, Kowalczyk AE, Jakubiec-Bartnik B, et al. Immunohistochemical visualization of pro-inflammatory cytokines and enzymes in ovarian tumors. *Folia Histochem Cytobiol.* 2014;52(2):124–37. doi:10.5603/FHC.2014.0015.

215. Jammal MP, DA Silva AA, Filho AM, et al. Immunohistochemical staining of tumor necrosis factor-α and interleukin-10 in benign and malignant ovarian neoplasms. *Oncol Lett.* 2015;9(2):979–83. doi:10.3892/ol.2014.2781.

216. Muthukumaran N, Miletti-González KE, Ravindranath AK, Rodríguez-Rodríguez L. Tumor necrosis factor-alpha differentially modulates CD44 expression in ovarian cancer cells. *Mol Cancer Res.* 2006;4(8):511–20. doi:10.1158/1541-7786.MCR-05-0232.

217. Massagué J. TGFbeta in cancer. *Cell.* 2008;134(2):215–30. doi:10.1016/j.cell.2008.07.001.

218. Ó hAinmhire E, Quartuccio SM, Cheng W, Ahmed RA, King SM, Burdette JE. Mutation or loss of p53 differentially modifies TGFβ action in ovarian cancer. *Plos One.* 2014;9(2):e89553. doi:10.1371/journal.pone.0089553.

219. Gao J, Zhu Y, Nilsson M, Sundfeldt K. TGF-β isoforms induce EMT independent migration of ovarian cancer cells. *Cancer Cell Int.* 2014;14(1):72. doi:10.1186/s12935-014-0072-1.

220. Yeung T-L, Leung CS, Wong K-K, et al. TGF-β modulates ovarian cancer invasion by upregulating CAF-derived versican in the tumor microenvironment. *Cancer Res.* 2013;73(16):5016–28. doi:10.1158/0008-5472.CAN-13-0023.

221. Kurman RJ, Shih I-M. Molecular pathogenesis and extraovarian origin of epithelial ovarian cancer—shifting the paradigm. *Hum Pathol.* 2011;42(7):918–31. doi:10.1016/j.humpath.2011.03.003.

222. Kurman RJ, Visvanathan K, Roden R, Wu TC, Shih I-M. Early detection and treatment of ovarian cancer: shifting from early stage to minimal volume of disease based on a new model of carcinogenesis. *Am J Obstet Gynecol.* 2008;198(4):351–56. doi:10.1016/j.ajog.2008.01.005.

223. Salvador S, Gilks B, Köbel M, Huntsman D, Rosen B, Miller D. The fallopian tube: primary site of most pelvic high-grade serous carcinomas. *Int J Gynecol Cancer.* 2009;19(1):58–64. doi:10.1111/IGC.0b013e318199009c.

224. Cancer Genome Atlas Research Network. Integrated genomic analyses of ovarian carcinoma. *Nature.* 2011;474(7353):609–15. doi:10.1038/nature10166.

225. Mayr D, Hirschmann A, Löhrs U, Diebold J. KRAS and BRAF mutations in ovarian tumors: a comprehensive study of invasive carcinomas, borderline tumors and extraovarian implants. *Gynecol Oncol.* 2006;103(3):883–87. doi:10.1016/j.ygyno.2006.05.029.

226. Singer G, Oldt R, Cohen Y, et al. Mutations in BRAF and KRAS characterize the development of low-grade ovarian serous carcinoma. *J Natl Cancer Inst.* 2003;95(6):484–86.

227. Gemignani ML, Schlaerth AC, Bogomolniy F, et al. Role of KRAS and BRAF gene mutations in mucinous ovarian carcinoma. *Gynecol Oncol.* 2003;90(2):378–81.

228. Murdoch WJ, Townsend RS, McDonnel AC. Ovulation-induced DNA damage in ovarian surface epithelial cells of ewes: prospective regulatory mechanisms of repair/survival and apoptosis. *Biol Reprod.* 2001;65(5):1417–24.

229. Fathalla MF. Incessant ovulation—a factor in ovarian neoplasia? *Lancet.* 1971;2(7716):163.

230. Collaborative Group on Epidemiological Studies of Ovarian Cancer, Beral V, Doll R, Hermon C, Peto R, Reeves G. Ovarian cancer and oral contraceptives: collaborative reanalysis of data from 45 epidemiological studies including 23,257 women with ovarian cancer and 87,303 controls. *Lancet.* 2008;371(9609):303–14. doi:10.1016/S0140-6736(08)60167-1.

231. Risch HA, Weiss NS, Lyon JL, Daling JR, Liff JM. Events of reproductive life and the incidence of epithelial ovarian cancer. *Am J Epidemiol.* 1983;117(2):128–39.

232. Purdie DM, Bain CJ, Siskind V, Webb PM, Green AC. Ovulation and risk of epithelial ovarian cancer. *Int J Cancer.* 2003;104(2):228–32. doi:10.1002/ijc.10927.

233. Bahar-Shany K, Brand H, Sapoznik S, et al. Exposure of fallopian tube epithelium to

follicular fluid mimics carcinogenic changes in precursor lesions of serous papillary carcinoma. *Gynecol Oncol.* 2014;132(2):322–27. doi:10.1016/j.ygyno.2013.12.015.

234. Lee Y, Miron A, Drapkin R, et al. A candidate precursor to serous carcinoma that originates in the distal fallopian tube. *J Pathol.* 2007;211(1):26–35. doi:10.1002/path.2091.

235. Saleemuddin A, Folkins AK, Garrett L, et al. Risk factors for a serous cancer precursor ("p53 signature") in women with inherited BRCA mutations. *Gynecol Oncol.* 2008;111(2):226–32. doi:10.1016/j.ygyno.2008.07.018.

236. Schildkraut JM, Bastos E, Berchuck A. Relationship between lifetime ovulatory cycles and overexpression of mutant p53 in epithelial ovarian cancer. *J Natl Cancer Inst.* 1997;89(13):932–38.

237. Risch HA. Hormonal etiology of epithelial ovarian cancer, with a hypothesis concerning the role of androgens and progesterone. *J Natl Cancer Inst.* 1998;90(23):1774–86.

238. Halme J, Hammond MG, Hulka JF, Raj SG, Talbert LM. Retrograde menstruation in healthy women and in patients with endometriosis. *Obstet Gynecol.* 1984;64(2):151–54.

239. Cibula D, Widschwendter M, Májek O, Dusek L. Tubal ligation and the risk of ovarian cancer: review and meta-analysis. *Hum Reprod Update.* 2011;17(1):55–67. doi:10.1093/humupd/dmq030.

240. Van Langendonckt A, Casanas-Roux F, Donnez J. Oxidative stress and peritoneal endometriosis. *Fertil Steril.* 2002;77(5):861–70.

241. Toyokuni S. Role of iron in carcinogenesis: cancer as a ferrotoxic disease. *Cancer Sci.* 2009;100(1):9–16. doi:10.1111/j.1349-7006.2008.01001.x.

242. Seidman JD. The presence of mucosal iron in the fallopian tube supports the "incessant menstruation hypothesis" for ovarian carcinoma. *Int J Gynecol Pathol.* 2013;32(5):454–58. doi:10.1097/PGP.0b013e31826f5ce2.

243. Lattuada D, Uberti F, Colciaghi B, et al. Fimbrial cells exposure to catalytic iron mimics carcinogenic changes. *Int J Gynecol Cancer.* 2015;25(3):389–98. doi:10.1097/IGC.0000000000000379.

244. Jung M, Mertens C, Brüne B. Macrophage iron homeostasis and polarization in the context of cancer. *Immunobiology.* 2015;220(2):295–304. doi:10.1016/j.imbio.2014.09.011.

245. Lousse J-C, Defrère S, Van Langendonckt A, et al. Iron storage is significantly increased in peritoneal macrophages of endometriosis patients and correlates with iron overload in peritoneal fluid. *Fertil Steril.* 2009;91(5):1668–75. doi:10.1016/j.fertnstert.2008.02.103.

246. Crichton RR, Wilmet S, Legssyer R, Ward RJ. Molecular and cellular mechanisms of iron homeostasis and toxicity in mammalian cells. *J Inorg Biochem.* 2002;91(1):9–18.

247. Yang G, Xiao X, Rosen DG, et al. The biphasic role of NF-kappaB in progression and chemoresistance of ovarian cancer. *Clin Cancer Res.* 2011;17(8):2181–94. doi:10.1158/1078-0432.CCR-10-3265.

248. Brinton LA, Sakoda LC, Sherman ME, et al. Relationship of benign gynecologic diseases to subsequent risk of ovarian and uterine tumors. *Cancer Epidemiol Biomark.* 2005;14(12):2929–35. doi:10.1158/1055-9965.EPI-05-0394.

249. Fukunaga M, Nomura K, Ishikawa E, Ushigome S. Ovarian atypical endometriosis: its close association with malignant epithelial tumours. *Histopathology.* 1997;30(3):249–55.

250. Ogawa S, Kaku T, Amada S, et al. Ovarian endometriosis associated with ovarian carcinoma: a clinicopathological and immunohistochemical study. *Gynecol Oncol.* 2000;77(2):298–304. doi:10.1006/gyno.2000.5765.

251. Jiang X, Hitchcock A, Bryan EJ, et al. Microsatellite analysis of endometriosis reveals loss of heterozygosity at candidate ovarian tumor suppressor gene loci. *Cancer Res.* 1996;56(15):3534–39.

252. Yamaguchi K, Mandai M, Toyokuni S, et al. Contents of endometriotic cysts, especially the high concentration of free iron, are a possible cause of carcinogenesis in the cysts through the iron-induced persistent oxidative stress. *Clin Cancer Res.* 2008;14(1):32–40. doi:10.1158/1078-0432.CCR-07-1614.

253. Wiegand KC, Shah SP, Al-Agha OM, et al. ARID1A mutations in endometriosis-associated ovarian carcinomas. *N Engl J Med.* 2010;363(16):1532–43. doi:10.1056/NEJMoa1008433.

254. Vander Heiden MG, Cantley LC, Thompson CB. Understanding the Warburg effect: the metabolic requirements of cell proliferation. *Science.* 2009;324(5930):1029–33. doi:10.1126/science.1160809.

255. Lisanti MP, Martinez-Outschoorn UE, Chiavarina B, et al. Understanding the "lethal" drivers of tumor-stroma co-evolution: emerging role(s) for hypoxia, oxidative stress and autophagy/mitophagy in the tumor micro-environment. *Cancer Biol Ther.* 2010;10(6):537–42. doi:10.4161/cbt.10.6.13370.

256. Koukourakis MI, Giatromanolaki A, Harris AL, Sivridis E. Comparison of metabolic pathways between cancer cells and stromal cells in colorectal carcinomas: a metabolic survival role for tumor-associated stroma. *Cancer Res.* 2006;66(2):632–37. doi:10.1158/0008-5472.CAN-05-3260.

257. Duechler M, Peczek L, Szubert M, Suzin J. Influence of hypoxia inducible factors on the immune microenvironment in ovarian cancer. *Anticancer Res.* 2014;34(6):2811–19.

258. Horiuchi A, Hayashi T, Kikuchi N, et al. Hypoxia upregulates ovarian cancer invasiveness via the binding of HIF-1α to a hypoxia-induced, methylation-free hypoxia response element of S100A4 gene. *Int J Cancer.* 2012;131(8):1755–67. doi:10.1002/ijc.27448.

259. Horiuchi A, Imai T, Shimizu M, et al. Hypoxia-induced changes in the expression of VEGF, HIF-1

alpha and cell cycle-related molecules in ovarian cancer cells. *Anticancer Res.* 2002;22(5):2697–702.

260. English DP, Roque DM, Santin AD. Class III b-tubulin overexpression in gynecologic tumors: implications for the choice of microtubule targeted agents? *Expert Rev Anticancer Ther.* 2013;13(1):63–74. doi:10.1586/era.12.158.

261. Parker AL, Kavallaris M, McCarroll JA. Microtubules and their role in cellular stress in cancer. *Front Oncol.* 2014;4:153. doi:10.3389/fonc.2014.00153.

262. Janke C, Bulinski JC. Post-translational regulation of the microtubule cytoskeleton: mechanisms and functions. *Nat Rev Mol Cell Biol.* 2011;12(12):773–786. doi:10.1038/nrm3227.

263. Kavallaris M. Microtubules and resistance to tubulin-binding agents. *Nat Rev Cancer.* 2010;10(3):194–204. doi:10.1038/nrc2803.

264. Kaira K, Takahashi T, Murakami H, et al. The role of βIII-tubulin in non-small cell lung cancer patients treated by taxane-based chemotherapy. *Int J Clin Oncol.* 2013;18(3):371–79. doi:10.1007/s10147-012-0386-8.

265. Tommasi S, Mangia A, Lacalamita R, et al. Cytoskeleton and paclitaxel sensitivity in breast cancer: the role of beta-tubulins. *Int J Cancer.* 2007;120(10):2078–85. doi:10.1002/ijc.22557.

266. Mariani M, Zannoni GF, Sioletic S, et al. Gender influences the class III and V β-tubulin ability to predict poor outcome in colorectal cancer. *Clin Cancer Res.* 2012;18(10):2964–75. doi:10.1158/1078-0432.CCR-11-2318.

267. Roque DM, Bellone S, Buza N, et al. Class III β-tubulin overexpression in ovarian clear cell and serous carcinoma as a maker for poor overall survival after platinum/taxane chemotherapy and sensitivity to patupilone. *Am J Obstet Gynecol.* 2013;209(1):62.e1–9. doi:10.1016/j.ajog.2013.04.017.

268. Roque DM, Buza N, Glasgow M, et al. Class III β-tubulin overexpression within the tumor microenvironment is a prognostic biomarker for poor overall survival in ovarian cancer patients treated with neoadjuvant carboplatin/paclitaxel. *Clin Exp Metastasis.* 2014;31(1):101–10. doi:10.1007/s10585-013-9614-5.

269. Carrara L, Guzzo F, Roque DM, et al. Differential in vitro sensitivity to patupilone versus paclitaxel in uterine and ovarian carcinosarcoma cell lines is linked to tubulin-beta-III expression. *Gynecol Oncol.* 2012;125(1):231–36. doi:10.1016/j.ygyno.2011.12.446.

270. Harper, Legasse T, Reader J, Rao GG, Staats P, Fulton A, Roque DM. EP4 receptor and class-III β-tubulin expression in smooth muscle tumors: implications for prognosis and treatment. International Gyencologic Cancer Society 16th Bienniel Meeting, Lisbon, Portrugal, October 29–31, 2016.

271. Roque DM, Bellone S, English DP, et al. Tubulin-β-III overexpression by uterine serous carcinomas is a marker for poor overall survival after platinum/taxane chemotherapy and sensitivity to epothilones. *Cancer.* 2013;119(14):2582–92. doi:10.1002/cncr.28017.

272. Raspaglio G, Filippetti F, Prislei S, et al. Hypoxia induces class III beta-tubulin gene expression by HIF-1alpha binding to its 3' flanking region. *Gene.* 2008;409(1–2):100–108. doi:10.1016/j.gene.2007.11.015.

273. Bordji K, Grandval A, Cuhna-Alves L, Lechapt-Zalcman E, Bernaudin M. Hypoxia-inducible factor-2α (HIF-2α), but not HIF-1α, is essential for hypoxic induction of class III β-tubulin expression in human glioblastoma cells. *FEBS J.* 2014;281(23):5220–36. doi:10.1111/febs.13062.

274. Fernández-Martínez AB, Jiménez MIA, Manzano VM, Lucio-Cazaña FJ. Intracrine prostaglandin E(2) signalling regulates hypoxia-inducible factor-1α expression through retinoic acid receptor-β. *Int J Biochem Cell Biol.* 2012;44(12):2185–93. doi:10.1016/j.biocel.2012.08.015.

275. Gao Y, Foster R, Yang X, et al. Up-regulation of CD44 in the development of metastasis, recurrence and drug resistance of ovarian cancer. *Oncotarget.* 2015;6(11):9313–26.

276. Ross JS, Sheehan CE, Williams SS, Malfetano JH, Szyfelbein WM, Kallakury BV. Decreased CD44 standard form expression correlates with prognostic variables in ovarian carcinomas. *Am J Clin Pathol.* 2001;116(1):122–28. doi:10.1309/KUK0-1M3D-LGNE-THXR.

277. Cho EY, Choi Y, Chae SW, Sohn JH, Ahn GH. Immunohistochemical study of the expression of adhesion molecules in ovarian serous neoplasms. *Pathol Int.* 2006;56(2):62–70. doi:10.1111/j.1440-1827.2006.01925.x.

278. Zagorianakou N, Stefanou D, Makrydimas G, et al. CD44s expression, in benign, borderline and malignant tumors of ovarian surface epithelium: correlation with p53, steroid receptor status, proliferative indices (PCNA, MIB1) and survival. *Anticancer Res.* 2004;24(3a):1665–70.

279. Berner HS, Davidson B, Berner A, et al. Expression of CD44 in effusions of patients diagnosed with serous ovarian carcinoma—diagnostic and prognostic implications. *Clin Exp Metastasis.* 2000;18(2):197–202.

280. Wang H, Tan M, Zhang S, et al. Expression and significance of CD44, CD47 and c-met in ovarian clear cell carcinoma. *Int J Mol Sci.* 2015;16(2):3391–404. doi:10.3390/ijms16023391.

281. Zou L, Yi T, Song X, Li S, Wei Y, Zhao X. Efficient inhibition of intraperitoneal human ovarian cancer growth by short hairpin RNA targeting CD44. *Neoplasma.* 2014;61(3):274–82.

282. Castells M, Milhas D, Gandy C, et al. Microenvironment mesenchymal cells protect ovarian cancer cell lines from apoptosis by inhibiting XIAP inactivation. *Cell Death Dis.* 2013;4:e887. doi:10.1038/cddis.2013.384.

283. Rafii A, Mirshahi P, Poupot M, et al. Oncologic trogocytosis of an original stromal cells induces chemoresistance of ovarian tumours. *Plos One.* 2008;3(12):e3894. doi:10.1371/journal.pone.0003894.

284. Touboul C, Vidal F, Pasquier J, Lis R, Rafii A. Role of mesenchymal cells in the natural history of ovarian cancer: a review. *J Transl Med.* 2014;12(1):271. doi:10.1186/s12967-014-0271-5.

285. Meads MB, Gatenby RA, Dalton WS. Environment-mediated drug resistance: a major contributor to minimal residual disease. *Nat Rev Cancer.* 2009;9(9):665–74. doi:10.1038/nrc2714.

5.

ADOPTIVE CELL IMMUNOTHERAPY FOR EPITHELIAL OVARIAN CANCER

Samir A. Farghaly

INTRODUCTION

The American Cancer Society estimates for ovarian cancer in the United States for 2017 are that about 22,440 women will receive a new diagnosis of ovarian cancer and about 14,080 women will die from ovarian cancer. Ovarian cancer ranks fifth in cancer deaths among women., accounting for more deaths than any other cancer of the female reproductive system. A woman's risk of getting ovarian cancer during her lifetime is about 1 in 75. Her lifetime chance of dying from ovarian cancer is about 1 in 100. In addition, ovarian cancer is the seventh most common cancer in women worldwide, with 239,000 new cases diagnosed in 2012. The five-year survival rate (which compares the five-year survival of people with the cancer to the survival of others at the same age who do not have cancer) ranges from approximately 30% to 50%. This rate has changed very little in the last 25 years, highlighting the need for novel therapies. Reprogramming the immune system cells to target and eradicate cancer cells represents a promising new treatment strategy. Immune T cells have the potential to control tumor growth without toxicity to healthy tissues when engineered to target proteins uniquely overexpressed in tumors. Evidence of the role of the immune system in human epithelial ovarian cancers (EOC) has come from epidemiologic and

clinical data demonstrating the presence of CD3[+] tumor-infiltrating T lymphocytes (TILs) and its association with good prognosis and longer survival.[1] Patients whose tumors contained TILs had a five-year overall survival (OS) rate of 38%, whereas patients whose tumors lacked TILs only had a rate of 4.5%. In addition, the five-year progression-free survival (PFS) rates for patients whose tumors lacked TILs were 31.0% and 8.7%, respectively. Several studies showed that the prognostic value is strongest for CD8[+] cytotoxic T lymphocytes that are localized within the epithelial component of tumors and that other factors associated with cytotoxic T lymphocyte activity are also associated with increased survival (e.g., IFNγ, IFNR, TNFα, and major histocompatibility complex [MHC] class I). Contrary, regulatory T cells, which suppress immune responses and maintain tolerance to self-antigens, are associated with decreased survival.[2] Further, the phenotype and composition of TIL subsets supports the premise that immune activation is associated with improved survival.[3] For example, CD8[+]CD103[+] T cells with an effector memory phenotype are present in large numbers in some high-grade serous ovarian cancers.[4] These findings provide the basis for possible therapeutic applications that enhance the number and functional activity of endogenous immune cells in high-grade serous ovarian cancer. The current immunotherapies for EOC fall into three categories: broad-acting immune checkpoint inhibitors and cytokines, therapeutic vaccines, and adoptive lymphocyte transfer.

ADOPTIVE T-CELL TRANSFER

T-cell receptors (TCRs) provide a recognition signal for T cells complemented by a co-stimulatory signal that can provide an on/off signal to regulate the activation of T cells (Figure 5.1).[5] Since Medawar et al.[6] carried out their seminal work, it has long been recognized that adoptively transferred T cells have the potential to target and kill cancer cells. However, in some cases transferred T cells lacked sufficient specificity to completely reject a tumor.[7-9] T cells genetically engineered to express novel receptors have enhanced tumor specificity. In addition,

advances in ex vivo expansion enable the production of clinically relevant doses of these therapeutic cells. Engineered T cells have also produced notable results in the clinic.

Adoptive T cell T lymphocytes transfer for cancer is an emerging concept. Engineering of T lymphocytes to express high-affinity antigen receptors can overcome immune tolerance. Advances in cell engineering to enable efficient gene transfer and ex vivo cell expansion have facilitated moving adoptive transfer to mainstream technology. The major challenge facing this technology is to increase the specificity of engineered T cells for tumors, as targeting shared antigens has the potential to lead to on target off-tumor toxicities. The major engineering challenge is the development of automated cell culture systems so that the approach can extend beyond specialized academic centers. The introduction adoptive T cell transfer involves

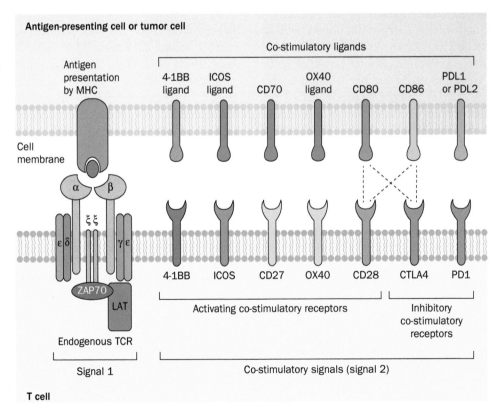

Figure 5.1 T cell receptor and costimulatory activation or inhibition of T cells. SOURCE: Fesnak AD, June CH, Levine BL. Engineered T cells: the promise and challenges of cancer immunotherapy. *Nat Rev Cancer* 2016 August 23;16(9): 566–81. Printed with permission of Springer Nature.

the isolation and reinfusion of T lymphocytes into patients to treat disease. The ultimate objective of this process is the stimulation and expansion of potent and antigen-specific T-cell immunity. Adoptive T-cell transfer to some extent overcomes limitations associated with vaccine-based strategies, such as the requirement to activate and expand a tumor antigen-specific T-cell response in patients who are often immune-compromised and deeply tolerant to cancer antigens.

Targeting of disease through the adoptive transfer of lymphocytes was first reported in rodent models.[10] Improved our understanding of T-cell biology, including the mechanisms for T-cells' activation and recognition of targets, the role of accessory surface molecules and signal transduction pathways involved in the regulation of T-cell function and survival has facilitated the ability to expand ex vivo large numbers of T cells for adoptive immunotherapy.[11–13]

The potential for adoptive T-cell transfer to treat various cancers have been evaluated, initially using T cells isolated from TILs.[14] Adoptive transfer of bulk T lymphocytes, obtained from the periphery and expanded ex vivo to generate large numbers prior to reinfusion into patients, is considered as an alternative strategy for adoptive T-cell therapy.[15] The initial approaches to apply this strategy involved leukapheresis of peripheral blood mononuclear cells from patients followed by bulk ex vivo expansion and reinfusion along with exogenous interleukin-2 (IL-2). This approach generates a population of activated T cells with lowered triggering thresholds. Also, clinical trials to evaluate the potential of adoptively transferred autologous activated T cells to augment stem cell transplants for hematologic malignancies showed that infusion of autologous co-stimulated T cells resulted in a rapid reconstitution of lymphocyte numbers.[16] Data from recent clinical trials using engineered antigen-specific T cells revealed the full potential of adoptive T-cell therapy to effectively target cancer, with objective clinical response in a number of cases[17,18,19] including patients with late-stage,

chemotherapy-resistant leukemias.[20,21] These recent results have shown that it is possible to achieve a long-standing objective of adoptive T-cell therapy.

The earliest clinical trials of engineered T cells in cancer relied on the expression of cloned TCRs with targeted affinity for tumor antigens. A TCR may recognize either intracellular or extracellular antigen in the context of MHC presentation. When designing a TCR to target tumor cells, having the option to target intracellular tumor antigen may be useful as this may expand the pool of potential targets. In addition, many tumors downregulate MHC class I expression, masking their presence from a TCR-engineered T cell. Recently, artificial receptors, such as chimeric antigen receptors (CARs), have been used to enhance engineered T-cell specificity (Figure 5.2). Unlike TCRs, CARs enable highly specific targeting of antigen in an MHC-independent fashion. CARs are formed from a combination of antibody-derived or ligand-derived domains and TCR domains. A CAR is composed of a specificity-conferring, B cell receptor–derived, extracellular antibody single-chain variable fragment, a TCR-derived CD3ζ domain and one or more intracellular co-stimulatory domains. CAR design has evolved to enhance efficacy and safety in the immunological settings (Figure 5.3). CAR T-cell targets, until recently, were limited to extracellular tumor antigens.

Most transgenic engineered TCRs also rely on recruitment of endogenous downstream signaling molecules such as linker for activation of T cell family member 1 (LAT) and ζ-associated protein of 70 kDa (ZAP70) to transduce the activation signal. Both endogenous and transgenic TCRs recognize intracellularly processed antigens and require co-stimulatory signals (Figure 5.1) for complete T-cell activation. CARs, on the other hand, lack TCR α and β chains. The extracellular portion of a CAR consists of single-chain variable fragments derived from immunoglobulin heavy chain variable (V_H) and Ig light chain variable (V_L) domains. Then these are fused to a transmembrane domain. Again,

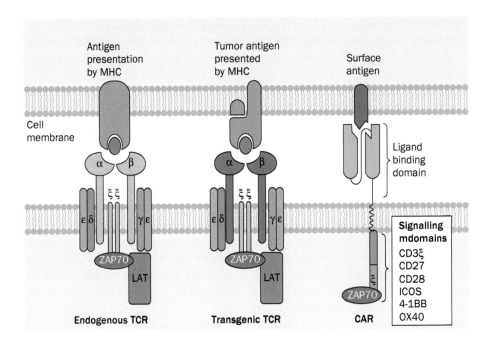

Figure 5.2 Comparing basic structure of engineered T-cell receptors and chimeric antigen receptors. SOURCE: Fesnak AD, June CH, Levine BL. Engineered T cells: the promise and challenges of cancer immunotherapy. *Nat Rev Cancer.* 2016 Aug 23;16(9): 566–81. Printed with permission of Springer Nature.

CARs must recruit endogenous downstream signaling molecules to transduce activating signal, but co-stimulation is provided in *cis* and in response to the same activating signal. CARs recognize cell surface antigens independently of the MHC and are therefore not tissue type restricted.

ADOPTIVE CELL THERAPY FOR EPITHELIAL OVARIAN CANCER

As noted, adoptive immunotherapy is based on the infusion of ex vivo expanded and/or activated immune effectors able to identify and destroy neoplastic cells.[22,23] Also, adoptive immunotherapy may be based either on Human Leukocyte Antigen (HLA)-restricted or unrestricted strategies.[21] The primary first focuses on T lymphocytes capable of recognizing tumor associated antigens (TAA) through their specific TCR; the second focuses on elements of the innate immune system which do not rely on HLA-mediated recognition of tumor targets; these effectors

are natural killer (NK) cells, lymphokine activated killer cells (LAKs), and cytokine induced killer (CIK) cells.[24] Anti-tumor lymphocytes may be adoptively infused unmodified or previously engineered with TAA-specific TCRs or CARs.[25,26] There are three sources of tumor-specific T cells for adoptive immunotherapy (Figure 5.4). TILs, which are naturally enriched for tumor-specific T cells, can be expanded nonspecifically in vitro then reinfused into their original host. For patients in whom TILs cannot be cultured, tumor-specific responses can be achieved by antigen-specific expansion or genetic engineering of polyclonal T-cell populations. Adoptive T-cell therapy, in contrast, creates a productive immune response. Through one of several techniques, T cells are harvested from a patient's blood or tumor and then stimulated to grow and expand in an in vitro culture system (Figure 5.5). After sufficient in vitro expansion, these cells are reinfused into the host, where they produce tumor destruction. This process is applicable to the majority of cancer patients who do not seem to possess

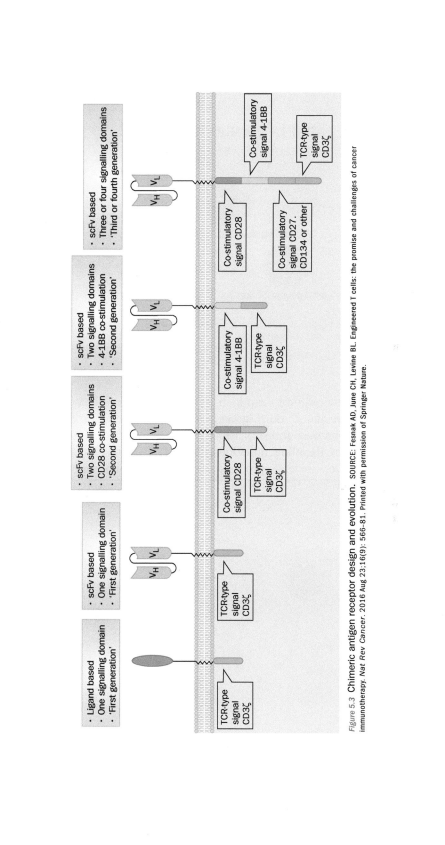

Figure 5.3 **Chimeric antigen receptor design and evolution.** SOURCE: Fesnak AD, June CH, Levine BL. Engineered T cells: the promise and challenges of cancer immunotherapy. *Nat Rev Cancer.* 2016 Aug 23;16(9): 566–81. Printed with permission of Springer Nature.

- Ligand based
- One signalling domain
- 'First generation'

- scFv based
- One signalling domain
- 'First generation'

- scFv based
- Two signalling domains
- CD28 co-stimulation
- 'Second generation'

- scFv based
- Two signalling domains
- 4-1BB co-stimulation
- 'Second generation'

- scFv based
- Three or four signalling domains
- 'Third or fourth generation'

TCR-type signal CD3ζ

TCR-type signal CD3ζ

Co-stimulatory signal CD28

TCR-type signal CD3ζ

Co-stimulatory signal 4-1BB

TCR-type signal CD3ζ

Co-stimulatory signal CD28

Co-stimulatory signal CD27, CD134 or other

Co-stimulatory signal 4-1BB

TCR-type signal CD3ζ

V_H V_L

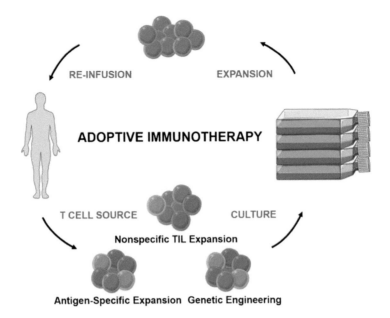

Figure 5.4 Process of adoptive T-cell immunotherapy. SOURCE: Perica K, Varela JC, Oelke M, Schneck J. Adoptive T-cell immunotherapy for cancer. *Rambam Maimonides Med J.* 2015 Jan 29;6(1): e0004.

a productive anti-cancer response prior to intervention. Tumor-specific T cells (green) can recognize overexpressed antigens, neo-antigens derived from germline mutations (Figure 5.5). However, several processes exist to suppress anti-cancer responses. T cell-intrinsic mechanisms such as loss of functionality and expression of checkpoint proteins (PD-1, CTLA-4) lead to T-cell exhaustion. Tumor-intrinsic mechanisms include secretion of suppressive factors such as TGF-B, or expression or checkpoint ligands.

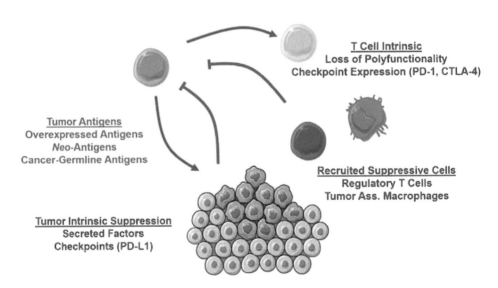

Figure 5.5 T-cell anti-cancer responses. SOURCE: Perica K, Varela JC, Oelke M, Schneck J. Adoptive T-cell immunotherapy for cancer. *Rambam Maimonides Med J.* 2015 Jan 29;6(1): e0004.

In addition, tumors recruit suppressive cells such as regulatory T cells and tumor-associated macrophages that further inhibit T-cell responses.

Currently, several TAAs have been described as potential targets in ovarian cancer[27] such as New York esophageal-1, p53; human epidermal growth factor 2/neu;[28] surviving, folate receptor α, sperm surface protein; Wilms tumor protein 1; Mucin 1; melanoma associated antigen-3; CA-125; and human telomerase reverse transcriptase.[29] Zhang et al. reported a correlation between the distribution of TILs and clinical outcome in EOCs. They analyzed 186 frozen specimens from advanced-stage EOCs and showed that the presence of CD3 + TILs was associated with a significant improvement in median PFS (22.4 vs. 5.8 months) and OS (50.3 vs. 18 months).[30]

Also, it has been shown that disease-free survival (DFS) was associated with the CD8, CD3, FoxP3, TIA-1, CD20, and MHC class I and class II expression in retrospective series of 500 patients.[31] A functional TAA targeting in EOC has been shown in vitro cultured T lymphocytes specific for human sperm protein 17 (Sp17).[32] Also, it was noted that adoptive infusion in nonobese diabetic/severe combined immunodeficiency mice, T lymphocytes were able to eradicate EOC tumor xenografts expressing high levels of Sp17.[33] There is emerging evidence suggests that TILs are not a monomorphic entity but are phenotypically and functionally different. Aoki et al. treated 17 patients with advanced or recurrent EOC. Seven patients were treated with TILs after a single infusion of cyclophosphamide. In this group, TILs represented the first line therapy in four patients ineligible of standard chemotherapy; three patients had a recurrent chemo-resistant tumor. Another group of 10 patients received TILs in association with chemotherapy. Eight patients with a previously untreated tumor received cisplatin, Adriamycin, 5-fluorouracil, and cyclophosphamide; two patients with a platinum-resistant tumor received an analogue of cisplatin (254-S) as a single agent.

One complete response and four partial responses were reported in the seven patients treated with TILs infusion alone. However, duration of response was only three to five months.[34] Mittica et al. noted that in a group of 10 patients, combination with chemotherapy, 7 patients had complete and 2 partial responses. The duration of response ranged from 13 to 26 months. It is worth noting that in the literature the response rate induced by chemotherapy is about 60%.[35,36]

In addition, Fujita et al. tested the efficacy of maintenance therapy with TILs. Thirteen patients (TILs group) with no residual tumor after primary cytoreduction and platinum-based chemotherapy received additional maintenance therapy with TILs obtained from cancer tissues. Eleven additional patients (control group) received standard treatment consisting in surgery followed by platinum-based chemotherapy. In this study, a significant difference both in three-year OS (100 vs. 67.5%; $p < 0.01$) and three-year DFS (82.1 vs. 54.5%; $p < 0.05$) was observed. The three-year DFS difference was also statistically significant in patients with macroscopic residual tumor after surgery (76.2 vs. 33.3%; $p < 0.05$). Overall, the treatment was well tolerated, with no severe complications reported.[37]

HLA UNRESTRICTED ADOPTIVE IMMUNOTHERAPY

NK cells are involved in innate immunity and tumor surveillance; they also have the ability to recognize MHC class I or class I-like molecules on target cells through a class of receptors, NK cell receptors (NKR), which can inhibit or activate NK cell function. NK cells represent about 10% of circulating lymphocytes, with a CD56 + CD3- mature phenotype and wield their activity through MHC-independent mechanisms.[38] NK cells can be divided in CD56bright CD16− population, which are characterized by low cytotoxicity but are able to produce high amounts of cytokines, and CD56dim CD16+ population which mediate antibody-dependent cellular cytotoxicity (ADDC) through CD16.[39,40] NK cells activation is dependent upon the activation of costimulatory NKR, including NKG2D, DNAX accessory molecule-1 (DNAM-1), 2B4, NTB-A, CRACC, CD2, CD59, NKp80, and CD94/NKG2C and of the natural cytotoxicity receptors ([NCR]: NKp30, NKp44, and NKp46).[41]

NK cells have a capacity to kill several tumors, such as sarcoma and leukemia, but in ovarian cancer disease the efficacy of NK cells to kill tumor is not clear. Carlsten et al. have shown that NKs derived from healthy donor can recognize and kill in vitro ovarian carcinoma cells, isolated from peritoneal effusions, through the activation of DNAM-1 signaling with complementary contributions of NKG2D and NCR receptors.[41] Also, NK cells derived ascites from patients affected by EOC did not have cytotoxic potential against autologous tumors and NK cells derived from same patients showed reduced cytotoxic activity against K-562 cell line.[42] It has been shown that CA 125 is a potent inhibitor of NK cell-mediated cytolysis of tumor cells[43] through the downregulation of CD16 and CD94/ NKG2A expression. Also, it was noted that NK cells incubated with CA 125 for 72 hours exhibited a 50% to 70% decrease in the lysis of K562 targets respect to control.[45] This group previously demonstrated that NK cells derived from ascites were enriched in CD56bright CD16– subset compared to NK cells derived from autologous peripheral blood (32% vs. 10%).[44] LAK cells are a mixture of ex vivo expanded and activated T, NK, and NKT cells which display major MHC non-restricted cytotoxicity that do not rely on HLA-mediated recognition of tumor targets. Some activity of LAK cells against several cancer cell lines was noted, such myelogenous leukemia line (K562) and colon cancer cell lines.[45]

Rosenberg et al. reported the use of LAK cells to treat 25 patients with advanced cancer: patients received both autologous LAK cells with high doses of IL-2. They observed objective regression in 11 of the 25 cases with pulmonary or hepatic metastases from melanoma, colon cancer, or renal-cell cancer, and complete tumor regression was observed in primary unresectable lung adenocarcinoma. However, the administration of high doses of IL2 was the cause of a strong toxicity limiting the use of LAK cell therapy.[46] Another group demonstrated that non-cytotoxic and sub lethal pretreatment of ovarian cancer cell line (Skov-3 cells that are not sensitive to NK cells) with paclitaxel enhance LAK cell-mediated killing.[47]

CIK cells are heterogeneous ex vivo expanded T lymphocytes, characterized by the presence of two main subsets: the first, with a CD3 + CD56+ phenotype, mainly responsible for the antitumor activity of CIKs and the second (CD3 + CD56-) more similar to conventional T lymphocytes.[48] The antitumor activity of CIKs is MHC-unrestricted and mediated by the interaction of CIKs' membrane receptor NKG2D with MHC class I polypeptide-related sequence MICA, MICB or members of the unique long 16-binding protein (ULBP) family (ULBP1, 2, and 3) on tumor cells.[50-52]

The expression of these proteins is induced by pathological stimuli, and it is associated with several tumor histotypes.[49] It was shown that CIKs had some clinical activity in solid tumors, such as non–small cell lung cancer, hepatocellular cancer, renal cell cancer, and gastric cancer, with reasonable safety profile.[53,54] Retrospective studies have shown that NKG2D ligands are expressed on the surface of ovarian cancer cells.[54,55] Also, McGillivray et al. showed that the expression of l RAET1 and ULBP2 NKG2D ligands correlates with a worse prognosis.[56] In addition, it was noted the possibility to expand CIK cells from peripheral blood of patients with ovarian cancer in the presence of appropriate cytokines such as IL2, IFNγ, and OCT3.[57] In other preclinical models, CIKs were able to kill 45% of SKOV-3 human ovarian cancer cells and were able to inhibit 73% of SK-OV-3 tumor growth in nude mice xenografts.[58]

Negrin et al. in another study, observed the killing of primary ovarian carcinoma with and without bispecific antibodies against cancer antigen-125 (BSAbxCA125 with affinity to both CD3 and CA 125) and Her2 (BSAbxHer2, with affinity to both CD3 and Her2). The addition of bispecific antibodies significantly enhanced the mean percentage of tumor-specific killing in in vitro models.[59]

In vivo expansion and efficacy of adoptively transferred allogeneic NKs was studied in 14 ovarian and 6 breast cancer patients after a lymphodepletion regimen.[60] The preparative regimen consisted of high-dose cyclophosphamide and fludarabine in seven cases followed by a 200 cGy total body irradiation.

In addition, lymphodepletion was previously shown to increase innate immunity through higher homeostatic cytokines exposure and reduction of the T regulatory and myeloid-derived suppressor cells number.[61,62] Stewart et al. reported the safety and activity of LAKs in 10 patients with chemoresistant ovarian cancers. Patients were previously treated with six intraperitoneal infusions of IL-2. Mononuclear cells were collected by leukaphereses and LAKs were reinfused in peritoneum with IL-2 followed by three additional doses of IL-2. The dose-limiting toxicity was the accumulation of ascites and the consequent abdominal pain; other adverse reactions were fever, nausea and vomiting, diarrhea, and anemia. The reported clinical response was poor.[63] Additionally, Liu et al. investigated the feasibility and efficacy of this therapy by measuring PFS and OS. Ninety-two patients with stage IIB–IV EOC were enrolled; all of them underwent cytoreductive surgery followed by six to eight courses of carboplatin and paclitaxel chemotherapy. One month after the last course, 46 patients received monthly infusion of 11.82 ± 1.61X 109 autologous CIK cells, while the other 46 patients received no further treatment. An increase in median PFS was noted in patients treated with CIKs as maintenance therapy (37.7 vs. 22.2 months, $p = 0.004$). OS did not reach statistical significance, except in stages IIB–IIIB subgroup.[47]

CONCLUSION

It has been established that ACT induces regression in a number of malignancies ranging from melanoma to certain types of leukemia, prostate cancer, and ovarian cancer. The initial studies are encouraging and provide proof-of-principle evidence. However, several aspects of ACT need to be optimized. In order to adoptive T-cell therapy to be effective it will have to be combined with other anti-tumor therapies. These are therapeutic vaccination, checkpoint inhibition, agonistic antibodies, small molecule inhibitors of tumors, and targeting of tumor stroma and neo-vasculature. It is worth noting that engineered T cells are an interesting technological advancement. The complexity of cells and the challenge of controlling T cells after the introduction of synthetically derived receptors in a therapeutic setting raise scientific, regulatory, economic, and cultural obstacles to the establishment of engineered T cells as a widespread and viable pharmaceutical platform. In addition, one of the hurdles that must be overcome for ACT to be more relevant to patients with cancer is its economic cost. These complex therapies require the development of literally a new drug for each patient, with several weeks of cell culture, skilled man-hours, and patient preparation.

REFERENCES

1. Zhang L, Conejo-Garcia JR, Katsaros D, et al. Intratumoral T cells, recurrence, and survival in epithelial ovarian cancer. N Engl J Med. 2003;348(3):203–13.
2. Curiel TJ, Coukos G, Zou L, et al. Specific recruitment of regulatory T cells in ovarian carcinoma fosters immune privilege and predicts reduced survival. Nat Med. 2004;10(9):942–49.
3. Milne K, Kobel M, Kalloger SE, et al. Systematic analysis of immune infiltrates in high-grade serous ovarian cancer reveals CD20, FoxP3 and TIA-1 as positive prognostic factors. PLoS ONE. 2009;4(7):e6412.
4. Webb JR, Milne K, Watson P, Deleeuw RJ, Nelson BH. Tumor-infiltrating lymphocytes expressing the tissue resident memory marker CD103 are associated

with increased survival in high-grade serous ovarian cancer. *Clin Cancer Res.* 2014;20(2):434–44.

5. Fesnak AD, June CH, Levine BL. Engineered T cells: the promise and challenges of cancer immunotherapy. *Nat Rev Cancer.* 2016 Aug 23;16(9): 566–81

6. Disis ML, Calenoff E, McLaughlin G, et al. Existent T-cell and antibody immunity to HER-2/neu protein in patients with breast cancer. *Cancer Res.* 1994;54:16–20.

7. Billingham RE, Brent L, Medawar PB. Quantitative studies on tissue transplantation immunity. II. The origin, strength and duration of actively and adoptively acquired immunity. *Proc R Soc Lond B Biol Sci.* 1954;143:58–80.

8. Yee C, Thompson JA, Byrd D, Riddell SR, Roche P, Celis E, Greenberg PD. Adoptive T cell therapy using antigen-specific CD8⁺ T cell clones for the treatment of patients with metastatic melanoma: *in vivo* persistence, migration, and antitumor effect of transferred T cells. *Proc Natl Acad Sci U S A.* 2002;99:16168–73.

9. Mackensen A, Meidenbauer N, Vogl S, Laumer M, Berger J, Andreesen R. Phase I study of adoptive T-cell therapy using antigen-specific CD8⁺ T cells for the treatment of patients with metastatic melanoma. *J Clin Oncol.* 2006;24:5060–69.

10. Mitchison NA. Studies of the immunological response to foreign tumor transplants in the mouse. 1. The role of lymph node cells in conferring immunity by adoptive transfer. *J Exp Med.* 1955 Aug 1;102(2):157–77.

11. Cheever MA, Chen W. Therapy with cultured T cells: principles revisited. *Immunol. Rev.* 1997;157:177–94.

12. Greenberg PD. Adoptive T cell therapy of tumors: mechanisms operative in the recognition and elimination of tumor cells. *Adv Immunol.* 1991;49:281–355.

13. Restifo NP, Dudley ME, Rosenberg SA. Adoptive immunotherapy for cancer: harnessing the T cell response. *Nat Rev Immunol.* 2012;12:269–81.

14. Dudley ME., Yang JC, Sherry R, et al. Adoptive cell therapy for patients with metastatic melanoma: evaluation of intensive myeloablative chemoradiation preparative regimens. *J Clin Oncol.* 2008;26:5233–39.

15. Rapoport AP, Stadtmauer EA, Aqui N, et al. Restoration of immunity in lymphopenic individuals with cancer by vaccination and adoptive T-cell transfer. *Nat Med.* 2005;11:1230–37.

16. Laport GG., Levine BL, Stadtmauer EA, et al. Adoptive transfer of costimulated T cells induces lymphocytosis in patients with relapsed/refractory non-Hodgkin lymphoma following CD34+-selected hematopoietic cell transplantation. *Blood.* 2003;102:2004–13.

17. Brentjens RJ, Davila ML, Riviere I, et al. CD19-targeted T cells rapidly induce molecular remissions in adults with chemotherapy-refractory acute lymphoblastic leukemia. *Sci Transl Med.* 2013;5:77ra38.

18. Johnson LA., Morgan RA, Dudley ME, et al. Gene therapy with human and mouse T-cell receptors mediates cancer regression and targets normal tissues expressing cognate antigen. *Blood.* 2009;114:535–46.

19. Kochenderfer JN, Dudley ME, Feldman SA, et al. B-cell depletion and remissions of malignancy along with cytokine-associated toxicity in a clinical trial of anti-CD19 chimeric-antigen-receptor transduced T cells. *Blood.* 2012;119:2709–20.

20. Grupp SA, Kalos M, Barrett D, et al. Chimeric antigen receptor-modified T cells for acute lymphoid leukemia. *N Engl J Med.* 2013;368:1509–18.

21. Kalos M, Levine BL, Porter DL, Katz S, Grupp SA, Bagg A, June CH. T cells with chimeric antigen receptors have potent antitumor effects and can establish memory in patients with advanced leukemia. *Sci Transl Med.* 2011;3:95ra73.

22. Schwab CL, English DP, Roque DM, et al. Past, present and future targets for immunotherapy in ovarian cancer. *Immunotherapy.* 2014;6:1279–93.

23. Perica K, Varela JC, Oelke M, Schneck J. Adoptive T cell immunotherapy for cancer. *Rambam Maimonides Med J.* 2015;6, e0004.

24. Farag SS, Caligiuri MA. Human natural killer cell development and biology. *Blood Rev.* 2006;20:123–37.

25. Srivastava S, Riddell SR. Engineering CAR-T cells: design concepts. *Trends Immunol.* 2015; 36:494–502.

26. Perica K, Varela JC, Oelke M, Schneck J. Adoptive T-cell immunotherapy for cancer. *Rambam Maimonides Med J.* 2015 Jan 9;6(1):e0004.

27. Zsiros E, Tanyi J, Balint K, Kandalaft LE. Immunotherapy for ovarian cancer: recent advances and perspectives. *Curr Opin Oncol.* 2014;26:492–500.

28. Valabrega G, Fagioli F, Corso S, et al. ErbB2 and bone sialoprotein as markers for metastatic osteosarcoma cells. *Br J Cancer.* 2003;88:396–400.

29. Reuschenbach M, von Knebel DM, Wentzensen N. A systematic review of humoral immune responses against tumor antigens. *Cancer Immunol Immunother.* 2009;58:1535–44.

30. Zhang L, Conejo-Garcia JR, Katsaros D, et al. Intratumoral T cells, recurrence, and survival in epithelial ovarian cancer. *N Engl J Med.* 2003;348:203–13.

31. Clarke B, Tinker AV, Lee CH, et al. Intraepithelial T cells and prognosis in ovarian carcinoma: novel associations with stage, tumor type, and BRCA1 loss. *Mod Pathol.* 2009;22:393–402.

32. Straughn JM, Shaw DR, Guerrero A, et al. Expression of sperm protein 17 (Sp17) in ovarian cancer. *Int J Cancer.* 2004;108:805–11.

33. Chiriva-Internati M, Weidanz JA, Yu Y, et al. Sperm protein 17 is a suitable target for adoptive T-cell-based immunotherapy in human ovarian cancer. *J Immunother.* 2008;31:693–703.

34. Aoki Y, Takakuwa K, Kodama S, et al. Use of adoptive transfer of tumor-infiltrating lymphocytes alone or in combination with cisplatin-containing

chemotherapy in patients with epithelial ovarian cancer. *Cancer Res.* 1991;51:1934–39.

35. Shelley WE, Carmichael JC, Brown LB, et al. Adriamycin and cisplatin in the treatment of stage III and IV epithelial ovarian carcinoma. *Gynecol Oncol.* 1988;29:208–21.

36. Kobayashi H, Maeda M, Hayata T, Kawashima Y. Clinical study of combination chemotherapy with CDDP, ADM and CPM for ovarian cancer. *Nihon Gan Chiryo Gakkai Shi.* 1988;23:829–36.

37. Fujita K, Ikarashi H, Takakuwa K, et al. Prolonged disease-free period in patients with advanced epithelial ovarian cancer after adoptive transfer of tumor-infiltrating lymphocytes. *Clin Cancer Res.* 1995;1:501–7.

38. Gammaitoni L, Leuci V, Mesiano G, et al. Immunotherapy of cancer stem cells in solid tumors: initial findings and future prospective. *Expert Opin Biol Ther.* 2014;14:1259–70.

39. Patankar MS, Jing Y, Morrison JC, et al. Potent suppression of natural killer cell response mediated by the ovarian tumor marker CA125. *Gynecol Oncol.* 2005;99:704–13.

40. Vivier E, Ugolini S, Blaise D, et al. Targeting natural killer cells and natural killer T cells in cancer. *Nat Rev Immunol.* 2012;12:239–52.

41. Carlsten M, Björkström NK, Norell H, et al. DNAX accessory molecule-1 mediated recognition of freshly isolated ovarian carcinoma by resting natural killer cells. *Cancer Res.* 2007;67:1317–25.

42. Ruggeri L, Mancusi A, Capanni M, et al. Exploitation of alloreactive NK cells in adoptive immunotherapy of cancer. *Curr Opin Immunol.* 2005;17:211–17.

43. Maggino T, Gadducci A. Serum markers as prognostic factors in epithelial ovarian cancer: an overview. *Eur J Gynaecol Oncol.* 2000;21:64–69.

44. Belisle JA, Gubbels JA, Raphael CA, et al. Peritoneal natural killer cells from epithelial ovarian cancer patients show an altered phenotype and bind to the tumour marker MUC16 (CA125). *Immunology.* 2007;122:418–29.

45. Phillips JH, Lanier LL. Dissection of the lymphokine-activated killer phenomenon: relative contribution of peripheral blood natural killer cells and T lymphocytes to cytolysis. *J Exp Med.* 1986;164:814–25.

46. Rosenberg SA, Lotze MT, Muul LM, et al. Observations on the systemic administration of autologous lymphokine-activated killer cells and recombinant interleukin-2 to patients with metastatic cancer. *N Engl J Med.* 1985;313:1485–92.

47. Law KS, Chen HC, Liao SK. Non-cytotoxic and sublethal paclitaxel treatment potentiates the sensitivity of cultured ovarian tumor SKOV-3 cells to lysis by lymphokine-activated killer cells. *Anticancer Res.* 2007;27:841–50.

48. Liu J, Li H, Cao S, et al. Maintenance therapy with autologous cytokine-induced killer cells in patients with advanced epithelial ovarian cancer after first-line treatment. *J Immunother.* 2014;37:115–22.

49. Sangiolo D. Cytokine induced killer cells as promising immunotherapy for solid tumors. *J Cancer.* 2011;2:363–68.

50. Verneris MR, Karami M, Baker J, et al. Role of NKG2D signaling in the cytotoxicity of activated and expanded CD8+ T cells. *Blood.* 2004;103:3065–72.

51. Kasahara M, Yoshida S. Immunogenetics of the NKG2D ligand gene family. *Immunogenetics.* 2012;64:855–67.

52. Bae DS, Hwang YK, Lee JK. Importance of NKG2D-NKG2D ligands interaction for cytolytic activity of natural killer cell. *Cell Immunol.* 2012;276:122–27.

53. Mesiano G, Todorovic M, Gammaitoni L, et al. Cytokine-induced killer (CIK) cells as feasible and effective adoptive immunotherapy for the treatment of solid tumors. *Expert Opin Biol Ther.* 2012;12:673–84.

54. Ma Y, Zhang Z, Tang L, et al. Cytokine-induced killer cells in the treatment of patients with solid carcinomas: a systematic review and pooled analysis. *Cytotherapy.* 2012;14:483–93.

55. Li K, Mandai M, Hamanishi J, et al. Clinical significance of the NKG2D ligands, MICA/B and ULBP2 in ovarian cancer: high expression of ULBP2 is an indicator of poor prognosis. *Cancer Immunol Immunother.* 2009;58:641–52.

56. McGilvray RW, Eagle RA, Rolland P, et al. ULBP2 and RAET1E NKG2D ligands are independent predictors of poor prognosis in ovarian cancer patients. *Int J Cancer.* 2010;127:1412–20.

57. Gritzapis AD, Dimitroulopoulos D, Paraskevas E, et al. Large-scale expansion of CD3(+)CD56(+) lymphocytes capable of lysing autologous tumor cells with cytokine-rich supernatants. *Cancer Immunol Immunother.* 2002;51:440–48.

58. Kim HM, Kang JS, Lim J, et al. Inhibition of human ovarian tumor growth by cytokine-induced killer cells. *Arch Pharm Res.* 2007;30:1464–70.

59. Chan JK, Hamilton CA, Cheung MK, et al. Enhanced killing of primary ovarian cancer by retargeting autologous cytokine-induced killer cells with bispecific antibodies: a preclinical study. *Clin Cancer Res.* 2006;12:1859–67.

60. Geller MA, Cooley S, Judson PL, et al. A phase II study of allogeneic natural killer cell therapy to treat patients with recurrent ovarian and breast cancer. *Cytotherapy.* 2011;13:98–107.

61. Muranski P, Boni A, Wrzesinski C, et al. Increased intensity lymphodepletion and adoptive immunotherapy—how far can we go? *Nat Clin Pract Oncol.* 2006;3:668–81.

62. Watanabe S, Deguchi K, Zheng R, et al. Tumor-induced CD11b + Gr-1+ myeloid cells suppress T cell sensitization in tumor-draining lymph nodes. *J Immunol.* 2008;181:3291–300.

63. Stewart JA, Belinson JL, Moore AL, et al. Phase I trial of intraperitoneal recombinant interleukin-2/lymphokine-activated killer cells in patients with ovarian cancer. *Cancer Res.* 1990;50:6302–10.

6.

ANTIBODY-BASED THERAPY FOR OVARIAN CANCER

Yousef Alharbi, Manish S. Patankar, and Rebecca J. Whelan

INTRODUCTION

Ovarian cancer is the fifth most common cancer in women and is often lethal because effective therapeutic strategies for its cure have not been developed.[1] Standard treatment for this disease includes surgical removal of the tumors coupled with several rounds of intravenous or intraperitoneal chemotherapy with cisplatin and paclitaxel. While a majority of patients respond well to this treatment regimen and experience significant reductions in tumor burden, complete elimination of the disease is not achieved. Patients not responding to this treatment are classified as platinum-refractory whereas patients experiencing an initial remission followed by recurrence within six months of the end of the last chemotherapy cycle are clinically categorized as those with platinum-resistant disease. Even though a significant percentage of patients are platinum sensitive (experiencing recurrence six months after the last cycle of chemotherapy), recurrent tumors are detected in most of these women within three years after administration of the last chemotherapy cycle. Even after extensive research and a strong focus on developing novel strategies for treatment, the five-year survival of patients is 25% to 35%, a number that has not changed significantly since the 1980s. Therefore, major efforts are currently underway in several laboratories around the world to develop novel therapeutics for the treatment of ovarian cancer. Prime candidates for novel treatment of ovarian cancer include small molecule agents that target specific signaling pathways as well as antibody and cell-based immunotherapies. This chapter reviews the literature on antibody-based immunotherapeutics for the treatment of ovarian cancer. To fully understand these immunotherapies, we first consider the biology of ovarian cancer and the interplay between tumor cells and peripheral blood and intratumoral immune cells. A brief review of this literature will provide the foundation for understanding antibody-based immunotherapeutic approaches for the treatment of ovarian cancer.

OVARIAN CANCER: INCIDENCE AND SUBTYPES

Ovarian cancer is the most lethal gynecological malignancy, and it is frequently diagnosed at an advanced stage when the tumor has already metastasized and the options for treatment are limited. Based on estimations published by the American Cancer Society in 2015, approximately 21,000 women in the United States will be diagnosed with ovarian cancer and about 14,000 will succumb to this disease. Ovarian cancer is a broad term that encompasses tumors of epithelial, stromal, and germ cell. Approximately 90% of ovarian cancers are of epithelial origin, and these are the focus of our discussion. In the past decade, modern understanding of the origins of epithelial ovarian cancer has emerged from genomic analysis of tumor samples obtained from patients. Based on this analysis, epithelial ovarian cancer is classified as Type I or Type II.[2] Clear cell, endometrioid, mucinous, and low-grade serous ovarian tumors are classified as Type I. On the other hand, high-grade serous tumors, which constitute 75% of all ovarian tumors, are classified as Type II.[3]

Each type and subtype of epithelial ovarian tumor displays a unique mutational signature that has been used for this modern classification of the disease. For example, while Type II ovarian tumors almost invariably exhibit mutations in the tumor suppressor p53, Type I tumors generally do not express mutant p53. Instead, the clear cell and endometrioid subtypes of Type I tumors carry mutations in ARID1A and PIK3CA.[3] The diversity in the mutational status indicates that each type and subtype of epithelial ovarian tumor likely has unique aspects to its biology that manifests in the form of severity of the disease.

High-grade serous ovarian cancer has high malignant potential compared to Type I tumors. The differences in the genetic alterations and the subsequent differences in the molecular makeup of the cancers contribute to differences in the prognosis of each type of cancer. Another difference between Type I and Type II ovarian cancer is the tissue from which each tumor is now thought to originate. Incidence of clear cell and endometrioid Type I tumors is positively associated with endometriosis, a benign disease that occurs following retrograde transfer of endometrial tissue in the peritoneum.[4] These abnormal endometrial lesions in the peritoneum acquire mutations that lead to clear cell or endometrioid tumors.

On the other hand, Type II high-grade serous tumors were thought to occur due to malignant transformation of epithelial cells surrounding the outer wall of the ovaries. While this may be the case in a subset of Type II tumors, it appears that at least 50% to 60% of Type II tumors originate in the epithelium of the distal end of the fallopian tubes. Transformed fallopian epithelial cells are

implanted on the surface of the ovaries as the fimbria rub against them during ovulation or other normal anatomical interactions.[3] The differences in mutational status as well as the tissue of origin of the different types of ovarian cancer indicate that therapies should be designed and modified to specific types of disease. In other words, a therapy against high-grade serous ovarian cancer may not be assumed to be successful for Type I tumors. This is especially true for immunotherapies as the antigens being targeted with antibodies will differ depending on the type and subtype of cancer. Therefore, if not individualized, the immunotherapies should at least be formulated by considering the exact diagnosis (Table 6.1).

Another important point to consider, particularly when designing immunotherapies, is the location of any metastases. Especially in Type II ovarian cancer, tumors are not only found on the surface of the ovaries but also on the peritoneal walls and surfaces lining peritoneal organs. Omentum is an especially favored site for metastasis of high-grade serous

TABLE 6.1 **MAJOR SUBTYPES OF OVARIAN CANCER**

Major Ovarian Cancer Subtypes	Major Precursor Lesion	Predominant Mutations
Type I		
Clear-cell carcinoma	Endometriosis	KRAS and ARID1A
Endometrioid carcinoma	Endometriosis	PTEN and ARID1A
Mucinous ovarian tumor	Mucinous cystadenomas	KRAS
Low-grade serous carcinoma	Serous cystadenomas and adenofribroma	BRAF and KRAS
Type II		
High-grade serous carcinoma	Serous tubal intra-epithelial carcinoma (STIC)	p53

tumors. Another feature of ovarian cancer is accumulation of ascites fluid. This fluid typically has a significant number of immune cells and also some cancer cells. Each site where tumor cells are located presents the potential of a diverse immune environment. For example, immune cells infiltrating at the primary tumor site can be different than those present in the peritoneum and omentum.

Ascites fluid is composed of immune cells that roughly approximate the distribution of peripheral blood mononuclear cells. However, the immune cells in ascites and the other locations where tumors are found are influenced by the cellular and molecular environment in which they reside. The immune cells are expected to be under the direct influence of immunosuppressive factors secreted by the tumor as well as by other cells in the tumor microenvironment. These interactions affect the biological activities of the infiltrating immune cells. Therefore, for immunotherapy to be successful, tumor location as well as the factors impacting the activities of the infiltrating immune cells should considered. This is especially important in designing immunotherapy clinical trials; patients with the appropriate molecular makeup and anatomical distribution should be enrolled to increase the chances of success.

IMMUNOTHERAPY AGAINST OVARIAN CANCER

In the majority of the cases, ovarian cancer is detected at a late stage when options for treatment are limited. The standard of care for ovarian cancer includes debulking surgery followed by chemotherapy with platinum compounds (cisplatin or carboplatin) and taxols (paclitaxel or docetaxel). Neoadjuvant therapy, in which patients are initially treated with chemotherapy followed by debulking surgery and additional chemotherapy, is widely used for treatment of ovarian cancer. In the majority of cases, patients respond well to this treatment and a reduction in cancer is achieved. A period of low tumor burden

persists for significant time, providing an extended temporal window when patients can be treated with a maintenance regimen to control the cancer. The development of a maintenance regimen is congruent with the goal of setting up cancer as a chronic disease.

The use of immunotherapy as a maintenance regimen is especially attractive during the period of low tumor burden, when the immune system can be considered to be under minimal influence of immunosuppressive mechanisms emanating from the cancer. Application during this time period also allows immunotherapy to act when the tumor load is low. An effective initial immune response against the cancer when developed during the period of low tumor load is expected to lead to a memory response against future tumor growth, thus potentially leading to long-term protection from the disease.

Immunohistological analysis of high-grade serous ovarian tumors has led to identification of tumor-infiltrating T cells. Several elegant studies conclusively show that the presence of cytotoxic T cells above a specific threshold in the ovarian cancer tumor microenvironment has a positive benefit on patient survival with approximately eight-fold increase in the five-year survival over patients that have no or minimal T-cell infiltration.[5-7] Conversely, increased infiltration of regulatory T cells (T_{reg}) negatively influences patient survival.

These considerations have driven the development of immunotherapies against ovarian cancer. The currently used immunotherapies can be categorized into three major approaches. The first is to develop vaccines against the disease. This is typically achieved by loading peptides from antigenic tumor-associated proteins on the antigen-presenting dendritic cells. The presented peptides are recognized by T cells, leading to an adaptive immune response against the cancer.

Various ovarian cancer associated antigenic peptides have been identified as targets for vaccine strategies. Prominent antigenic targets include NY-ESO, a cancer-testis antigen that is overexpressed by ovarian tumors.[8] Other targets for vaccines include the tumor suppressor p53 and the epidermal growth factor receptor Her2. Finally, there are also reports of whole tumor lysates used to develop vaccines. The presumed advantage of using whole tumor lysates is the potential of developing immune responses against multiple antigens in an unbiased manner.

The second approach involves development of cell-based therapies against the tumor. This approach is embodied by the development of the chimeric antigen receptor (CAR) expressing T cells. In this approach, autologous T cells isolated from patients are engineered to express chimeric receptors that contain extracellular domains that bind to antigens on the surface of cancer cells and intracytoplasmic domains that contain signaling units of CD28 and 4-1BB. The binding of the chimeric receptors to the antigen on the cancer cell surface results in activation of the signaling domains and subsequent activation of the T cells and response against the tumors. Mesothelin, MUC16, and folate receptor-α (FR–α) are prominent antigens against which CAR T cells have been developed. Studies are currently underway to determine if these CAR T cells can be used for the treatment of ovarian cancer. It should also be noted that Charles Sentman and colleagues have previously proposed the development of engineered natural killer (NK) cells that express CAR and similar to the CAR T cells can produce cytolytic responses against tumors that express the targeted antigens.[9] While CAR NK cells have not been studied in clinical trials in ovarian cancer, the initial data available with these engineered immune cells in mouse models has been very promising.

The final approach to immunotherapy against ovarian tumors involves the development of antibodies that specifically bind antigens expressed by cancer cells. The result of this binding is the activation of innate immune cells—primarily NK cells and macrophages—to develop an immune response against the cancer. We next discuss the antibodies that have been developed to target ovarian tumors. Our discussion includes a description of antibody production and the mechanism by which antibodies produce an immune response against cancer cells. Following this discussion, we identify specific antibodies that have prominently been studied as agents against ovarian tumors. Finally, we discuss the potential for coupling antibody-based immunotherapy with chemotherapy to produce an augmented therapeutic effect against ovarian cancer.

DEVELOPMENT OF THERAPEUTIC ANTIBODIES

The discovery by Kohler and Milstein of a technique to generate monoclonal antibodies against a specific antigen was a milestone achievement that led to major advances in the biological sciences.[10] The impact of monoclonal antibodies is most observed in the medical industry where these reagents have transformed health-care diagnostics, allowing the development of assays that can accurately detect and quantify specific biomarkers and diagnose benign and malignant disease. While the use of antibodies as therapeutic agents has not achieved the same level of success as diagnostic assays, steady progress has been maintained, and now with a better understanding of the immune system and new gene editing techniques, the development of therapeutic antibodies is expected to achieve greater success.

The development of therapeutic antibodies typically follows a similar pathway. In most cases the process is initiated with the identification of a murine monoclonal antibody that binds a specific cancer antigen. After careful characterization of the antibody sequence and its exact molecular epitope, the antibody is further investigated for its potential therapeutic effects using in vitro assays and animal models. After a certain level of maturity of the data is achieved, further development of the antibody requires humanization. This process is achieved by including the variable domains of the antibody into the backbone of a human antibody. The murine monoclonal antibody is a foreign protein and hence when administered causes a human anti-murine antibody (HAMA) response. The HAMA response results in a side reaction that negates or at least attenuates the therapeutic action of the antibody against the target antigen.

There is literature suggesting that the HAMA response is sometimes beneficial in increasing the level of overall immune activation, resulting in the possibility of increasing immune response against the tumor. However, it is generally believed that HAMA responses are detrimental to the therapeutic efficiency of the antibody. Therefore, humanization of the antibodies is essential before an antibody can be approved for clinical use. Humanized antibodies (huMAb) only have relatively small portion (the variable regions) of the original murine monoclonal antibodies. As a result the development of HAMA responses is significantly decreased and the therapeutic antibodies can therefore target the intended antigen with high efficacy.

Another important point to consider is the type of immune responses triggered by the huMAb. Two cell types involved in the immune response are NK cells and macrophages, both of which express Fc receptors, activating receptors that bind the Fc portion of antibodies. After antibodies engage their target antigens, immune cells bind the antigen-antibody complex via Fc receptors. Binding results in activation of NK cells and macrophages, which trigger a cytolytic response against the cancer cells. Recruitment of perforin granules, granzymes, and other proteolytic factors to the immune synapse (contact site between the cancer and immune cells) results in initiation of the cytolytic response. The proteolytic enzymes cause damage of the cancer cells and eventual cell death via programmed cell death, also known as apoptosis.

The targeted cell death caused by the binding of antibodies is termed antibody-dependent cell-mediated cytotoxicity (ADCC; Figure 6.1). It should be noted that the therapeutic antibodies are only effective if immune cells are available to make physical contact with the targeted cancer cells so that cell death can be initiated through ADCC. In other words, infiltration of immune cells into the tumor microenvironment is essential for the therapeutic antibodies to be effective against the cancer. Therapeutic antibodies

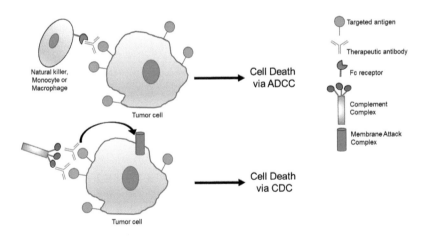

Figure 6.1 The two major immune mechanisms that allow therapeutic antibodies to kill targeted cancer cells are shown. In ADCC, the therapeutic antibody binding to antigen on the cancer cell surface leads to recruitment of immune effector cells that express Fc receptors (NK cells, monocytes, and macrophages). The Fc receptor is an activating receptor that upon binding to the Fc portion of the therapeutic antibody triggers the effectors to mediate cancer cell death via apoptosis. In CDC, antibody binding to antigen leads to binding of complement proteins. Successive recruitment of the complement proteins results in formation of the complement complex and eventually the membrane attack complex leading to cancer cell death.

can also mediate cancer cell lysis through complement-dependent cytotoxicity (CDC; Figure 6.1). In this case, upon binding of the antibodies to their antigens, C1q, a small protein synthesized by hepatocytes, is recruited. This event triggers the additional recruitment and formation of a complement cascade. If the antibody is binding to an antigen on the surface of cancer cells, the complement cascade matures to form a membrane attack complex and ultimately results in cancer cell death.

A requirement for the therapeutic antibodies to be effective is the selection of the appropriate antigen. The minimum requirement is for the antigens to be expressed in sufficient density on the cancer cells. An important aspect in choosing the appropriate antigen is whether the molecule is expressed selectively or at least expressed at higher levels on cancer cells. An antigen that is also expressed at high levels on normal tissues and cells is not desirable because of the potential to increase toxicity. Typically, the antigens that are chosen are either cell surface glycoproteins or oligosaccharides that are expressed on either glycoproteins or glycolipids.

Another factor to consider while choosing the antigen is whether the antigen can be shed from the cancer cell surface. Shed antigens are problematic because they can bind therapeutic antibody and attenuate its ability to mediate ADCC, because fewer immune cells can be recruited to form immune synapses with the cancer cells.

THERAPEUTIC ANTIBODIES AGAINST OVARIAN CANCER

Various antibodies have been developed and are being tested for treatment of ovarian cancer. The therapeutic antibodies we discuss can be categorized into three groups (Figure 6.2). The first group is the one that has been most studied and involves antibodies against specific antigens on the surface of ovarian cancer cells. The second group has been developed against CTLA-4 and PD1, two molecules responsible for controlling T-cell activation. Antibodies against T cell regulatory molecules result in amplification of the T-cell response by negating naturally occurring regulatory mechanisms. As a result, in the presence of these therapeutic antibodies, a strong immune reaction is mediated against the tumors. The third type of therapeutic antibodies tested against ovarian cancer recognize interleukin-6 (IL-6) and other cytokines. These antibodies

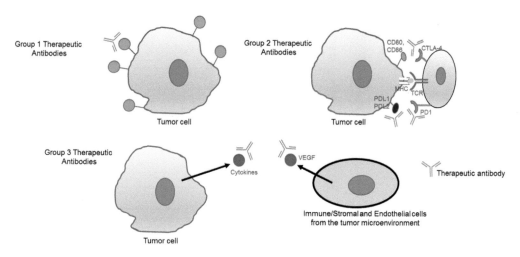

Figure 6.2 The three groups of therapeutic antibodies. Group 1 antibodies target antigens expressed on the surface of cancer cells. Group 2 antibodies are directed against immune checkpoints. Group 3 antibodies target tumor growth-promoting factors secreted by the tumor or cells in the tumor microenvironment.

scavenge circulating cytokines and prevent them from mediating their responses. In this sense, the third group of antibodies does not target the tumor directly but instead amplifies the immune response against the tumor. However, the antibodies in this third group differ from those in the second group because they do not bind to regulatory molecules expressed on the surface of the T cells but instead bind to soluble proteins in systemic circulation.

GROUP 1: THERAPEUTIC ANTIBODIES

Therapeutic antibodies belonging to this group target antigens on the surface of ovarian cancer cells. Their mode of action is to elicit ADCC against tumors via NK or macrophages.

Four major ovarian cancer antigens— MUC16, mesothelin, epithelial cell adhesion molecule (EpCAM), and FR-α—have been targeted with therapeutic antibodies.

Anti-MUC16 Antibodies

Type II high-grade serous ovarian tumors overexpress MUC16. This mucin is a Type I transmembrane glycoprotein with a postulated molecular weight of 3-5 million Da.[11] The protein backbone of this mucin is composed of approximately 24,000 amino acids decorated with hundreds of asparagine-linked (N-linked) and serine/threonine-linked (O-linked) oligosaccharide chains. The protein backbone is divided into a large N-terminal domain, a tandem repeat region, and a short cytoplasmic tail.[12–14] The tandem repeat domain is composed of up to 60 repeats each comprising 156 amino acids (Figure 6.3).

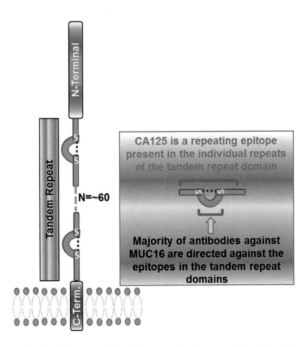

Figure 6.3 The molecular organization of MUC16. A short C-terminal region (256 amino acids) contains a cytoplasmic tail and a single transmembrane region. The tandem repeat domain is composed of up to 60 repeats, each containing156 amino acids. The repeats are not homologous, but a significant number contain the peptide that is defined as the CA125 biomarker. The N-terminal is over 12,000 amino acids long. The molecule is extensively glycosylated with N- and O-linked oligosaccharides. Inset shows an expanded view of an individual repeat from the tandem repeat domain. Disulfide bridges form the 21 amino acid loop.

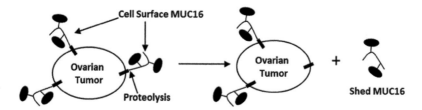

Figure 6.4 Cell surface and shed forms of MUC16. MUC16 is overexpressed by ovarian tumors. This type I transmembrane glycoprotein is expressed on the cell surface. However, proteolytic cleavage in the acidic Golgi compartment also may lead to shedding of the mucin. The shed MUC16 molecules are detected in the serum of cancer patients as the tumor biomarker CA125.

MUC16 is expressed on the surface of cancer cells. Proteolytic cleavage occurring in the Golgi complex[15] likely results in a form of MUC16 that is shed from the surface (Figure 6.4). Shed MUC16 is released from the cancer cells and is detected as the CA125 serum antigen. CA125 is a repeating peptide epitope present in the tandem repeat region of MUC16.

The exact role of MUC16 is under intense investigation. Recent reports show that MUC16 is involved in intracellular signaling that promotes proliferation of cancer cells.[16,17] On the other hand, the extracellular portion of MUC16, by binding to mesothelin (a glycosylphosphatidylinositol linked surface glycoprotein expressed on mesothelial and ovarian cancer cells) promotes peritoneal migration of ovarian tumor cells and formation of ovarian tumor spheroids.[18,19]

In addition, MUC16 serves as immunosuppressive role, preventing NK cells and macrophages from attacking cancer cells.[20,21] MUC16 expressed on the cancer cells may act as a physical and electrostatic barrier (because of its bulk and negative charge), preventing the formation of immunological synapses between NK cells and cancer cells. Additionally, cell surface bound as well as shed MUC16 can act as a ligand of the NK and macrophage inhibitory receptor Siglec-9 (Figure 6.5). MUC16/Siglec-9 binding triggers an inhibitory response that prevents the NK cells and macrophages from cytolysing cancer cells.

As mentioned, MUC16 contains an extensive tandem repeat domain (Figure 6.3). The primary significance of the tandem repeats

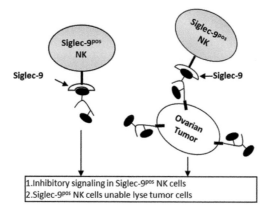

Figure 6.5 MUC16 suppresses NK cell activity by serving as a ligand of the inhibitory receptor Siglec-9. The α-2,3 linked sialic acids of MUC16 (closed circles) bind to Siglec-9. Shed and surface-bound MUC16 contain these sialic acids, and both can serve as ligands of Siglec-9. Binding of Siglec-9 to its ligand results in activation of the phosphatases SHP-1 and SHP-2, precluding the formation of an activating immune synapse between the NK cells and cancer cells. As a result the NK cells are unable to lyse cancer cells.

is that, in the majority of the 60 repeats, there is a peptide epitope defined as CA125, a biomarker used to monitor progression of ovarian cancer. Each patient with Type II ovarian cancer is monitored for serum levels of CA125. A decrease or a stable reading of CA125 level indicates a stable disease whereas elevation of this biomarker indicates recurrence. Thus the clinical significance of CA125—and, by inference, of MUC16—as a biomarker for high-grade serous ovarian cancer is well established.

Considering the overexpression of MUC16 on Type II tumors and its limited expression in other tissues, this mucin was considered a strong candidate for developing anti-cancer antibodies. One of the first attempts to this end resulted in the development of the MAB-B43.13 murine monoclonal antibody.[22-28] Biochemical studies demonstrated that this antibody specifically recognized CA125. Initially technicium labeled MAB-B43.13 was developed with the intended use to image ovarian tumor foci. In the initial clinical trial to determine efficacy of this imaging strategy, an unexpected side outcome was the delayed recurrence of ovarian cancer in some patients. Encouraged by this result, efforts were undertaken to determine if the MAB- B43.13 antibody could be used as a therapeutic reagent. In vitro experiments and data from mouse models showed that treatment with the MAB-B43.13 antibody produced strong immunological responses that delayed progression of tumor growth, decreased ascites formation, and prolonged overall survival of tumor-bearing mice. These results led to clinical testing of this antibody, which at that time was renamed Oregovomab. An initial single-arm Phase II trial conducted in 20 patients showed that Oregovomab was well tolerated.[29] HAMA responses against Oregovomab were detected in 79% of patients. Anti-CA125 antibody and anti-CA125 T cell responses were observed in 11% and 39% of the patients recruited in this trial, respectively. Patients who developed anti-CA125 immune responses showed significant improvement in their survival and time to progression of the disease.

Encouraged by these results, a larger clinical trial of 145 women with ovarian cancer was conducted with 73 patients receiving Oregovomab and 72 administered placebos.[30,31] In this two-arm trial, however, no significant benefit was observed following treatment with Oregovomab.

Secondary data analysis suggested that patients with successful primary therapy showed a significant increase in time to relapse of the tumor upon treatment with Oregovomab, as compared to the placebo-treated cohort (24 months vs. 10.8 months). Here, successful primary therapy was defined as microscopic or small diameter—less than or equal to 2 cm—residual tumors following debulking surgery, favorable response to chemotherapy as assessed by a decrease in serum CA125 levels to below 65 U/ml after third cycle of chemotherapy, and a normalized but detectable CA125 concentration following initial therapy. While the results did not bear out the promise of the earlier trial, a benefit of the Oregovomab therapy was detected in a subset of the population.

A Phase III trial recruited 373 ovarian cancer patients where Oregovomab was administered as a maintenance regimen.[32] The results of this trial were also disappointing because there was no benefit in overall survival of the patients in the treatment cohort. The negative results from these last two clinical trials have prevented further development of Oregovomab for treatment of ovarian cancer.

Abagovomab is an anti-idiotypic antibody developed against the variable region of the anti-CA125 monoclonal antibody, OC125. When administered in mice, and subsequently when tested in clinical trials, it was demonstrated that anti-idiotypic responses develop against CA125 following administration of Abagovomab.[33-36] Data suggest the development of cytotoxic T cell responses against CA125 in addition to the anti-idiotypic responses. Based on these results, Abagovomab was tested in clinical trials as a therapeutic against ovarian cancer.

In an initial Phase I/II trial, Abagovomab was administered to 119 patients with tumors in the ovary, fallopian tubes, and peritoneal cavity. This trial suggested an increase in overall survival of 23.4 months in patients who developed anti-idiotypic responses following administration of Abagovomab as compared to control cohorts where the overall survival was only 4 months. These positive results were however, not reproduced in a subsequent Phase III double-blind, placebo-controlled trial where Abagovomab was administered as a maintenance regimen. No improvement in overall survival of patients receiving Abagovomab was observed in this trial. Thus both anti-CA125 antibody approaches have not resulted in positive benefits to patients.

There are attempts being made to combine Oregovomab with chemotherapy.[37] However, the lack of success in the major clinical trials is disheartening and suggests the need to develop other approaches to antibody-based immunotherapy against ovarian cancer.

One potential complication with using anti-CA125 antibodies is the fact that this antigen is not only expressed on the surface of the cancer cells but is also released from the tumor cells into peripheral circulation.[11] As a result Oregovomab and the anti-idiotypic antibodies developed following administration of Abagovomab result in the formation of complexes of the antibodies with circulating CA125. Complex formation lowers the effective concentration of antibody available for direct binding to tumors. As explained earlier, since ADCC of tumors by NK cells and macrophages requires direct contact between the tumor and immune cells, the low level of actual tumor targeting by the antibodies likely hinders the therapeutic efficacy of Oregovomab and Abagovomab.

Anti-Folate Receptor-α Antibodies

Folic acid or folate is one of eight members of the Vitamin B family; folate is Vitamin B9.[38] Tetrahydrofolate is the reduced, biologically active form of folate. Tetrahydrofolate is essential for DNA and RNA synthesis, amino acid metabolism, and several methylation reactions. Through these actions, tetrahydrofolate promotes cell growth, proliferation, and survival. Folic acid is absorbed by the small intestines from diet. Metabolism of absorbed folate in the liver leads to synthesis of methyltetrahydrofolate, which is released into the peripheral blood thereby allowing its uptake in tissues.

At the tissue level, there are four folate receptors—α, β γ, and δ—responsible for cellular uptake of circulating tetrahydrofolate. Of these four receptors, the α and β receptor are linked via a glycosylphosphatidylinositol anchor to the surface of the cells. FR-α is an interesting molecule because of its restricted expression on normal tissue and its several-fold increase in expression on a variety of tumors.[39-42] In normal tissues, FR-α is expressed on kidney epithelia (where it plays a role in reabsorption of folate from urine) and the placenta, and on some immune cells. FR-α is expressed at high levels on tumors of ovarian, lung, kidney, endometrial, colorectal, breast, pancreas, and other cancers. In ovarian cancer, over 80% of patients show up to 90-fold increase in FR-α expression levels compared to normal ovarian surface epithelium.[43] This striking observation has identified FR-α as a potential target molecule for therapies against ovarian cancer.

Attempts are being made to chemically couple folate to chemotherapeutic drugs (vinca alkaloids, for example).[44-49] The goal is to use folate to selectively deliver the chemotherapeutic agent to the cancer cells. Clinical trials are currently underway to test if the vinca alkaloid-folate conjugate (Vintafolide), when administered in combination with existing chemotherapeutic drugs, can increase progression-free survival (PFS) in ovarian cancer patients. A Phase II trial of Vintafolide in platinum-resistant ovarian cancer patients has shown only a minor increase in PFS (5 months for the Vintafolide treatment group vs. 2.7 months for patients in the control arm).[50]

In an alternate approach, an antibody, Farletuzumab, has been developed against FR-α.[51] This therapeutic antibody has been shown to induce cancer cell death via ADCC as well as complement-dependent cancer cell death. In a Phase II clinical trial in platinum-sensitive ovarian cancer patients, Farletuzumab administered in combination with carboplatin and paclitaxel resulted in an over 70% objective response rate compared to historical outcomes. Approximately 20% of the patients in this trial also showed an increase in PFS.[52] The positive results of this initial study led to a Phase III trial where Farletuzumab, carboplatin, and a taxol derivative were administered. The control group received the same chemotherapeutic drugs except that Farletuzumab was replaced by placebo. No significant increase in PFS of patients in the Farletuzumab arm of the study was observed.

Success of anti-FR-α therapy most likely depends on FR-α expression levels on the tumor cells of each patient. Thus patients with FR-α levels above a specific threshold may likely benefit from FR-α-targeted treatments. Alternatively, it may be possible to induce ovarian tumors to express FR-α by treatment with estrogen or other agents. Tumors primed using these approaches to express higher levels of FR-α may serve as better candidates for FR-α-targeted therapies.

Anti-Mesothelin Antibodies

Another important antigen overexpressed on the majority of ovarian tumors is mesothelin, a glycosylphosphatidyl inositol-linked glycoprotein.[53] A precursor of mesothelin is initially expressed as a 69 kDa protein that is processed and cleaved into the 40 kDa mesothelin and a 31 kDa protein designated as megakaryocyte-potentiating factor (MPF).[54] The MPF is released from the cell whereas mesothelin is anchored to the cell membrane via a glycosylphosphatidylinositol linkage. Elevated expression of mesothelin is observed in mesothelioma and in ovarian and pancreatic cancer.

The biological role of mesothelin is not fully understood. However, one of the binding partners of mesothelin is MUC16.[55-57] Studies have suggested that mesothelin interacts with the N-linked glycan chains of MUC16.[55] This molecular interaction has been shown to mediate attachment of ovarian tumor cells to the mesothelium, which is also known to express mesothelin.

The MUC16-mesothelin interaction likely allows ovarian cancer cells to metastasize to the peritoneal walls. Additionally, both mesothelin and MUC16 are overexpressed on ovarian cancer cells. Studies have shown that ovarian cancer cells can bind to each other via interactions between mesothelin and MUC16 on adjacent cells. It is likely that MUC16-mesothelin interactions allow ovarian cancer cells from the primary tumor site to attach to already metastasized tumors in the peritoneum.

Considering the higher expression levels of mesothelin and its importance in metastasis of ovarian tumors, this glycoprotein has been identified as an important molecule for antibody-based immunotherapy. MORAB-009 (Amatuximab) is a chimeric antibody that has been developed against mesothelin. This antibody is being investigated as a therapeutic agent for mesothelioma, ovarian, and pancreatic tumors. Results from a Phase I trial were published in 2010. In this trial a total of 24 patients were recruited.[58] Of these, 13 patients were diagnosed with mesothelioma, 7 with pancreatic cancer, and 4 with ovarian cancer. Patients received a median of four infusions of MORAB-009. The therapy was well tolerated with an observed dose-dependent increase in circulating levels of therapeutic antibody. Importantly, 11 of the 24 patients enrolled in this study had stable disease at the end of the trial. There are no reports of a Phase II trial of MORAB-009 in ovarian cancer patients. Phase II trials are currently underway in patients with malignant pleural mesothelioma.

Apart from MORAB-009, there are also attempts made to conjugate anti-mesothelin antibody to cytotoxic agents. SS1P is a chimeric molecule composed of anti-mesothelin Fv fragment coupled to PE38, a truncated portion of Pseudomonas exotoxin A. This reagent has been tested in a Phase I trial of patients with mesothelioma.[59] SS1P fused to IL-12 has also been developed.[60] These reagents are novel and have the potential to be used as therapeutic agents for ovarian cancer.

A conjugate of anti-mesothelin antibody with the cytotoxic drug monomethyl aurastatin-e has also been developed.[61] This agent has shown significant anti-tumor activity in mouse model studies of mesothelioma, pancreatic cancer, and ovarian cancer. The data are especially promising because the reagent has also shown inhibition of tumor growth in a patient-derived tumor model. A Phase I trial of this drug is currently underway.

Anti-EpCAM Antibodies

EpCAM functions in homotypic epithelial cell adhesion and in cell signaling, proliferation, and migration. EpCAM is a 39-42 kDa glycoprotein comprising a large extracellular domain, a single transmembrane region, and a short cytoplasmic tail.[62] Originally identified as a highly expressed antigen on colon cancers, it is also expressed in ovarian cancers. Uniquely among candidate biomarkers, EpCAM is highly expressed across all subtypes of ovarian carcinoma.[63] It is significantly overexpressed in primary, metastatic, and recurrent epithelial ovarian carcinoma, compared with non-cancerous ovarian epithelium,[64] and its overexpression correlates with reduced patient survival.[65] In contrast with its expression on epithelial-derived cells, EpCAM is not expressed on cells of mesothelial origin, such as those that line the peritoneal cavity; this differential expression pattern makes EpCAM a tumor-specific marker in the peritoneum that may be fruitfully targeted by functional antibodies.

Catumaxomab is a bispecific, trifunctional antibody that through two different Fab regions simultaneously binds EpCAM (present on tumor cells) and CD3 (expressed on T cells). Through an Fc region composed of two different isotypes (mouse IgG2a and rat IgG2b), it also binds the human FcRγI and FcRγIII receptors on accessory cells such as macrophages, dendritic cells, and NK cells.[66] The effect of this trifunctionality is to recruit different immune cell types to the tumor cell and then activate those immune cells, forming a multicellular complex that facilitates T-cell mediated lysis and antibody-dependent cell-mediated cytotoxicity of the tumor cell.

Clinical trials of catumaxomab have demonstrated success in the management of malignant ascites in patients with ovarian and other cancers. In an initial prospective study,[66] eight patients with peritoneal carcinomatosis were given intraperitoneal application of the trifunctional antibody. Treatment eliminated ascites accumulation, with a mean paracentesis-free interval of 38 weeks and the elimination of tumor cells, with no severe adverse side effects. A subsequent Phase I/II multicenter study involved 23 women with recurrent ascites resulting from advanced, refractory ovarian cancer.[67] As in the prospective study, intraperitoneal application of the trifunctional antibody (now called catumaxomab) significantly reduced ascites flow rate. Twenty-two of 23 enrolled patients did not require paracentesis from the last infusion through the end of the study. A prospective Phase II/III trial randomized 258 cancer patients to paracentesis plus catumaxomab (treatment) or paracentesis alone (control); patients were also stratified by cancer type, 129 ovarian and 129 non-ovarian.[68] The primary end point was puncture-free survival.

Treatment significantly increased puncture-free survival (median 46 days vs. median 11 days for the control group), and the treatment group also displayed fewer

TABLE 6.2 MAJOR ANTIGENS OF OVARIAN
TUMORS TARGETED BY IMMUNOTHERAPY

Antigen	Molecular Characteristic	Site of Expression in Cancer Cell
NY-ESO1	18 kDa protein/ cancer-testis antigen	Intracellular
p53	53 kDa protein	Intracellular
EGFR	180 kDa glycoprotein	Transmembrane
Her2	185 kDa protein	Transmembrane
Mesothelin	40 kDa glycoprotein	GPI-anchored cell surface
MUC16	3-5 million Da mucin	Transmembrane and shed from cell surface

NOTE: EGFR = epidermal growth factor receptor.

signs and symptoms of ascites. Although it was not the primary end point for the study, overall survival also showed a positive trend in the treatment group (71 days vs. 44 days). The conclusion of the study was that catumaxomab shows clear clinical benefit for patients with malignant ascites, with tolerable side effects.

Solitomab is a recently reported bispecific antibody that, like catumaxomab, binds both EpCAM and CD3. In a study of chemotherapy-refractive cell lines in vitro and fresh tumor cells ex vivo, incubation with solitomab heightened the sensitivity of tumor cells to T-cell toxicity and reduced the number of viable ovarian tumor cells present in ascites.[69] No clinical trial data have yet been reported for solitomab (Table 6.2).

GROUP 2: THERAPEUTIC ANTIBODIES

Whereas antibodies in the first group directly target antigens on the surface of cancer cells, those in the second group enhance T-cell mediated recognition of tumors. T-cell activity is tightly regulated via an interplay of activating and inhibitory receptors, allowing regulation of activated T cells and avoiding damage of normal self tissues. Activation of T cells occurs upon recognition of aberrant peptides presented on the major histocompatibility complex (MHC) antigens of antigen presenting cells. The T cell receptor engagement with the MHC-peptide complex results in activation of the T-cell response. Maintenance of this activated response requires co-stimulation by several receptor systems such as CD28, OX40, CD137, and others. The co-stimulatory receptors interact with their respective ligands on the antigen-presenting cells to produce a strong T-cell response. The inhibitory receptors, on the other hand, provide a critical role in attenuating the T-cell responses. Cytotoxic T-lymphocyte antigen-4 (CTLA-4; CD152) and programmed cell death protein-1 (PD1; CD279) are examples of prominent inhibitory receptors expressed on T cells. CTLA-4 and CD28 both bind to CD80 and CD86, which are expressed on the antigen-presenting cells and cancer cells. This is one way cancer cells can evade the immune system. By recognizing the same ligands, CTLA-4 competes with CD28 and thereby attenuates T cell co-stimulation.

While CTLA-4 attenuates T cell activation, PD1 upon binding to its ligands, PDL1 and PDL2, controls the activity of T cells in peripheral tissues when there is an inflammatory response and thereby prevents autoimmunity. Both CTLA-4 and PD1, because of their regulatory roles, are known as immune checkpoint receptors. Binding of CTLA-4 and PD1 to their ligands triggers activation of intracellular phosphatases (SHP2, PP2A, for example) that decrease the activation of kinases involved in the mediation of stimulatory and co-stimulatory T-cell responses. By expressing PDL1 and PDL2, tumor cells are able to inhibit T-cell responses via PD1.

The inhibitory roles of CTLA-4 and PD1 led to the knowledge that these checkpoint inhibitory mechanisms interfere with the development of robust T cell-mediated immunity against a variety of tumors. Efforts have therefore been made to develop strategies that will limit or eliminate the inhibitory activities of CTLA-4 and PD-1. The most successful strategies have been the development of monoclonal antibodies that bind to these two inhibitory molecules or their ligands to neutralize checkpoint blockade of the T cell-mediated anti-cancer response. Here we discuss the data obtained from clinical trials of anti-CTLA-4 and anti-PD1 antibodies.

Ipilimumab is an anti-CTLA-4 humanized monoclonal antibody that has been approved by the Food and Drug Administration (FDA) for treatment of melanoma. Data from preclinical studies suggest that ipilimumab may also be effective against ovarian tumors. In one clinical trial two patients with ovarian cancer were recruited along with melanoma patients.[70] For one ovarian cancer patient, administration of ipilimumab led to decreased levels of CA125. In the second patient, CA125 levels stabilized. Data from both patients suggested that ipilimumab treatment resulted in control of ovarian tumor progression. Ipilimumab is currently being tested in a Phase II clinical trial for safety and efficacy in patients with residual disease after completion of multiple rounds of chemotherapy. Results of this trial are awaited. In a Phase I/II trial involving 11 patients with stage IV ovarian cancer pretreated with chemotherapy, ipilimumab was well tolerated, and significant anti-tumor effects were observed in patients who had a dramatic fall in CA125 due to the treatment of mesenteric lymph nodes or hepatic metastasis.[71]

Preclinical studies with anti-PD1 antibodies have shown promising results against ovarian cancer. In one clinical trial testing safety and efficacy of anti-PDL1 antibodies, of the 17 ovarian cancer patients recruited to the study, 3 patients had stable disease for 24 weeks.[72] Additional clinical trials are needed to further prove therapeutic efficiency of these checkpoint blockade antibodies for treatment of ovarian cancer. Data from a recent anti-PD1 therapy trial is encouraging, however. Nivolumab is a fully IgG4 monoclonal antibody that targets PD-1 receptor. In a Phase II study involving 20 patients with platinum-resistant and advanced ovarian cancer, two doses of nivolumab (1 and 3 mg/kg; 10 patients per treatment group) were administered intravenously every two weeks for up to one year.[73] The patients were assessed every eight weeks and patients with disease progression were taken off the study. The response rate was low in the low dose (1 mg/kg) cohort; two patients showed partial response (10% response) and two showed stable disease. In the 3mg/kg dose cohort, two patients experienced a complete response. The 3mg/kg dose had better efficacy without increased toxicity. In conclusion, the results from this trial are encouraging, with nivolumab showing some efficacy and manageable toxicity.

GROUP 3: THERAPEUTIC ANTIBODIES

While the therapeutic antibodies classified in Groups 1 and 2 are targeted against cell surface proteins expressed either on the surface of immune cells or ovarian tumors, a third class of biologic reagents have been developed against secreted factors known to play tumor-promoting roles. The secreted factors targeted increase tumor angiogenesis or are cytokines and chemokines that induce intratumoral infiltration of regulatory immune cells (T_{regs}, for example).

Bevacizumab (Avastin), an Anti-VEGF Antibody

The concept of treating cancer by preventing angiogenesis (the growth of new vasculature) within solid tumors was originally proposed by Judah Folkman in 1972.[74] Vascular endothelial growth factor (VEGF) promotes angiogenesis. By binding to tyrosine kinase receptors, VEGF causes proliferation and migration of endothelial cells and the formation of new blood vessels; it serves this role in normal processes—such as wound healing and the female reproductive cycle—and in tumor growth.[75] VEGF is recognized by bevacizumab (Avastin), a humanized mouse monoclonal antibody developed by Genentech. Bevacizumab has been approved by the FDA for several metastatic cancers, including colorectal, lung, kidney, cervix, and ovarian (approval for breast cancer was granted in 2008 and revoked in 2011).

An initial Phase II study evaluating the safety and efficacy of bevacizumab in patients with platinum-resistant ovarian cancer showed single-agent activity, with a median PFS of 4.4 months. The study was terminated early, however, because of a higher incidence of gastrointestinal (GI) perforation (11.4%) compared to other cancer types.[76] The results of four major randomized control trials for bevacizumab have been since published, two (Gynecologic Oncology Group [GOG 218] and International Collaboration on Ovarian Neoplasms [ICON7]) using bevacizumab as a first-line therapeutic and the others (Ovarian Cancer Study Comparing Efficacy and Safety of Chemotherapy and Anti-Angiogenic Therapy in Platinum-Sensitive Recurrent Disease [OCEANS] and Avastin Use in Platinum-Resistant Epithelial Ovarian Cancer [AURELIA]) using it in second-line therapy. The results of these clinical trials have recently been reviewed[77,78] and are summarized briefly here.

A GOG study reported in 2007 assessed the efficacy and tolerability of single-agent bevacizumab in patients with recurrent epithelial ovarian cancer. Twenty-one percent of enrolled patients showed clinical response to an intravenous treatment administered every 21 days. Median PFS was 4.7 months; median overall survival was 17 months. Adverse effects were considered tolerable, and the authors concluded that Phase III investigation of bevacizumab was merited.[79] In a double-blind, placebo-controlled, Phase III trial, women with newly diagnosed epithelial ovarian cancer (stage III or IV) who had undergone surgical debulking were assigned to one of three experimental treatments. All treatment groups received paclitaxel and carboplatin in 22 treatment cycles. The control

group also received placebo in all treatment cycles. One test group ("bevacizumab-initiation") received bevacizumab in treatment cycles 2 through 6 with placebo replacing bevacizumab in cycles 7 through 22; the other test group ("bevacizumab-throughout") received bevacizumab in treatment cycles 2 through 22.

PFS was the primary end point of the study. The shortest PFS was observed in the control group (10.3 months), followed by the bevacizumab-initiation group (11.2 months) and then the bevacizumab-throughout group (14.1). The authors concluded that the use of bevacizumab with carboplatin and paclitaxel prolonged median PFS by about four months. No significant differences in overall survival were reported at the time of the study's publication.[80] The ICON7 reported the results of an 11-nation Phase III trial in 2011.[81] In this study, women with ovarian cancer were randomly assigned to either a standard therapy regimen (carboplatin plus paciltaxel) or to the standard regimen plus bevacizumab. PFS for all patients was 22.4 months in the standard therapy group and 24.1 months in the group that received bevacizumab; in patients at high risk for progression, the PFS benefit conferred by bevacizumab was greater (14.5 months for standard therapy and 18.1 months with added bevacizumab). In 2015 the overall survival results of ICON7 were reported.[82] The authors found no overall improvement in survival with the addition of bevacizumab. They reported, however, that in a high-risk subset of study participants—those with inoperable or suboptimally debulked stage III or stage IV disease—an overall survival benefit was observed (34.5 months on chemotherapy alone vs. 39.0 months with added bevacizumab). These conclusions have been met with skepticism from others in the field[83] to which the authors have responded.[84]

The OCEANS was a randomized, double-blind Phase III trial comparing chemotherapy with and without addition of bevacizumab.[85] Patients in this study had platinum-sensitive recurrent ovarian, primary peritoneal, or fallopian tube cancer and were randomly assigned to either gemcitabine and carboplatin (GC) treatment with placebo or to GC treatment with bevacizumab. Median PFS (the study's primary end point) was 8.4 months in the GC group and 12.5 months in the GC with bevacizumab group. The final survival and safety data from the OCEANS study was reported in 2015[86] and showed no significant difference in overall survival in the two treatment groups.

AURELIA was a randomized Phase III trial evaluating the combination of bevacizumab with chemotherapy in platinum-resistant ovarian cancer.[87] Patients were randomly assigned to single-agent chemotherapy alone or combined with bevacizumab. Median PFS with chemotherapy alone was 3.4 months versus 6.7 months with the addition of bevacizumab; this improvement was significant. Improvement in overall survival was not observed, though the permission of cross-over during the study complicates the interpretation of survival data. The study also tracked GI perforation and found its occurrence in only 2.2% of patients treated with bevacizumab.

Siltuximab, an Anti-IL-6 Antibody

Tumor necrosis factor- α (TNF-α), CXCL12, and IL-6 constitute a cytokine network that is overexpressed by ovarian tumors. Several lines of evidence show that these cytokines produce chronic effects that promote tumor angiogenesis and increased infiltration of regulatory immune cells in the tumor microenvironment. Inhibition of TNF-α production is clearly linked with a decrease in tumor growth because of attenuation of angiogenesis. IL-6 is also implicated in tumor-associated thrombocytosis. Tumor-derived IL-6 stimulates the release of thrombopoietin from the liver.

Thrombopoietin is a hormone that increases platelet biogenesis from megakaryocytes. The platelets formed as a result have been conclusively shown to promote angiogenesis of ovarian and other tumors. This data supports the development of an IL-6 blocking antibody as a therapeutic for the treatment of ovarian and other IL-6-producing tumors. Siltuximab is an antibody targeting IL-6. This antibody forms a complex with circulating IL-6, preventing the cytokine from mediating its pro-tumor effects.

In a Phase II clinical trial, 18 women with ovarian cancer were administered siltuximab.[88] One patient showed partial response as defined by the RECIST/CA125 criteria and decreased uptake of [^{18}F]-Fluorodeoxy glucose by PET/CT imaging, indicating decreased tumor load. In three other patients there was a significant decrease in CA125 levels, and in one patient serum CA125 concentration doubling time decreased. In a more recent dose escalation Phase I trial of siltuximab, 84 patients (35 colorectal, 29 ovarian, 9 pancreatic, and 11 other) were recruited. Data from ovarian cancer patients in this trial showed no major improvement in objective responses. The authors of the study suggest that the lack of response indicated that siltuximab therapy may have limited clinical benefit in patients with advanced stage solid tumors, which unfortunately constitutes the majority of the patients with Type II ovarian cancer (Table 6.3).

Antibody-Drug Conjugates

The high antigen specificity of antibodies is being used not only to drive immune responses against tumors as described previously but also to deliver cytotoxic drugs to cancer cells. In this case, chemotherapeutic drugs are chemically attached to a tumor-targeting antibody. Upon attachment of the antibody-drug conjugate to its intended receptor, the cancer cell internalizes the antigen-antibody complex. The complex then traffics through acidic lysosomal compartments where typically the chemotherapeutic drug detaches from the antibody to produce its cytotoxic effect. Antibody-drug conjugates therefore rely more on the tumor-targeting potential of the antibodies rather than their

Immunotherapeutic Antibody	Reference	Major Findings from Clinical Trial
Group 1		
Anti-MUC16 (Oregovomab)	32	There was no benefit in overall survival of the patients in the treatment cohort.
Anti-MUC16 (Abgovomab)	36	No improvement in overall survival of patients receiving Abagovomab was observed in Phase II.
Anti-folate receptor (Farletuzumab)	51 and 52	No significant increase in progression-free survival of patients in the Farletuzumab arm of the study was observed in Phase III.
Anti-mesothelin (Amatuximab)	58	In a Phase I trial, therapy was well tolerated with an observed dose-dependent increase in circulating levels of therapeutic antibody. Some patients in this study had stable disease at the end of the trial. There are no reports of a Phase II trial in ovarian cancer patients.
Anti-EpCAM (Catumaxomab)	68	Phase II and III showed the treatment significantly increased progression-free survival; patients displayed fewer signs and symptoms of ascites. Overall, catumaxomab shows clear clinical benefit for patients with malignant ascites, with tolerable side effects.
Group 2		
Anti-CTLA4 (Ipilimumab)	70 and 71	In Phase I/II, decrease or stabilized the level of CA125. In a Phase I/II trial involving 11 patients with stage IV ovarian cancer pretreated with chemotherapy, Ipilimumab was well tolerated, and significant antitumor effects were observed in patients who had a dramatic fall in CA125 due to the treatment of mesenteric lymph nodes or hepatic metastasis.
Group 3		
Anti-VEGF (Bevacizumab)	80	Phase III trial showed that bevacizumab with carboplatin and paclitaxel prolonged median progression-free survival by about four months.
Anti-IL-6 antibody (Siltuximab)	88	In a Phase II trial, the lack of response indicated that Siltuximab therapy may have limited clinical benefit in patients with advanced stage solid tumors, which constitutes the majority of the patients with Type II ovarian cancer.

ability to elicit an immune response against the cancer. A caveat is that although the chemotherapeutic drug is likely the major driver of the therapeutic effect, potential contribution of an immune response (via ADCC or CDC and a subsequent adaptive response) should not be completely discounted. The combination of chemotoxic effects and potential for development of an immune response against the tumor is a desirable feature of the antibody-drug conjugates. An advantage of these drugs is decreased toxicity because the chemotherapy is more likely to be selectively internalized by cancer cells than normal tissues, provided the antibody targets a molecule that is either exclusively expressed or overexpressed by tumors versus healthy tissues. An important example of antibody-drug conjugate developed for treatment of ovarian cancer is described next.

MUC16-Targeting Antibodies Coupled to Cytotoxic Drugs

In a study published in 2007, researchers at Genetech developed antibody-drug conjugates based on Mabs with affinity for different binding sites on MUC16: one (11D10) recognized a non-repeating epitope and the other (3A5) recognized an epitope in the repeat domain, thereby binding multiple independent sites on each MUC16 molecule.[89] The antibody-drug conjugate formed from 3A5 exhibited superior cellular toxicity in vitro and in tumor xenograft models. Circulating CA125 levels did not alter overall toxicity of the antibody-drug conjugate, and in a primate model, the 3A5 drug conjugate was well tolerated at levels exceeding the therapeutic dose. This promising preliminary study prompted efforts to improve the conjugation chemistry, through the introduction of cysteine substitutions to serve as drug conjugation sites.[90] A Phase I clinical trial (NCT01335958) was conducted to assess safety, pharmacokinetics, and pharmacodynamic activity of DMUC5754A, an antibody-drug conjugate containing a humanized MUC16 antibody and the cytotoxic drug MMAE; promising preliminary results from this study were reported at the 2013 meeting of the American Association of Cancer Research, with tolerable side effects

and evidence of toxicity to MUC16 expressing cells.[91] Another clinical trial (NCT02146313) will evaluate the safety and pharmacokinetics of another another antibody-drug conjugate (DMUC4064A) in patients with platinum-resistant ovarian cancer.

Immunocytokines: Antibody-Cytokine Conjugates

Another strategy to enhance the therapeutic potential of antibodies is their conjugation to cytokines. The resulting chimeric molecules display cytokines on both chains of a therapeutic antibody. The cytokines are typically attached to the heavy chain of the antibody, although novel constructs with the antibody attached to the light chain of the antibody have also been developed and are being tested in preclinical and clinical settings (Figure 6.6).[92-94] IL-2 and IL-12 are examples of cytokines that are commonly conjugated to the therapeutic antibody.

Immunocytokines provide an opportunity to locally deliver immune activating cytokines to the tumor surface through the targeting enabled by the antibody. The immunocytokines promote killing of cancer cells via ADCC. At the same time the cytokines locally activate infiltrating immune cells and thereby amplify the immune response against the cancer.

Hu14.18-IL2 is an immunocytokine that has been studied in a Phase I clinical trial in ovarian cancer patients.[95,96] This chimeric

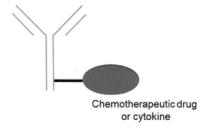

Chemotherapeutic drug or cytokine

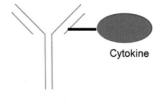

Cytokine

Figure 6.6 Chemotherapeutic drug or immune activating cytokine conjugated tumor-targeting antibodies. Antibodies conjugated to chemotherapeutic drugs deliver cytotoxic agents to cancer cells. Cytokine-conjugated therapeutic antibodies are also known as immunocytokines. In immunocytokines the cytokines may be linked to the Fc domain or the light chain of the targeting antibody.

molecule is composed of humanized 14.18 antibody that recognizes EpCAM. The IL-2 molecules are attached to each of the two heavy chains of 14.18 antibody. An initial Phase I trial of hu14.18-IL2 showed that this immunocytokine is well tolerated. A subsequent trial of this therapeutic reagent has not been conducted.

An important point to consider is that immunocytokines facilitate the formation of immune synapses between tumor cells and NK cells.[97,98] These immune synapses are unique because they not only result from the engagement of Fc receptors on the NK cells but also result in polarization of the IL-2 receptor of the NK cells to the site of contact between tumor and immune cells. The contribution of polarized IL-2 receptor at the immunocytokine-mediated synapse is not clear. However, it has been found that even in NK cell lines lacking Fc receptors, polarization of IL-2 receptor at the synapse is associated with increased killing of EpCAM- expressing targets by the hu14.18-IL2 immunocytokine.

COMBINING CHEMOTHERAPY WITH ANTIBODY-BASED IMMUNOTHERAPY

There is increasing evidence that treatment of tumors with chemotherapeutic agents can result in increased infiltration of immune cells in the tumor microenvironment.[99] In addition to T cells, macrophages and NK cells are recruited to the tumor microenvironment following treatment with platinum and taxol-based drugs and with doxorubicin and other agents. Efforts are now underway to utilize immune infiltration to therapeutic advantage by appropriately administering anti-tumor antibodies that will result in further increasing immunologic recognition and lysis of the tumors. Attempts have already been made to combine chemotherapy with Oregovomab.[37] Although data on such a combinatorial approach to therapy has not matured at this time, such a therapeutic

approach carries significant potential and will be studied exhaustively in future trials. The cancer death caused by chemotherapeutic drugs results in exposure and recognition of a wide array of tumor antigens by the immune system, thus the immune system is already being primed by the cancer cell apoptosis and necrosis caused by chemotherapy. An additional boost to the immune response with an appropriate combination of antibodies is therefore expected to produce a complementary therapeutic effect. A challenge with this approach, however, will be the deleterious effect of the chemotherapeutic drugs on the immune cells. It will be important to administer therapeutic antibodies when the level of chemotherapeutic drugs in peripheral circulation and within the tumor can be tolerated by the immune system. Alternatively, targeted delivery of chemotherapeutic agents (either through development of agents selectively taken up by tumors or by encapsulation of drugs in tumor-targeting nanoparticles) will also help reduce adverse effects on the immune cells. The coming decade is likely to see major advances in such approaches. The hope is that these new strategies will lead to the development of effective strategies against ovarian cancer when the majority of the existing experimental approaches have shown only limited benefit in curing this fatal cancer.

REFERENCES

1. Siegel R, Ma J, Zou Z, Jemal A. Cancer statistics, 2014. *CA Cancer J Clin*. 2014;64(1):9–29.
2. Nik NN, Vang R, Shih Ie M, Kurman RJ. Origin and pathogenesis of pelvic (ovarian, tubal, and primary peritoneal) serous carcinoma. *Annu Rev Pathol*. 2014;9:27–45.
3. Kurman RJ, Shih Ie M. Molecular pathogenesis and extraovarian origin of epithelial ovarian cancer—shifting the paradigm. *Hum Pathol*. 2011;42(7):918–31.
4. Anglesio MS, Bashashati A, Wang YK, et al. Multifocal endometriotic lesions associated with cancer are clonal and carry a high mutation burden. *J Pathol*. 2015;236(2):201–9.
5. Zhang L, Conejo-Garcia JR, Katsaros D, et al. Intratumoral T cells, recurrence, and

survival in epithelial ovarian cancer. *N Engl J Med.* 2003;348(3):203–13.

6. Curiel TJ, Coukos G, Zou L, et al. Specific recruitment of regulatory T cells in ovarian carcinoma fosters immune privilege and predicts reduced survival. *Nat Med.* 2004;10(9):942–49.

7. Sato E, Olson SH, Ahn J, et al. Intraepithelial CD8+ tumor-infiltrating lymphocytes and a high CD8+/regulatory T cell ratio are associated with favorable prognosis in ovarian cancer. *Proc Natl Acad Sci U S A.* 2005;102(51):18538–43.

8. Odunsi K, Qian F, Matsuzaki J, et al. Vaccination with an NY-ESO-1 peptide of HLA class I/II specificities induces integrated humoral and T cell responses in ovarian cancer. *Proc Natl Acad Sci U S A.* 2007;104(31):12837–42.

9. Barber A, Zhang T, DeMars LR, Conejo-Garcia J, Roby KF, Sentman CL. Chimeric NKG2D receptor-bearing T cells as immunotherapy for ovarian cancer. *Cancer Res.* 2007;67(10):5003–8.

10. Kohler G, Milstein C. Continuous cultures of fused cells secreting antibody of predefined specificity. *Nature.* 1975;256(5517):495–97.

11. Felder M, Kapur A, Gonzalez-Bosquet J, et al. MUC16 (CA125): tumor biomarker to cancer therapy, a work in progress. *Mol Cancer.* 2014;13(1):129.

12. O'Brien TJ, Beard JB, Underwood LJ, Dennis RA, Santin AD, York L. The CA 125 gene: an extracellular superstructure dominated by repeat sequences. *Tumour Biol.* 2001;22(6):348–66.

13. O'Brien TJ, Beard JB, Underwood LJ, Shigemasa K. The CA 125 gene: a newly discovered extension of the glycosylated N- terminal domain doubles the size of this extracellular superstructure. *Tumour Biol.* 2002;23(3):154–69.

14. Yin BW, Lloyd KO. Molecular cloning of the CA125 ovarian cancer antigen. identification as a new mucin, MUC16. *J Biol Chem.* 2001;276(29):27371–75.

15. Das S, Majhi PD, Al-Mugotir MH, Rachagani S, Sorgen P, Batra SK. Membrane proximal ectodomain cleavage of MUC16 occurs in the acidifying Golgi/post-Golgi compartments. *Sci Rep.* 2015;5:9759.

16. Das S, Rachagani S, Torres-Gonzalez MP, et al. Carboxyl-terminal domain of MUC16 imparts tumorigenic and metastatic functions through nuclear translocation of JAK2 to pancreatic cancer cells. *Oncotarget.* 2015;6(8):5772–87.

17. Lakshmanan I, Ponnusamy MP, Das S, et al. MUC16 induced rapid G2/M transition via interactions with JAK2 for increased proliferation and anti-apoptosis in breast cancer cells. *Oncogene.* 2012;31(1):805–17.

18. Gubbels JA, Belisle J, Onda M, et al. Mesothelin-MUC16 binding is a high affinity, N- glycan dependent interaction that facilitates peritoneal metastasis of ovarian tumors. *Mol Cancer.* 2006;5(1):50.

19. Rump A, Morikawa Y, Tanaka M, et al. Binding of ovarian cancer antigen CA125/MUC16 to mesothelin mediates cell adhesion. *J Biol Chem.* 2004;279(10):9190–98.

20. Gubbels JA, Felder M, Horibata S, et al. MUC16 provides immune protection by inhibiting synapse formation between NK and ovarian tumor cells. *Mol Cancer.* 2010;9:11.

21. Belisle JA, Horibata S, Gubbels JA, et al. Identification of Siglec-9 as the receptor for MUC16 on human NK cells, B cells, and monocytes. *Mol Cancer.* 2010;9(1):118.

22. Madiyalakan R, Yang R, Schultes BC, Baum RP, Noujaim AA. OVAREX MAb-B43.13:IFN-gamma could improve the ovarian tumor cell sensitivity to CA125-specific allogenic cytotoxic T cells. *Hybridoma.* 1997;16(1):41–45.

23. Reinsberg J, Krebs D. Are human anti-idiotypic anti-OC125 antibodies formed after immunization with the anti-CA125 antibody B43.13? *Hybridoma.* 1997;16(1):59–63.

24. Wagner U, Schlebusch H, Kohler S, Schmolling J, Grunn U, Krebs D. Immunological responses to the tumor-associated antigen CA125 in patients with advanced ovarian cancer induced by the murine monoclonal anti-idiotype vaccine ACA125. *Hybridoma.* 1997;16(1):33–40.

25. Ma J, Samuel J, Kwon GS, Noujaim AA, Madiyalakan R. Induction of anti-idiotypic humoral and cellular immune responses by a murine monoclonal antibody recognizing the ovarian carcinoma antigen CA125 encapsulated in biodegradable microspheres. *Cancer Immunol Immunother.* 1998;47(1):13–20.

26. Schultes BC, Baum RP, Niesen A, Noujaim AA, Madiyalakan R. Anti-idiotype induction therapy: anti-CA125 antibodies (Ab3) mediated tumor killing in patients treated with Ovarex mAb B43.13 (Ab1). *Cancer Immunol Immunother.* 1998;46(4):201–12.

27. Schultes BC, Zhang C, Xue LY, Noujaim AA, Madiyalakan R. Immunotherapy of human ovarian carcinoma with OvaRex MAb-B43.13 in a human-PBL-SCID/BG mouse model. *Hybridoma.* 1999;18(1):47–55.

28. Noujaim AA, Schultes BC, Baum RP, Madiyalakan R. Induction of CA125-specific B and T cell responses in patients injected with MAb-B43.13—evidence for antibody-mediated antigen- processing and presentation of CA125 in vivo. *Cancer Biother Radiopharm.* 2001;16(3):187–203.

29. Gordon AN, Schultes BC, Gallion H, et al. CA125- and tumor-specific T-cell responses correlate with prolonged survival in oregovomab-treated recurrent ovarian cancer patients. *Gynecol Oncol.* 2004;94(2):340–51.

30. Berek JS. Immunotherapy of ovarian cancer with antibodies: a focus on oregovomab. *Expert Opin Biol Ther.* 2004;4(7):1159–65.

31. Berek JS, Taylor PT, Gordon A, et al. Randomized, placebo-controlled study of oregovomab for consolidation of clinical remission in patients with advanced ovarian cancer. *J Clin Oncol.* 2004;22(17):3507–16.

32. Berek J, Taylor P, McGuire W, Smith LM, Schultes B, Nicodemus CF. Oregovomab maintenance monoimmunotherapy does not improve outcomes in advanced ovarian cancer. *J Clin Oncol.* 2009;27(3):418–25.

33. Reinartz S, Boerner H, Koehler S, Von Ruecker A, Schlebusch H, Wagner U. Evaluation of immunological responses in patients with ovarian cancer treated with the anti-idiotype vaccine ACA125 by determination of intracellular cytokines—a preliminary report. *Hybridoma.* 1999;18(1):41–45.

34. Reinartz S, Wagner U, Giffels P, Gruenn U, Schlebusch H, Wallwiener D. Immunological properties of a single-chain fragment of the anti-idiotypic antibody ACA125. *Cancer Immunol Immunother.* 2000;49(4–5):186–92.

35. Wagner U, Kohler S, Reinartz S, et al. Immunological consolidation of ovarian carcinoma recurrences with monoclonal anti-idiotype antibody ACA125: immune responses and survival in palliative treatment. *Clin Cancer Res.* 2001;7(5):1154–62.

36. Reinartz S, Kohler S, Schlebusch H, et al. Vaccination of patients with advanced ovarian carcinoma with the anti-idiotype ACA125: immunological response and survival (phase Ib/II). *Clin Cancer Res.* 2004;10(5):1580–87.

37. Braly P, Nicodemus CF, Chu C, et al. The immune adjuvant properties of front-line carboplatin-paclitaxel: a randomized phase 2 study of alternative schedules of intravenous oregovomab chemoimmunotherapy in advanced ovarian cancer. *J Immunother.* 2009;32(1):54–65.

38. Assaraf YG, Leamon CP, Reddy JA. The folate receptor as a rational therapeutic target for personalized cancer treatment. *Drug Resist Update.* 2014;17(4-6):89–95.

39. Weitman SD, Lark RH, Coney LR, et al. Distribution of the folate receptor GP38 in normal and malignant cell lines and tissues. *Cancer Res.* 1992;52(12):3396–401.

40. Brown Jones M, Neuper C, Clayton A, et al. Rationale for folate receptor alpha targeted therapy in "high risk" endometrial carcinomas. *Int J Cancer.* 2008;123(7):1699–703.

41. Hartmann LC, Keeney GL, Lingle WL, et al. Folate receptor overexpression is associated with poor outcome in breast cancer. *Int J Cancer.* 2007;121(5):938–42.

42. Parker N, Turk MJ, Westrick E, Lewis JD, Low PS, Leamon CP. Folate receptor expression in carcinomas and normal tissues determined by a quantitative radioligand binding assay. *Anal Biochem.* 2005;338(2):284–93.

43. Kalli KR, Oberg AL, Keeney GL, et al. Folate receptor alpha as a tumor target in epithelial ovarian cancer. *Gynecol Oncol.* 2008;108(3):619–26.

44. Reddy JA, Dorton R, Bloomfield A, et al. Rational combination therapy of vintafolide (EC145) with commonly used chemotherapeutic drugs. *Clin Cancer Res.* 2014;20(8):2104–14.

45. Leamon CP, Vlahov IR, Reddy JA, et al. Folate-vinca alkaloid conjugates for cancer therapy: a structure-activity relationship. *Bioconjug Chem.* 2014;25(3):560–68.

46. Reddy JA, Dorton R, Westrick E, et al. Preclinical evaluation of EC145, a folate-vinca alkaloid conjugate. *Cancer Res.* 2007;67(9):4434–42.

47. Leamon CP, Reddy JA, Vlahov IR, et al. Comparative preclinical activity of the folate- targeted Vinca alkaloid conjugates EC140 and EC145. *Int J Cancer.* 2007;121(7):1585–92.

48. Leamon CP, Reddy JA, Vlahov IR, Kleindl PJ, Vetzel M, Westrick E. Synthesis and biological evaluation of EC140: a novel folate-targeted vinca alkaloid conjugate. *Bioconjug Chem.* 2006;17(5):1226–32.

49. Leamon CP, Reddy JA, Vlahov IR, et al. Synthesis and biological evaluation of EC72: a new folate-targeted chemotherapeutic. *Bioconjug Chem.* 2005;16(4):803–11.

50. Naumann RW, Coleman RL, Burger RA, et al. PRECEDENT: a randomized phase II trial comparing vintafolide (EC145) and pegylated liposomal doxorubicin (PLD) in combination versus PLD alone in patients with platinum-resistant ovarian cancer. *J Clin Oncol.* 2013;31(35):4400–406.

51. Kalli KR. MORAb-003, a fully humanized monoclonal antibody against the folate receptor alpha, for the potential treatment of epithelial ovarian cancer. *Curr Opin Invest Drugs.* 2007;8(12):1067–73.

52. Armstrong DK, White AJ, Weil SC, Phillips M, Coleman RL. Farletuzumab (a monoclonal antibody against folate receptor alpha) in relapsed platinum-sensitive ovarian cancer. *Gynecol Oncol.* 2013;129(3):452–58.

53. Chang K, Pastan I. Molecular cloning of mesothelin, a differentiation antigen present on mesothelium, mesotheliomas, and ovarian cancers. *Proc Natl Acad Sci U S A.* 1996;93(1):136–40.

54. Hassan R, Bera T, Pastan I. Mesothelin: a new target for immunotherapy. *Clin Cancer Res.* 2004;10(12 Pt 1):3937–42.

55. Gubbels JA, Belisle J, Onda M, et al. Mesothelin-MUC16 binding is a high affinity, N- glycan dependent interaction that facilitates peritoneal metastasis of ovarian tumors. *Mol Cancer.* 2006;5(1):50.

56. Rump A, Morikawa Y, Tanaka M, et al. Binding of ovarian cancer antigen CA125/MUC16 to mesothelin mediates cell adhesion. *J Biol Chem.* 2004;279(10):9190–98.

57. Scholler N, Garvik B, Hayden-Ledbetter M, Kline T, Urban N. Development of a CA125- mesothelin cell adhesion assay as a screening tool for biologics discovery. *Cancer Lett.* 2006;247(1):130–36.

58. Hassan R, Cohen SJ, Phillips M, et al. Phase I clinical trial of the chimeric anti-mesothelin monoclonal antibody MORAb-009 in patients with mesothelin-expressing cancers. *Clin Cancer Res.* 2010;16(24):6132–38.

59. Hassan R, Sharon E, Thomas A, et al. Phase 1 study of the antimesothelin immunotoxin SS1P in combination with pemetrexed and cisplatin for

front-line therapy of pleural mesothelioma and correlation of tumor response with serum mesothelin, megakaryocyte potentiating factor, and cancer antigen 125. *Cancer.* 2014;120(21):3311–19.

60. Kim H, Gao W, Ho M. Novel immunocytokine IL12-SS1 (Fv) inhibits mesothelioma tumor growth in nude mice. *PLoS One.* 2013;8(11):e81919.

61. Scales SJ, Gupta N, Pacheco G, et al. An antimesothelin-monomethyl auristatin e conjugate with potent antitumor activity in ovarian, pancreatic, and mesothelioma models. *Mol Cancer Ther.* 2014;13(11):2630–40.

62. Patriarca C, Macchi RM, Marschner AK, Mellstedt H. Epithelial cell adhesion molecule expression (CD326) in cancer: a short review. *Cancer Treat Rev.* 2012;38:68–75.

63. Köbel M, Kalloger, SE, Boyd N, et al. Ovarian carcinoma subtypes are different diseases: implications for biomarker studies. *PLoS Med.* 2008;5:e232.

64. Bellone S, Siegel ER, Cocco E, et al. Overexpression of epithelial cell adhesion molecule in primary, metastatic, and recurrent/chemotherapy-resistant epithelial ovarian cancer: implications for epithelial cell adhesion molecule-specific immunotherapy. *Int J Gynecol Cancer.* 2009;19(5):860–66.

65. Spizzo G, Went P, Dirnhofer S, et al. Overexpression of epithelial cell adhesion molecule (Ep-CAM) is an independent prognostic marker for reduced survival of patients with epithelial ovarian cancer. *Gynecol Oncol.* 2006;103(2):483–88.

66. Heiss MM, Ströhlein MA, Jäger M, et al. Immunotherapy of malignant ascites with trifunctional antibodies. *Int J Cancer.* 2005;117(3):435–43.

67. Burges A, Wimberger P, Kümper C, et al. Effective relief of malignant ascites in patients with advanced ovarian cancer by a trifunctional anti-EpCAM ´ anti-CD3 antibody: a phase I/II study. *Clin Cancer Res.* 2007;13(13):3899–905.

68. Heiss MM, Murawa P, Koralewski P, et al. The trifunctional antibody catumaxomab for the treatment of malignant ascites due to epithelial cancer: results of a prospective randomized phase II/III trial. *Int J Cancer.* 2010;127(9):2209–21.

69. English DP, Bellone S, Schwab CL, et al. Solitomab, an epithelial cell adhesion molecule/CD3 bispecific antibody (BiTE), is highly active against primary chemotherapy-resistant ovarian cancer cell lines in vitro and fresh tumor cells ex vivo. *Cancer.* 2015;121(3):403–12.

70. Hodi FS, Mihm MC, Soiffer RJ, et al. Biologic activity of cytotoxic T lymphocyte-associated antigen 4 antibody blockade in previously vaccinated metastatic melanoma and ovarian carcinoma patients. *Proc Natl Acad Sci U S A.* 2003;100(8):4712–17.

71. Tse BW, Collins A, Oehler MK, Zippelius A, Heinzelmann-Schwarz VA. Antibody-based immunotherapy for ovarian cancer: where are we at? *Ann Oncol.* 2014;25(2):322–31.

72. Brahmer JR, Tykodi SS, Chow LQ, et al. Safety and activity of anti-PD-L1 antibody in patients with advanced cancer. *N Engl J Med.* 2012;366(26):2455–65.

73. Hamanishi J, Mandai M, Ikeda T, et al. Safety and antitumor activity of anti-PD-1 antibody, nivolumab, in patients with platinum-resistant ovarian cancer. *J Clin Oncol.* 2015;33(34):4015–22.

74. Folkman J. Anti-angiogenesis: new concept for therapy of solid tumors. *Ann Surg.* 1972;175(3):409–16.

75. Hoeben A, Landuyt B, Highley MS, Wildiers H, Van Oosterom AT, De Bruijn EA. Vascular endothelial growth factor and angiogenesis. *Pharmacol Rev.* 2004;56(4):549–80.

76. Cannistra SA, Matulonis UA, Penson RT, et al. Phase II study of bevacizumab in patients with platinum-resistant ovarian cancer or peritoneal serous cancer. *J Clin Oncol.* 2007;25(33):5180–86.

77. Shu CA, Konner JA. Breaking down the evidence for bevacizumab in ovarian cancer. *Oncologist.* 2015;20(2):91–93.

78. Li J, Zhou L, Chen X, Ba Y. Addition of bevacizumab to chemotherapy in patients with ovarian cancer: a systematic review and meta-analysis of randomized trials. *Clin Transl Oncol.* 2015;17(9):673–83.

79. Burger RA, Sill MW, Monk BJ, Greer BE, Sorosky JI. Phase II trial of bevacizumab in persistent or recurrent epithelial ovarian cancer or primary peritoneal cancer: a gynecologic oncology group study. *J Clin Oncol.* 2007;25(33):5165–71.

80. Burger RA, Brady MF, Bookman MA, et al. Incorporation of bevacizumab in the primary treatment of ovarian cancer. *N Engl J Med.* 2011;365:2473–83.

81. Perren TJ, Swart AM, Pfisterer J, et al. A phase 3 trial of bevacizumab in ovarian. *N Engl J Med.* 2011;365:2484–96.

82. Oza AM, Cook AD, Pfisterer J, et al. Standard chemotherapy with or without bevacizumab for women with newly diagnosed ovarian cancer (ICON7): overall survival results of a phase 3 randomised trial. *Lancet Oncol.* 2015;16(8):928–36.

83. Gyawali B, Shimokata T, Ando Y. Discordance between the results and conclusions of ICON7. *Lancet Oncol.* 2015;16: e478.

84. Oza AM, Cook AD, Kaplan R, Parmar MKB, Perren TJ. Authors' reply. *Lancet Oncol.* 2015; 16:e478.

85. Aghajanian C, Blank SV, Goff BA, et al. OCEANS: a randomized, double-blind, placebo- controlled phase III trial of chemotherapy with or without bevacizumab in patients with platinum-sensitive recurrent epithelial ovarian, primary peritoneal, or fallopian tube cancer. *J Clin Oncol.* 2012;30(17):2039–45.

86. Aghajanian C, Goff B, Nycum LR et al. Final overall survival and safety analysis of OCEANS, a phase 3 trial of chemotherapy with or without bevacizumab in patients with platinum-sensitive recurrent ovarian cancer. *Gynecol Oncol.* 2015;139(1):10–16.

87. Pujade-Lauraine E, Hilpert F, Weber B, et al. Bevacizumab combined with chemotherapy for platinum-resistant recurrent ovarian cancer: the

AURELIA open-label randomized phase III trial. *J Clin Oncol.* 2014;32(13):1302–11.

88. Coward J, Kulbe H, Chakravarty P, et al. Interleukin-6 as a therapeutic target in human ovarian cancer. *Clin Cancer Res.* 2011;17(18):6083–96.

89. Chen Y, Clark S, Wong T, et al. Armed antibodies targeting the mucin repeats of the ovarian cancer antigen, MUC16, are highly efficacious in animal tumor models. *Cancer Res.* 2007;67(10):4924–32.

90. Junutula JR, Raab H, Clark S, et al. Site-specific conjugation of a cytotoxic drug to an antibody improves the therapeutic index. *Nat Biotechnol.* 2008;26(8):925–32.

91. Liu J, Moore K, Birrer M, et al. Targeting MUC16 with the antibody-drug conjugate (ADC) DMUC5754A in patients with platinum-resistant ovarian cancer: a phase I study of safety and pharmacokinetics. *Cancer Research.* 2013;73(8, Suppl. 1).

92. Yang RK, Kalogriopoulos NA, Rakhmilevich AL, et al. Intratumoral hu14.18-IL-2 (IC) induces local and systemic antitumor effects that involve both activated T and NK cells as well as enhanced IC retention. *J Immunol.* 2012;189(5):2656–64.

93. Lode HN, Xiang R, Becker JC, Gillies SD, Reisfeld RA. Immunocytokines: a promising approach to cancer immunotherapy. *Pharmacol Ther.* 1998;80(3):277–92.

94. Reisfeld RA, Becker JC, Gillies SD. Immunocytokines: a new approach to immunotherapy of melanoma. *Melanoma Res.* 1997;7(Suppl 2):S99–106.

95. Connor JP, Felder M, Hank J, et al. Ex vivo evaluation of anti-EpCAM immunocytokine huKS-IL2 in ovarian cancer. *J Immunother.* 2004;27(3):211–19.

96. Connor JP, Cristea MC, Lewis NL, et al. A phase 1b study of humanized KS-interleukin-2 (huKS-IL2) immunocytokine with cyclophosphamide in patients with EpCAM-positive advanced solid tumors. *BMC Cancer.* 2013;13:20.

97. Gubbels JA, Gadbaw B, Buhtoiarov IN, et al. Ab-IL2 fusion proteins mediate NK cell immune synapse formation by polarizing CD25 to the target cell-effector cell interface. *Cancer Immunol Immunother.* 2011;60(12):1789–800.

98. Buhtoiarov IN, Neal ZC, Gan J, et al. Differential internalization of hu14.18-IL2 immunocytokine by NK and tumor cell: impact on conjugation, cytotoxicity, and targeting. *J Leukoc Biol.* 2011;89(4):625–38.

99. Galluzzi L, Buque A, Kepp O, Zitvogel L, Kroemer G. Immunological effects of conventional chemotherapy and targeted anticancer agents. *Cancer Cell.* 2015;28(6):690–714.

7.

EPITOPE/PEPTIDE-BASED MONOCLONAL ANTIBODIES FOR IMMUNOTHERAPY OF OVARIAN CANCER

Gregory Lee

INTRODUCTION

According to recent cancer statistics in 2015, the annual occurrence of ovarian cancer can be as many as 240,000 in women worldwide. This cancer can result in the annual death of more than 150,000.[1-4] Therefore, ovarian cancer has become the seventh most common cancer and the eighth most common cause of death from cancer among women, especially in North America and Europe.[4,5] One of the most common characteristics for this type of cancer is the absence of signs and symptoms during the early stages of disease occurrence. In spite of extensive research during the last several decades, no effective treatments including immunotherapy and chemotherapy are available for ovarian cancer. However, antibody-based target-oriented anti-cancer drugs have been proven to be successful in immunotherapy of many other types of cancer[1,6,7] such as that of lung and breast.[6-8]

Newly discovered pan cancer biomarker-based monoclonal antibodies might be final alternatives for the immunotherapy of ovarian cancer. These monoclonal antibodies may be specific to epitopes or peptides of the commonly found cancer-associated antigens which are abundantly or overexpressed on the surface of ovarian cancer as well as many other types of cancer.[9,10] They can be subsequently developed into effective antibody-based drugs targeting ovarian cancer cells as well as others.[9,10]

Recently, two such monoclonal antibodies have been generated and selected for effectively targeting cancer of multi-tissue origins,[9,10] including that of the ovary.[9,10] During the early stages of these two anti-cancer drugs development, about a decade ago, the ovarian cancer cell line was selected as a model for such investigations with encouraging progress.[11] They may be developed eventually as effective anti-cancer drugs following required systematic preclinical and clinical studies.

RP215 is a monoclonal antibody out of a total of 3,000 generated against OC-3-VGH ovarian cancer cell line in 1987.[11] Following MALDI-TOF MS analysis of the purified antigen, CA215, and loss of epitope activity upon the periodate treatment, it was clearly established that RP215 reacts with a carbohydrate-associated epitope located in the variable region of mainly immunoglobulin heavy chains expressed by most of cancer cells.[11,12] This antibody and its humanized form were shown in an ovarian cancer study model to inhibit the growth/proliferation of cancer cells in vitro or in vivo.[13-15] The molecular mechanisms of action have been elucidated regarding the targeting of ovarian cancer by RP215 and are summarized in this chapter.

GHR106 is a peptide-based monoclonal antibody which was generated against a N1-29 amino acid residues corresponding to the oligopeptide in the extracellular domains of the human GnRH receptor highly expressed on the surface of many cancer types including that of the ovary. Furthermore, for ovarian cancer, the incidence of positive staining for the surface-expressed GnRH receptor can range from 70% to 100% during extensive immunohistochemical studies to be described later.[16-20] By using OC-3-VGH ovarian cancer cell line on the study model, the mechanisms of action of GHR106 in targeting ovarian cancer have been elucidated. Surface expressions of GnRH receptor in cancer cells have been generally considered critical for the growth/proliferation of cancer cells in vitro and in vivo. GHR106 has been shown to serve as the long-acting bioequivalent analog of GnRH decapeptide analogs which have a relatively short half-life in circulation (minutes/hours vs. 15–20 days for antibodies).[17-20] The results of such comprehensive studies are summarized in this review to highlight the possibility of using peptide-based GHR106 in humanized forms in targeting ovarian cancer, as well as several others. It may become an alternative and effective immunotherapeutic application in the future for the treatment of ovarian and other types of cancer.

Due to the pan cancer nature of the target antigens of these two monoclonal antibodies, they are highly expressed by almost all types of cancer cells including that of ovary. However, the data presented in this review was derived from a well-established ovarian cancer cell line, OC-3-VGH (established in 1985 by Department OBS/GYN VGH, Taipei, Taiwan). This ovarian cancer cell line was used as a study model to elucidate the molecular mechanisms of action of these two unique epitope/peptide-based antibodies

for immunotherapy of ovarian cancer in the future.

MECHANISMS OF ACTION OF RP215 IN TARGETING OVARIAN CANCER

IMMUNOHISTOCHEMICAL STUDIES AND TISSUE SPECIFICITY

As mentioned, RP215 was one of 3,000 monoclonal antibodies generated and selected against the OC-3-VGH ovarian cancer cell line. Immunohistochemical studies were performed with cancerous tissue sections from ovarian cancer patients.[10,12] The positive staining rate can be as high as 64% (n = 87).[12] Other types of cancer with epithelial origins such as esophagus (76%, n = 56), lung (31%, n = 58), breast (32%, n = 59), stomach (50%, n = 93), colon (44%, n = 87), and cervix (84%, n = 51) were also found to be expressed at high levels among cancerous tissues.[11,12] Immunohistochemical studies were also performed with sections of more than 20 different tissues from normal individuals. It was generally observed that the cross-reactivity of RP215 with normal tissues was limited to those of hyperplastic epithelial cells such as skin (epidermis), cervix, and esophagus but not in any others.[10,12]

ELUCIDATION OF EPITOPE STRUCTURE RECOGNIZED BY RP215

The epitope structure of RP215 was investigated with affinity-purified CA215 which is recognized specifically by RP215. Due to the fact that RP215-specific epitope is sensitive to mild periodate treatment, it was generally believed that RP215-specific epitope in CA215 is carbohydrate-associated. Through analysis by MALDI-TOF MS, it was generally concluded that the majority of RP215-specific "sugar" epitope is localized on the heavy chains of immunoglobulins expressed by cancer cells.[10-12] CA215 also consists of other types of glycoproteins, generally classified as immunoglobulin superfamily proteins (IgSF) including T-cell receptors,[15,21] as well as other unrelated ones such as mucin.[21,22]

To elucidate the basic glycan structure recognized by RP215, glycopeptide mapping and glycolinkage analysis were performed. In view of the fact that RP215-binding activity is not affected upon treatments with tunicamycin (N-linked glycan biosynthesis inhibitor),[15,21] it was judged that O-linked glycan may be involved in the formation of RP215-epitope. Furthermore, RP215 binding to CA215 is not affected by competitive binding with anti-human IgG (Fc) but strongly inhibited by anti-Fab. This led us to conclude that RP215-specific carbohydrate-associated epitope should be located in the Fab, or variable region of immunoglobulin heavy chains. Following extensive glycoanalysis, primary Core I-linked trisaccharide structure was deduced as part of RP215-specific epitope. It was further assumed that amino acid residues might also be involved in the epitope formation for RP215.

TARGETING OVARIAN CANCER CELL WITH RP215

In vitro Evaluations with OC-3-VGH Ovarian Cancer Cell

Through immunohistochemical studies, and RP215-specific epitope structural analysis, it was generally concluded that RP215 recognize the carbohydrate-associated epitope localized in the variable regions of immunoglobulin heavy chains expressed by cancer cells in general.[11,14] In fact, immunoglobulins expressed by cancer cells have been known for decades, although little is known regarding their molecular basis of expressions. Early studies with immunoglobulin gene-related SiRNA seem to suggest that cancerous immunoglobulins may be essential for the growth/proliferation of cancer cells.[23,24] Therefore, during

the last decade, RP215 has been used as a unique probe to replace anti-human IgG to study the mechanisms of action of cancerous immunoglobulins for the growth/proliferation of cancer cells. Induced apoptosis by TUNEL assay was employed to study the detrimental effect on cancer cells in vitro/in vivo. Both RP215 and anti-human IgG were found to induce apoptosis to cultured OC-3-VGH ovarian cancer cells and strongly influenced the growth/proliferation of cancer cells.[12,14]

RP215 of murine origin (mRP215) was modified into humanized form (hRP215). Both mRP215 and hRP215[16] were found to be bioequivalent functionally in inducing apoptosis to cultured ovarian cancer cells. Results of TUNEL apoptosis assay with treatments of mRP215, hRP215, and anti-human IgG on cultured cancer cells are presented in Figure 7.1A. In view of the binding of RP215 to surface immunoglobulins expressed by cultured ovarian cancer cells, complement-dependent cytotoxicity (CDC) reactions were induced to result in lysis of cancer cells in culture. mRP215 and hRP215 were found to be bioequivalent in inducing CDC reactions to cultured cancer cells. Results of comparative CDC studies are summarized in Figure 7.1B with OC-3-VGH ovarian cancer cells as the model.

Tumor Growth Inhibition by RP215 by Nude Mouse Experiments

Nude mouse experiments were performed for "proof of concept" in anti-cancer efficacy of RP215 in vivo. The results of these studies revealed that RP215 significantly inhibits tumor growth or reduces the volume of implanted tumor (OC-3-VGH ovarian cancer cells) in a dose-dependent manner with nude mouse animal models.[10,12] Typical results with implanted OC-3-VGH ovarian cancer cells are presented in Figure 7.2.

In addition, nude mouse experiments with low, medium, and high concentrations

A

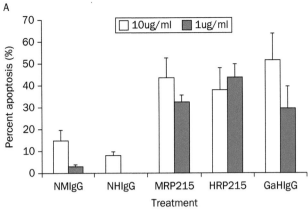

B

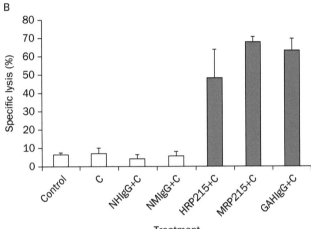

Figure 7.1 (A) Percent induced apoptosis of cultured OC-3-VGH ovarian cancer cells following 24 hours incubation with various antibodies by TUNEL assay. Antibodies were added separately for 24 hours incubation and include 10 μg/mL and 1 μg/mL of normal mouse IgG (NMIgG), normal human IgG (NHIgG), murine RP215 (mRP215), respectively. Cancer cell lines tested include DU-145 (prostate), A549 (lung), C33A (cervix), and OC-3-VGH (ovary). (B) Complement-dependent cytotoxicity assay to demonstrate complement-dependent lysis of OC-3-VGH ovarian cancer cells with different treatments in the presence or absence of complement. C represents complement. Negative controls include no treatment (control), complement only (C), normal human IgG plus complement (NHIgG+C), and normal mouse IgG plus complement (NMIgG+C), respectively. Treatments which resulted in a significant percentage of lysis included humanized RP215 plus complement (HRP215+C), murine RP215 plus complement (MRP215+C), and goat anti-human IgG plus complement (GAHIgG+C), respectively. Modified from Lee G, Cheung AP, Ge B, et al. Monoclonal anti-idiotype antibodies against carbohydrate-associate epitope for anti-cancer vaccine development. *J Vaccines Vaccination.* 2010; 1(2): 1–7, and Holmberg MT, Blom AM, Mei S. Regulation of complement classical pathway by association of C4b-binding protein to the surfaces of SK-OV-3 and Caov-3 ovarian adenocarcinoma cells. *J Immunol.* 2001; 167(2): 935–39. with permission.

of I[131]-labeled RP215 were also performed with implanted OC-3-VGH ovarian cancer cells. The reduction in tumor volume with injection of I[131]-labeled RP215 is even more dramatic as compared to the negative control. The results clearly indicated that RP215 demonstrates potential as an anti-cancer drug for the immunotherapy of ovarian cancer and other human cancers as well.[10]

Comparative Effects of RP215 on Gene Regulation of Ovarian Cancer Cells

RP215 is known to react mainly with a carbohydrate-associated epitope located in the variable regions of cancer cell-expressed immunoglobulin heavy chains and other types of IgSF designated in general as CA215.[25] Therefore, RP215 should

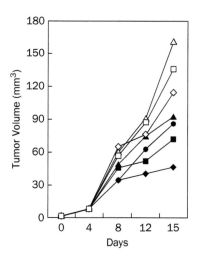

Figure 7.2 Effects of various treatments on the growth of implanted OC-3-VGH ovarian cancer cells in nude mice from day 1 to day 15. Δ, Negative control (NC); ▲, positive control (PC); ●, RP215 high dose (AH); ○, RP215 low dose (AL); ◆, I131-labeled RP215 high dose (I-AH); ■, I131-labeled RP215 medium dose (I-AM); □, I131-labeled RP215 low dose (I-AL). Reprinted from Lee G, Ge B. Inhibition of in vitro tumor cell growth by RP215 monoclonal antibody and antibodies raised against its anti-idiotype antibodies. *Cancer Immunol Immunother.* 2010; 59(9): 1347–56, Lee G. Cancerous immunoglobulins and CA215: implications in cancer immunology. *Amer J Immunol.* 2012; 8: 101–16, with permission.

examined. The results of this study are consistent with the potential roles of TLRs in carciogenesis as well as the growth/proliferation of ovarian cancer cells, and perhaps other types of cancer. TLR-3 was significantly upregulated, whereas TLR-6 and TLR-9 were downregulated. High correlations of gene expression changes of TLRs as well as the others following treatment of OC-3-VGH ovarian cancer cells with RP215 or anti-human IgG were observed, and the correlation curve is presented in Figure 7.3.

HUMANIZATION OF RP215 FOR CANCER IMMUNOTHERAPY: DEMONSTRATION OF BIOEQUIVALENCE

Since cancer cell-surface expressed immunoglobulins are essential for the growth/proliferation of cancer cells, epitope-based RP215 can be used to specifically target cancerous immunoglobulins and cancer cells as well. Therefore, RP215 in humanized forms can serve as a suitable candidate for anti-cancer drug development and immunotherapeutic applications.[16] Through CRO service by LakePharma Inc., the humanized versions of RP215 were constructed and demonstrated to have affinity and specificity to CA215, comparable or equivalent to the original murine RP215. The resulting humanized (hRP215) and murine (mRP215) were found to have very similar or identical CDR regions. Certain amino acid substitutions would be required in the FR domains of hRP215 to avoid undesirable immunogenicity arising from the inherited structure of mRP215.[16]

Substantial bioequivalence between hRP215 and mRP215 can be demonstrated by sandwich or binding assay with either form of RP215 as the capturing or detecting antibody for the quantitation of CA215. Both mRP215 and hRP215 were shown to have comparable affinity constants (4.2 nM vs. 4.4 nM) to CA215. Neither was shown to cross-react with normal human IgG. Based on the available biochemical and

functionally act like antibodies against antigen receptors including cancer cell-expressed immunoglobulins and T-cell receptors on the surface.[25] Through detailed gene regulation analysis, it was generally observed that genes related to the growth/proliferation of cancer cells are affected similarly upon treatment of cultured ovarian cancer cells with either RP215 or anti-antigen receptors (anti-immunoglobulins). Through gene regulation studies by using a semi-quantitative RT-PCR method, similar gene level changes with high correlations by these ligands were observed. Among the genes studied, upregulation of genes including NFαB1, IgG, TCR, p21, and ribosomal proteins P1 and downregulations of other genes such as cyclin D1 and c-fos were observed. Consistently, changes in gene expression levels of toll-like receptors (TLR) following treatments with RP215 or antibodies against IgG or TCR were also

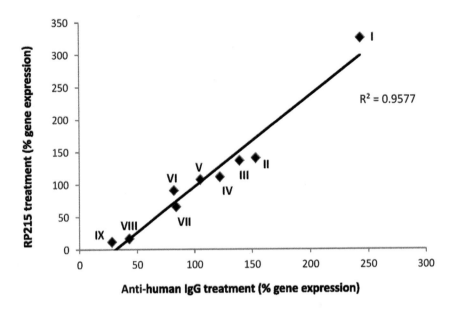

Figure 7.3 Correlation analysis of the changes in gene expression levels of selected genes involved in cellular growth/ proliferation and the innate immune response following separate treatments of RP215 and anti-human IgG of the OC-3-VGH ovarian cancer cell line. The data represent the relative gene expression levels of TLR-3 (I), NFκB-1 (II), P21 (III), P1 (IV), IgG (V), c-fos (VI), cyclin D1 (VII), TLR-9 (VIII), and TLR-4 (IX) in the OC-3-VGH ovarian cancer cells following separate treatments with RP215 and anti-human IgG and have been plotted for correlation analysis. The correlation coefficient between these two antibody ligands was determined to be $R^2 = 0.9577$. Reprinted from Holmberg MT, Blom AM, Mei S. Regulation of complement classical pathway by association of C4b-binding protein to the surfaces of SK-OV-3 and Caov-3 ovarian adenocarcinoma cells. *J Immunol.* 2001; 167(2): 935–39, with permission.

immunological criteria, both mRP215 and hRP215 are bioequivalent. Furthermore, hRP215 and mRP215 were judged to be bioequivalent in inducing apoptosis (by TUNEL assay) to cultured OC-3-VGH ovarian cancer cells, even at a concentration of as low as 1 µg/mL. Therefore, the bioequivalent hRP215 can be utilized for the development of anti-cancer drugs in the subsequent preclinical and clinical studies.[16]

IMMUNODIAGNOSTIC APPLICATIONS OF RP215 FOR MONITORING OF OVARIAN CANCER AND OTHERS

Since RP215 reacts specifically with a carbohydrate-associated epitope in CA215, which is widely expressed in almost all cancer cells of many tissue origins including that of

the ovary,[26] RP215-based sandwich enzyme immunoassay may have potential applications in the monitoring of patients with ovarian cancer, similar to those of CA215. RP215 was used simultaneously as the detection and capturing antibodies in a sandwich enzyme immunoassay for monitoring serum levels of CA215 in patients with ovarian cancer.[26,27] Serum levels of CA215 (in Au/ mL) from normal individuals and from patients with different stages of ovarian carcinoma are shown in Table 7.1. Serum levels of CA215 were also found to correlate with clinical treatments. For example, significantly decreased serum CA215 levels were detected following seven days after surgical removal of the cancer or treatment with radiation or chemotherapy.[26,27] Therefore, our results strongly support the use of CA215 as a suitable pan cancer biomarker for the monitoring of early

TABLE 7.1 **SERUM LEVELS OF CA215 (IN AU/ML) FROM NORMAL INDIVIDUALS AND FROM PATIENTS WITH DIFFERENT STAGES OF OVARIAN OR CERVICAL CARCINOMA**

	Normal Control	Ovarian Carcinoma[a]			Cervical Carcinoma[b]		
		Stage 1	Stage 2	Stage 3	Stage 1	Stage 2	Stage 3
Number of cases (n)	59	24	7	40	35	18	7
Mean (Au/mL)	5.47	36.2	60.2	55.0	48.0	78.6	75.7
Standard deviation	10.37	27.2	27.0	44.7	44.7	61.8	83.9

[a] For normal control vs. any of the stages 1, 2, or 3 of ovarian carcinoma, $P < 0.001$. For stage 1 vs. stage 2 and 3 ovarian carcinoma, $P < 0.05$. For stage 2 vs. stage 3 ovarian carcinoma, $P > 0.05$.

[b] For normal control vs. any of the stages 1, 2, or 3 of cervical carcinoma, $P < 0.001$. For stage 1 vs. stage 2 and 3 cervical carcinoma, $P < 0.01$. For stage 2 vs. stage 3 cervical carcinoma, $P > 0.05$.

Reprinted from Lee G. Cancer cell-expressed immunoglobulins: CA215 as a pan cancer marker and its diagnostic applications. *Cancer Biomark.* 2009; 5(3): 137–42 with permission.

stages of ovarian cancer or other types of cancers as well.

DUAL ROLES OF RP215-RECOGNIZED CANCEROUS IMMUNOGLOBULINS IN CANCER CELLS IN HUMAN CIRCULATION

Through years of in vitro/in vivo studies, it has been shown that cancerous immunoglobulins play crucial roles in the growth/proliferation of cancer cells.[23] Results from recent studies also suggested that cancerous immunoglobulins are capable of binding both pro-cancer and anti-cancer serum proteins or components within human circulation. Therefore, it can be hypothesized that cancerous immunoglobulins play dual roles in cancer cells by serving to preserve the growth/proliferation of cancer cells while at the same time by neutralizing harmful human serum proteins components to cancer cells within the human circulation. Based on our recent biochemical analysis, the anti-cancer and pro-cancer human serum proteins components have been identified.[28–30] Based on this assumption, RP215 can be used to target cancerous immunoglobulins on the cancer cell surface by blocking its functional activities which can result in induction of apoptosis of cancer cells in vitro or in vivo. Therefore, RP215 in humanized form can be a suitable candidate for anti-cancer drug developments.

Human Serum Protein Components Interacting with CA215 and/or Cancerous Immunoglobulins and Exhibiting Pro-Cancer and Pro-Cancer Activities

Judging from experimental evidence, human serum protein components revealed binding interactions with either cancerous immunoglobulins or RP215-specific CA215 derived from cancer cells. Attempts were made to elucidate the potential mechanisms of action regarding the functional roles of these cancerous CA215 or immunoglobulins by analyzing the molecular nature of the isolated protein components in pool human serum specimens. Approximately 72% of the 50 serum protein components/fragments were found to be commonly detected with LC-MS/MS analysis[28–30] by either ligands. More than half were found to be associated with pro- or anti-cancer activities which were previously reported by others. Notably, the commonly recognized anti-cancer components by these two sets of cancerous ligands including 35 kDa inter-α-trypsin inhibition heavy chain 4, anastellin, apolipoprotein A1, fibrinogen β chain, and keratin type 1 cytoskeletal 9.[31-36] On the other hand, some pro-cancer serum components which were detected by the same methodology exhibit known pro-cancer properties to promote growth/proliferation of cancer cells. Among these are C4b-binding protein, complement C3, complement factor H, serotranferrin, and vitronectin.[37-42]

In summary, we believe that cancerous immunoglobulins and/or CA215 expressed by cancer cells serve play two important but opposite functional roles by interacting with certain human serum proteins either with anti-cancer or pro-cancer properties in the human circulation.

IMMUNODOMINANT RP215-SPECIFIC EPITOPE AND ANTI-IDIOTYPIC ANTI-CANCER VACCINE

Immunodominance of RP215-Specific Epitope

The carbohydrate-associated epitope(s) recognized by RP215 was shown to be immunodominant in mice. When mice were immunized with affinity-purified CA215 derived from the shed medium of OC-3-VGH ovarian cancer cells, the monoclonal antibodies generated were shown to react with the same carbohydrate-associated epitope recognized by RP215.[43] Judging from comparisons of the primary structure of these antibodies, three distinct groups were classified. Group I shows identical amino acid sequences as those of RP215. Groups II and III were found to correspond to the linear and conformational structures, respectively, of the same and unique carbohydrate-associated epitope. All the new antibodies were shown to induce apoptosis to OC-3-VGH ovarian cancer cells even at a concentration of as low as 1 μg/mL. The immunodominance of this carbohydrate-associated epitope remains to be elucidated.

Anti-Idiotypic Monoclonal Antibodies as Anti-Cancer Vaccine

Since RP215 recognized a specific carbohydrate-associated epitope of CA215, monoclonal antibodies can be generated specifically against Fab idiotypes domains of RP215 in rats.[44] These anti-RP215 idiotypic antibodies were shown to carry internal image of RP215-specific epitope. Following immunization with these anti-idiotypic monoclonal antibodies in mice, the resulting anti-aid or Ab3 antibodies were found to behave like RP215 in many biochemical and immunological properties. Similar to those observed with RP215, Ab3 antisera were shown to induce apoptosis. Therefore, it was hypothesized that anti-idiotypic monoclonal antibodies or its Fab fragments bear the internal image of RP215-specific epitope.[14,44] These monoclonal antibodies may be suitable as anti-cancer vaccines to induce Ab3 responses in humans for the immunotherapy of human cancer in the future.[44]

DEMONSTRATION OF EFFECTIVE IMMUNOTHERAPY TO OVARIAN CANCER BY PRECLINICAL PROOF OF CONCEPT STUDIES

Since the initial generation of RP215, numerous biochemical, immunological, and functional studies have been performed to elucidate the mechanisms of action of RP215 in targeting cancer cells including that of the ovary.[10-12] With the OC-3-VGH cancer cell line as the study model, RP215 and its humanized form of RP215 were shown to be bioequivalent in targeting mainly immunoglobulins expressed on the surface of ovarian cancer. Therefore, apoptosis and CDC reactions can be induced in the presence of RP215. Therefore, the target antigen on the cancer cell surface, designated as CA215, can be a specific target for immunotherapy of ovarian cancer cells. Furthermore, in vivo, nude mouse experimental models with implanted OC-3-VGH ovarian tumor resulted in a significant reduction of tumor volume upon dose-dependent treatment of RP215. Further experiments with bioequivalent hRP215 are required to provide proof of concept for the efficacy of immunotherapy to ovarian cancer.[10-12]

MECHANISMS OF ACTION OF GHR106 TARGETING OVARIAN CANCER

BINDING SPECIFICITY/AFFINITY AND IMMUNOHISTOCHEMICAL STUDIES

Demonstration of Binding Specificity and Affinity of GHR106 or Humanized GHR106 to Human GnRH Receptor and Its Bioequivalence to GnRH Peptide Analogs

It has been known for decades that GnRH receptor in the human anterior pituitary serves to stimulate the release of gonadotropin, LH, and FSH upon its specific binding to GnRH decepeptide (both type I and II).[45] Subsequent studies revealed that GnRH and its receptor also play extra-pituitary roles on normal and malignant cells or tissues,[46-48] the mechanisms of which are still being actively explored. Anti-proliferation effects of GnRH or its peptide analogs on cancer cells of different human tissue origins have been reported and have been the basis of cancer therapy.[20] However, the half-lives of GnRH peptide analogs are relatively short, ranging from minutes to hours. As an alternative, monoclonal antibodies were generated against a synthetic oligopeptide corresponding to N1-29 amino acid residues of the extracellular domains of human GnRH receptor.[17,18] Among these antibodies, GHR106 was shown to have affinity and specificity similar to those of GnRH or GnRH peptide analogs. By using microwells coated with OC-3-VGH ovarian cancer cells or with N1-29 synthetic peptide, the affinity constants (expressed in Kd) were determined. Kds of GnRH peptide analogs and GHR106 were found to be in the range

of 1 to 5 nM. Following humanization of GHR106, humanized GHR106 (hGHR106) were found to have comparable affinity to the GnRH receptor with that of GHR106 of murine origin. Furthermore, in view of the sequence homology of N1-29 synthetic peptides between human GnRH receptor and monkey GnRH receptor, GHR106, or hGHR106, were found to have a high degree of cross-reactivity with those of human and monkey but not with that of mouse origin.[19,49]

Immunohistochemical Studies of Normal and Cancerous Tissues for Expression of GnRH Receptor

The normal expression of GnRH receptor is limited to the human pituitary and a few tissues of gonadal origins such as testis and ovary. However, it is widely expressed in cancerous tissues of many origins, especially in ovary, pancreas, and liver[20] based on results of immunohistochemical analysis and RT-PCR. The positive high expression levels in different cancerous tissues can be as high as 50% to 100%.[20] Similar studies were also performed with more than 20 cancer cell lines of different tissue origins. Positive cell stainings as well as Western blot assay were observed with few exceptions, when using GHR106 as the probe.[17,18]

BIOEQUIVALENT FUNCTIONAL ROLES BETWEEN GHR106 AND GNRH ANTAGONIST, ANTIDE

Assessment by Induced Apoptosis

Previous studies revealed that GnRH analogs such as Antide was shown to induce apoptosis of cultured cancer cells upon incubation. Therefore, TUNEL assay was employed as a tool to compare the relative apoptosis-inducing efficacy of different GnRH peptide analogs and murine GHR106 (mGHR106), as well as hGHR106. Following 48 hours of inoculation with OC-3-VGH ovarian cancer cells in the presence of GnRH peptide analogs, Antide (0.1 µg/mL), mGHR106 (2, 4 and 10 µg/mL), and hGHR106 (10 µg/mL), a 40% to 65% increase in apoptosis of treated cancer cells was found (Figure 7.4) as compared to that of the negative control by using normal mouse IgG of the same concentration. The induction of apoptosis is not limited to OC-3-VGH ovarian cancer cells. PC-3 (prostate), A549 (lung), and MDA-MV-415 (breast) were also affected upon similar treatment with either Antide or mGHR106. When mGHR106 and hGHR106 were compared for efficacy in inducing apoptosis, they were found to be equally effective in inducing apoptosis to different cultured cancer cells, as demonstrated in the histograms shown in Figure 7.4B.

Lysis of Cancer Cells by Complement-Dependent Cytotoxicity Reactions

It was commonly known that specific binding interactions between the GnRH receptor on the surface of OC-3-VGH ovarian cancer cells and anti-GnRH receptor monoclonal antibodies such as mGHR106 and hGHR106 can result in the cell lysis in the presence of a complement. Therefore, both mGHR106 and hGHR106 at 10 µg/mL were demonstrated to induce CDC to OC-3-VGH ovarian cancer cells to a similar and significant extent. Results are summarized in Figure 7.4C. By comparison, when normal mouse IgG or normal human IgG were used as the negative control, little effect on complement-dependent lysis was observed. Furthermore, no CDC reactions were induced when the GnRH decapeptide analog, such as Antide, was used instead for incubation under the same assay conditions as those of GHR106 antibody.[17,19]

SIMILAR EFFECTS ON GENE REGULATION TO CULTURED OVARIAN CANCER CELL

Significant changes in gene regulations of cultured OC-3-VGH ovarian cancer cells were observed upon treatment with either GnRH peptide analog, Antide, or GHR106. A number of genes involved in growth/proliferation were analyzed for changes and assessed by semi-quantitative RT-PCR method. Among these are GnRH, GnRH receptor, $P_0/P_1/P_2$ (cell cycle regulation), L37 (protein synthesis), epidermal growth factor, c-fos (oncogene) as well as P21/Cyclin D1 (cell cycle regulation). GnRH peptide analog, Antide, and mGHR106 revealed identical gene regulation patterns upon their respective incubation with OC-3-VGH cultured cancer cells. This observation seems to suggest that both GnRH peptide analog Antide and the monoclonal antibody GHR106 have identical or very similar mechanisms of action to the cultured cancer cells. The results of such semi-quantitative studies with OC-3-VGH ovarian cancer cells are summarized in Table 7.2 for comparison.

DEMONSTRATION OF BIOEQUIVALENCE BETWEEN MGHR106 AND HGHR106

Through CRO service from LakePharma Inc. (Belmont, CA), mGHR106 was humanized by altering the amino acid sequences on the Fab regions of both heavy and light chains for mGHR106. With the use of special software programs for humanization, the affinity and specificity of GHR106 to human GnRH receptor were preserved. The overall substitution homolog in amino acid sequence can only be 80% and 85% between mGHR106 and hGHR106 for heavy and light chains, respectively. In contrast, 100% homology is required to preserve the binding affinity and specificity of hGHR106 in the CDR domains. Therefore, the overall homology between mGHR106 and hGHR106 in Fab regions was estimated to be 93% and 89%, respectively, for heavy and light chains.

Binding immunoassays were performed with microwells-coated OC-3-VGH ovarian cancer cells. The affinity constants (Kds) for the binding between mGHR106/hGHR106 and GnRH receptor on the well-coated

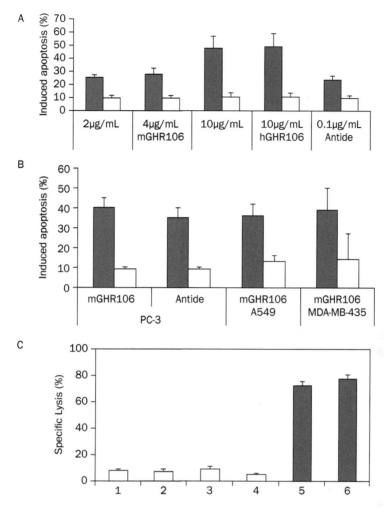

Figure 7.4 Experiments to reveal induced apoptosis and cell lysis by complement-dependent cytotoxicity reactions.

(A) Effects of GnRH decapeptide antagonist, Antide, and anti-GnRH receptor Mabs, mGHR106 and hGHR106, on induced apoptosis to OC-3-VGH ovarian cancer cells by TUNEL assay after 48 hours incubation. Data are presented in histograms and listed as followed in the x-axis: 2 µg/mL, 4 µg/mL, and 10 µg/mL mGHR106, 10 µg/mL hGHR106, and 0.1 µg/mL Antide. represents the negative control with either 10 µg/mL normal mouse IgG or 10 µg/mL human IgG for each corresponding set of experiments. (B) Effects of GnRH decapeptide antagonist, Antide, and anti-GnRH receptor Mab, mGHR106, on induced apoptosis to different cultured cancer cells by TUNEL assay after 48 hours incubation. Data are presented in histograms and listed as followed in the x-axis: mGHR106 (10 µg/mL) and Antide (0.1 µg/mL) with PC-3 prostate cancer cells; mGHR106 (10 µg/mL) with A549 lung cancer cells; mGHR106 (10 µg/mL) with MDA-MB-435 breast cancer cells. represents the negative control with either 10 µg/mL normal mouse IgG or 10 µg/mL human IgG for each corresponding set of experiments. (C) Lanes 1 to 4 represent negative controls. Lane 1: no treatment (negative control); Lane 2: 3 µL freshly prepared rabbit baby complement (negative control); Lane 3: normal human IgG (10 µg/ml plus complement) (negative control); Lane 4: normal mouse IgG (10 µg/ml) (negative control plus complement); Lane 5: hGHR106 (10 µg/ml plus complement) (2-hour incubation); Lane 6: mGHR106 (10 µg/ml plus complement) (2-hour incubation). Reprinted from [49] with permission.

TABLE 7.2 EFFECTS OF GNRH DECAPEPTIDE ANTAGONIST, ANTIDE, AND MGHR106 MAB ON THE EXPRESSION LEVEL CHANGES OF GENES INVOLVED IN CELL PROLIFERATION, PROTEIN SYNTHESIS, AND CELL CYCLE REGULATIONS OF CULTURED OC-3-VGH OVARIAN CANCER CELLS

	Relative Gene Expression Levels[a]	
Gene	mGHR106 (10 or 20µg/mL)[b]	Antide (GnRH Decapeptide Antagonist) (0.1 µg/mL)
GnRH	Up (60% ±10%)	Up (45% ± 15%)
GnRH receptor	NC	NC
P_0	Down	Down
P_1	Up	Up
P_2	NC	NC
L37	Down	Down
EGF	Down	Down
c-fos	NC	NC
P21	Up	Up
Cyclin D1	Down	Down

NOTE: EGF = epidermal growth factor; NC = no change.

[a] Following ligand incubation with cancer cells, relative expression level changes: up means increase by 20% or more (unless otherwise indicated); down means decrease by 20% or more or no change (less than 20% increase or decrease), with either 10 µg/mL or 20 µg/mL mGHR106 incubation, or 0.1 µg/mL Antide, are shown. The GAPDH gene was used as the internal reference.

[b] Changes in gene regulation do not vary significantly with either 10 or 20 µg/mL mGHR106 treatment of cancer cells.

Reprinted from Lee G, Chow SN, Chien CH, Liu S. Anti-GnRH receptor monoclonal antibodies, first-in-class GnRH analog. *J Gynecol Res.* 2015; 1(1): 102, with permission.

cancer cells were determined to be on the order of 1 to 5 nM. hGHR106 was found to inhibit the dose-dependent binding of mGHR106 to N1-29 synthetic peptide of human or monkey GnRH receptor coated on microwells but not to that of mouse GnRH receptor peptides. Based on these studies, the bioequivalence between mGHR106 and hGHR106 to human GnRH receptor were clearly demonstrated through the humanization strategy.

PROOF OF CONCEPT PRECLINICAL STUDIES TO DEMONSTRATE THE EFFICACY OF IMMUNOTHERAPY IN TARGETING HUMAN OVARIAN CANCER

Numerous biochemical and immunological studies have been performed to demonstrate bioequivalence between mGHR106 monoclonal antibodies and GnRH decapeptide analogs, Antide, in terms of binding to the GnRH receptor on the surface of OC-3-VGH ovarian cancer cells with comparable affinity and specificity and biological functions in inducing apoptosis to cultured ovarian cancer cells. However, for GHR106 or anti-GnRH receptor antibodies, CDC reactions can be functional to ovarian cancer cells in vitro and in vivo. However, this will not work with GnRH peptide analogs.[17] Furthermore, the monoclonal antibody GHR106 has a much longer half-life in circulation (5–15 days) as compared to those of GnRH peptide analogs (minutes to hours). The humanized form of GHR106 was shown to be virtually identical to murine GHR106 in terms of binding to the surface bound GnRH receptor of ovarian cancer cells as well as their ability to induce apoptosis or CDC reactions to cultured cancer cells.[10,17] Further experiments related to proof of concept of hGHR106 for effective immunotherapy of ovarian cancer would be required during preclinical studies.

CONCLUSION

In this review, two monoclonal antibody-based anti-cancer drugs candidates were reported for the immunotherapy of ovarian cancer. They are either epitope or peptide-based antibodies. RP215 was initially generated against OC-3-VGH ovarian cancer cell extract and was found to react specifically with the carbohydrate-associated epitope located mainly on the variable regions of immunoglobulin heavy chains expressed by almost all cancer cells including that of the ovary, which can be detected with relatively high incidence ($\geq$ 65%) through immunohistochemical analysis.[12] On the other hand, GHR106 was generated against a N1-29 synthetic peptide corresponding to the extracellular domains of human GnRH receptor which is expressed in high incidence (50%–100%) on the surface of almost all cancer cells including that of the ovary.[10,17] It can serve as the high molecular weight analogs of GnRH decapeptide analogs but with a much longer half-life. In the case of RP215, the target antigen CA215 was found to consist of cancerous immunoglobulins and many other minor glycoproteins such as IgSF, each of which is attached with RP215-specific "sugar" epitope. Our subsequent studies revealed that cancerous immunoglobulins on the cancer cell surface not only interact with human serum components which were shown previously to support the growth/proliferation of cancer cells but also serve to neutralize or interact with undesirable or hostile minor human serum proteins in circulation.[28-30] With RP215 as a unique probe to target ovarian cancer, it was observed that apoptosis as well as CDC reactions can be induced to inhibit the growth/proliferation of cancer cells following RP215 treatments.[14,23] Furthermore, dose-dependent volume reductions of implanted OC-3-VGH cancer cells were observed in response to injection of RP215 in a nude mouse animal model (Figure 7.2). Humanized form of RP215 (hRP215) has been successfully developed and was found to be highly bioequivalent to RP215 of murine origin, in many aspects of biochemical, immunological, biological, and functional properties.[16]

Compared to GnRH peptide analogs, GHR106 is the first-in-class monoclonal antibody which reacts specifically with the human GnRH receptor on OC-3-VGH cancer cells in a manner biosimilarly to the decapeptide GnRH analogs. However, GHR106 has a much longer half-life (days) as compared to those of GnRH peptide analogs (minutes to hours). Bioequivalence between GHR106 or its humanized form, hGHR106, and GnRH decapeptide analogs have been demonstrated through their respective binding as well as affinity/specificity to human GnRH receptor on the cancer cell surface as well as several other biochemical, immunological, and functional criteria.[16,19,20] The data presented in this review have clearly demonstrated that GHR106 can be a substitute to the GnRH decapeptide analog currently used in the clinical market.[20,46] The relatively long half-life of GHR106 may represent a major advantage in immunotherapy of human cancer including that of the ovary.[9,10] GHR106 may also be advantageous in clinical treatments of fertility regulations to replace the currently available GnRH peptide analogs.[45-48]

Lastly, the data presented in this review also suggest that mGHR106 and hGHR106 are virtually identical or bioequivalent in many biochemical, immunological, and functional studies.[16,19] Proof of concept experiments with hGHR106 may be required in the subsequent preclinical study to document the relative efficacy in the immunotherapy of ovarian cancer and possibly other types of cancer. The epitope/peptide-based monoclonal antibodies are characteristic of their targeting antigens as pan cancer biomarkers in nature. RP215 and GHR106 introduced in this review are targeting specifically CA215 and GnRH receptors, respectively, which are highly expressed in cancer cells of many tissue origins as described in this chapter.

Our initial objective is to develop antibody-based anti-cancer drugs for the immunotherapy of ovarian cancer. However, the clinical applications of these two antibody-based drug candidates should not be limited to the therapy of only one type of cancer but also others as well, provided that the target antigens are abundantly expressed on the surface of the cancer cells under consideration. Therefore, we believe that epitope/peptide-based monoclonal antibodies may be used for the immunotherapy of many different types of cancer in the future.

REFERENCES

1. World Cancer Report 2014. World Health Organization, 2014. Chapter 5.12.
2. Siegel R, Ma J, Zou Z, Jemal A. Cancer statistics 2014. *CA Cancer J Clin.* 2014; 64(1): 9–29.
3. Siegel RL, Miller KD, Jemal A. Cancer statistics 2015. *CA Cancer J Clin.* 2015; 65(1): 5–29.
4. Mørch LS, Løkkegaard E, Andreasen AH, Krüger-Kjær S, Lidegaard O. Hormone therapy and ovarian cancer. *JAMA.* 2009; 302(3): 298–305.
5. Jemal A, Murray T, Samuels A, Ghafoor A, Ward E, Thun MJ. Cancer statistics. *Cancer J Clin.* 2003; 53(1): 5–26.
6. Leffers N, Daemen T, Helfrich W, Boezen HM, Cohlen BJ, Nijman HW. Antigen-specific active immunotherapy for ovarian cancer. *Cochrane Database Sys Rev.* 2010; 9: CD007287. doi:10.1002/146518588.CD007287.pub3.
7. Cannistra SA. Cancer of the ovary. *N Eng J Med.* 2004; 351(24): 2519–29.
8. Borghaei H, Robinson MK, Adams GP, Weiner LM. Monoclonal antibodies. In: DeVita VT, Lawrence TS, Rosenberg SA, eds. *DeVita, Hellman, and Rosenberg's Cancer: Principles & Practice of Oncology.* 10th ed. Philadelphia, PA: Lippincott Williams & Wilkins; 2015.
9. Lee G, Zhu M, Ge B. Potential monoclonal antibody therapy for the treatment of ovarian cancer. In: Farghaly SA, ed. *Ovarian Cancer—Basic Science Perspective.* Vancouver, Canada: InTech; 2012: 385–406.
10. Lee G, Cheung A, Ge B, et al. CA215 and GnRH receptor as targets for cancer therapy. *Cancer Immunol Immunother.* 2012; 61(10): 1805–17.
11. Lee G, Laflamme E, Chien C-H, Ting HH. Molecular identity of a pan cancer marker, CA215. *Cancer Biol Ther.* 2008; 7(12): 2007–14.
12. Lee G, Chu R-A, Ting HH. Preclinical assessment of anti-cancer drugs by using RP215 monoclonal antibody. *Cancer Biol Ther* 2009; 8(2): 161–66.
13. Lee G. Functional roles of cancerous immunoglobulins and potential applications in cancer immunodiagnostics and immunotherapy. In: Khan WA, ed. *Innovative Immunology.* Monroe Township, NJ: Austin Publishing Group 2015; in press.
14. Lee G, Ge B. Inhibition of in vitro tumor cell growth by RP215 monoclonal antibody and antibodies raised against its anti-idiotype antibodies. *Cancer Immunol Immunother.* 2010; 59(9): 1347–56. doi:10.1007/s00262-010-0864-7.
15. Lee G. Cancerous immunoglobulins and CA215: implications in cancer immunology. *Amer J Immunol.* 2012; 8: 101–16.
16. Lee G, Huang C-Y, Ge B. Two distinct humanized monoclonal antibodies for immunotherapy of ovarian cancer. *J Cancer Sci Ther.* 2014; 6: 110–16. doi: 10.4172/1948-5956.1000258.
17. Lee G, Ge B. Growth inhibition of tumor cells in vitro by using monoclonal antibodies against gonadotropin-releasing hormone receptor. *Cancer Immunol Immunother.* 2010; 59(7): 1011–19.
18. Lee G, Ho J, Chow SN, Yasojima K, Schwab C, McGeer PL. Immunoidentification of gonadotropin releasing hormone receptor in human sperm, pituitary and cancer cells. *Am J Reprod Immunol.* 2000; 44: 170–77.
19. Lee G, Zhang H, Tang Y. Anti-GnRH receptor monoclonal antibodies as bioequivalent analogs of GnRH. In: Sills ES, editor. *Gonadotropin-Releasing Hormone (GnRH): Production, Structure and Function.* Los Angeles: Nova Biomedical; 2013; 10: 157–74.
20. Nagy A, Schally AV. Targeting of cytotoxic luteinizing hormone-releasing hormone analogs to breast, ovarian, endometrial and prostate cancers. *Biol Reprod.* 2005; 73(5): 851–59.
21. Lee G, Wu Q, Li CH, Ting HH, Chien C-H. Recent studies of a new carbohydrate-associated pan cancer marker, CA215. *J Clin Ligand Assay* 2006; 29(1): 47–51.
22. Lee G, Azadi P. Peptide mapping and glycoanalysis of cancer cell–expressed glycoproteins CA215 recognized by RP215 monoclonal antibody. *J Carbohydrate Chem.* 2012; 31(1): 10–30.
23. Qiu X, Zhu X, Zhang L, et al. Human epithelial cancers secrete immunoglobulin G. with undefined specificity to promote growth and survival of tumor cells. *Cancer Res.* 2003; 63(19): 6488–95.
24. Hu D, Zheng H, Liu H, et al. Immunoglobulin expression and its biological significance in cancer cells. *Cell Mol Immunol.* 2008; 5(5): 319–24.
25. Tang Y, Zhang H, Lee G. Similar gene regulation patterns for growth inhibition of cancer cells by RP215 or anti-antigen receptors. *J Cancer Sci Ther.* 2013; 5(6): 200–208.
26. Lee G. Cancer cell-expressed immunoglobulins: CA215 as a pan cancer marker and its diagnostic applications. *Cancer Biomark.* 2009; 5(3): 137–42.
27. Lee G, Ge B, Huang T-K, et al. Positive identification of CA215 pan cancer biomarker from serum specimens of cancer patients. *Cancer Biomark.* 2009; 6(2): 111–17.
28. Lee G, Huang C-Y, Liu S. Human serum proteins recognized by CA215 and cancerous immungobulins and implications in cancer immunology. *J Cancer Clin Oncol.* 2014; 3(2): 51–69.
29. Lee G, Huang C-Y, Liu S, Zhang H. The immunology of cancer cells. *Symbiosis Open J Immunol.* 2013; 1(1): 4–7.
30. Lee G, Huang C-Y, Liu S, Chien C-H, Chow S-N. Dual roles of cancer cell-expressed immunoglobulins in cancer immunology. *Am J Immunol.* 2014; 10(3): 156–65.
31. Hamm A, Veeck J, Bektas N, et al. Frequent expression loss of Inter-alpha-trypsin inhibitor heavy chain (ITIH) genes in multiple human solid tumors: a systematic expression analysis. *BMC Cancer.* 2008; 8(1): 25.

32. Pasqualini R, Bourdoulous S, Koivunen E, Woods VL Jr, Ruoslahti E. A polymeric form of fibronectin has antimetastatic effects against multiple tumor types. *Nat. Med.* 1996; 2(11): 1197–203.

33. Yi M, Ruoslahti E. A fibronectin fragment inhibits tumor growth, angiogenesis, and metastasis. *Proc Nat Acad Sci U S A.* 2001; 98(2): 620–24.

34. Zamanian-Daryoush M, Lindner D, Tallant TC, et al. The cardioprotective protein apolipoprotein A1 promotes potent anti-tumorigenic effects. *J Biol Chem.* 2013; 288(29): 21237–52.

35. Krajewska E, Lewis CE, Chen YY, et al. A novel fragment derived from the β chain of human fibrinogen, β43–63, is a potent inhibitor of activated endothelial cells *in vitro* and *in vivo*. *Br J Cancer.* 2010; 102(3): 594–601.

36. Yi W, Peng J, Zheng Y, et al. Differential protein expressions in breast cancer between drug sensitive tissues and drug resistant tissues. *Gland Surgery.* 2013; 2(2): 62–68.

37. Holmberg MT, Blom AM, Mei S. Regulation of complement classical pathway by association of C4b-binding protein to the surfaces of SK-OV-3 and Caov-3 ovarian adenocarcinoma cells. *J Immunol.* 2001; 167(2): 935–39.

38. Ajona D, Castano Z, Garayoa M, et al. Expression of complement factor H by lung cancer cells: effects on the activation of the alternative pathway of complement. *Cancer Res.* 2004; 64(17): 6310–18.

39. Ajona D, Hsu YF, Corrales L, Montuenga LM, Pio R. Down-regulation of human complement factor H sensitizes non-small cell lung cancer cells to complement attack and reduces *in vivo* tumor growth. *J Immunol.* 2007; 178(9): 5991–98.

40. Laskey J, Webb J, Schulman HM, Ponka P. Evidence that transferrin supports cell proliferation by supplying iron for DNA synthesis. *Exp Cell Res.* 1988; 176(1): 87–95.

41. Rossi MC, Zetter BR. Selective stimulation of prostatic carcinoma cell proliferation by transferrin. *Proc Natl Acad Sci U S A.* 1992; 89(13): 6197–201.

42. Hurt EM, Chan K, Duhagon Serrat MA, Thomas SB, Veenstra TD. Identification of vitronectin as an intrinsic inducer of cancer stem cell differentiation and tumor formation. *Cancer Cells.* 2010; 28(3): 390–98.

43. Lee G, Zhu M, Ge B, et al. Carbohydrate-associated immunodominant epitope(s) of CA215. *Immunol Invest.* 2012; 41(3): 317–36.

44. Lee G, Cheung AP, Ge B, et al. Monoclonal anti-idiotype antibodies against carbohydrate-associate epitope for anti-cancer vaccine development. *J Vaccines Vaccination.* 2010; 1(2): 1–7.

45. Yang-Feng TL, Seeburg HH, Franke U. Human luteinizing hormone-releasing gene (LHRH) is located on the short arm of chromosome 8 (region 8p11.2—p21). *Somat Cell Mol Genet.* 1986; 12(1): 95–100.

46. Hazum E, Conn PM. The molecular mechanism of GnRH action. I. The GnRH receptor. *Endocr Rev.* 1988; 9(4): 379–86.

47. Chi L, Zhou W, Prikhozhan A. Cloning and characterization of the human GnRH receptor. *Mol Cell Endocrinol.* 1993; 91(1–2): R1–R6.

48. Chien CH, Chen CH, Lee G, Chang TC, Chen RJ, Chow SN. Detection of gonadotropin-releasing hormone receptor and its mRNA in primary human epithelial ovarian cancers. *Int J Gynecol Cancer.* 2004; 14(3): 451–58.

49. Lee G, Chow SN, Chien CH, Liu S. Anti-GnRH receptor monoclonal antibodies, first-in-class GnRH analog. *J Gynecol Res.* 2015; 1(1): 102.

8.

DENDRITIC CELL VACCINE THERAPY FOR OVARIAN CANCER

Caitlin Stashwick, Brian J. Czerniecki, and Janos L. Tanyi

INTRODUCTION

Standard therapy for patients with epithelial ovarian cancer (EOC) consists of cytoreductive surgery combined with chemotherapy. Despite advances in aggressive cytoreductive surgery and new chemotherapeutic as well as antiangiogenic agents, the overall survival (OS) has not changed significantly. Over the past two decades, EOC has been recognized to be immunogenic, evidenced by the finding that ovarian cancer patients with tumor-infiltrating lymphocytes have significantly improved survival over those that do not.[1] This recognition supports the benefit of immune-based therapy in ovarian cancer. Goals of successful immunotherapy are to break self-tolerance and induce CD8+ cytotoxic T cells and CD4+ T-helper cells. Dendritic cell (DC) vaccine therapy holds promise as a successful mode of immunotherapy. The first clinical trial published using DCs for vaccination for cancer treatment was in melanoma in 1998 showing clinical responses in 5 of 16 patients with 2 complete remissions.[2] The first publication in ovarian cancer was in 1999,[3] and the Food and Drug Administration approved the first antitumor DC vaccine sipuleucel-T (Provenge) for prostate cancer in 2010. To fully understand the clinical applications, we first review DC biology.

BIOLOGY OF DCS

The DC was first discovered 1972.[4] DCs recognize and respond to microbes in the innate immune system but are also the most important antigen-presenting cells (APCs) for activating naïve T cells and therefore link innate immune reactions to adaptive immune responses.[5] DCs are a type of APC that present antigenic peptides to B and T cells. DCs reside in virtually all tissues, with the highest concentrations in skin, mucosa, and lymphoid organs.[4]

DC SUBSETS

Human DC are characterized by expression of high amounts of major histocompatibility complex (MHC) class II molecules and the absence of lineage markers such as CD14 (monocytes/macrophages), CD3 (T cells), CD19, CD20 and CD24 (B cells), CD56 (natural killer cells), and CD66b (granulocytes), classified in MHC II+ Lin cells. In the blood, DC are divided into myeloid or classical DC (cDC) and plasmacytoid DC (pDC).[6] Human DC and surface markers are summarized in Table 8.1 and cells derived from DC population and the proteins they produce in Table 8.2.

TABLE 8.1 HUMAN DC SUBSETS AND SURFACE MARKERS

Surface Markers

	HLA-DR	CD11c	CD123	CD1c (BDCA1)	CD141 (BDCA3)	CLEC9A (DNGR-1)	CD1a	CD14
CD1c+ cDC (Blood/resident)	+	++	–	+	+Immature	–	–	–
CD141+ cDC (Blood/resident)	+	+	–	–	++	+Immature Low mature	–	–
CD141+ CLEC9A cDC (Tissue/migratory)	+	+	–	–	++	+	–	–
pDC	+	–	+	–	–	–	–	–
Inflammatory DC	+	++	–	+	?	–	+	+
Langerhans cells	+	+	–	+	–	–	++	–

NOTE: DC = dentritic cell; cDC = classical dentritic cell; pDC = plasmacytoid dentritic cell; +/−, reported to be expressed or not in some tissues; ?, not reported, no data available. Modified from Durand M & Segura E (2015) The known unknowns of the human dendritic cell network. *Frontiers in Immunology* 6:129.

	Surface Markers	Proteins Produced
Immature DC	MHC class I/II low, CD11c high, CD80 low, CD86 low	
Mature/ activated cDC	MHC class I/II high, CD11c high, CD80 high, CD86 high	IL-12
Regulatory cDC	MHC class I/II low, CD11c high, CD40 low, B7-H1 high	IL-10, TFG-β
pDC	MHC class I/II low, CD11c low/int, CD19, BDCA-4	INF-α
Regulatory pDC	MHC class I/II low, CD11c low/int, CD19, BDCA-4, ICOS-L	IDO
MDSC	MHC class II low, CD11b, CD14 -/+	iNOS, IDO
TAM	CD11b, CD14, CD68, CD115,	VEGF, TGF-β, IL-10

NOTE: DC = dentritic cell; MHC = major histocompatibility; cDC = classical dentritic cell; IL = interleukin; TFG = transforming growth factor; pDC = plasmacytoid dentritic cell; INF = interferon; IDO = Indoleamine 2,3-dioxygenase; iNOS = inducible nitric oxide synthase; MDSC = myeloid-derived suppressor cells; TAM = tumor associated macrophages; VEGF = vascular endothelial growth factor.

Modified from Hargadon KM (2013) Tumor-altered dendritic cell function: implications for anti-tumor immunity. *Frontiers in Immunology* 4:192.

Classical DCs

Classical DCs in addition to being present in blood and secondary lymphoid organs are also present in skin, mucosa, and organs and respond to microbes by migrating to lymph nodes and display antigens to T cells.[5] DCs in this subset can produce interleukin (IL)-12 which enables production of interferon-gamma (INF-γ) secreting type 1 CD4+ T (Th1) cells. Maturation is very important step in DC antitumor immunity. Antigens presented by a DC in the immature state actually promote tumor tolerance and regulatory T (Treg) cell production.[7,8] cDC are separated into further subsets: CD1c+(BDCA1) DC and CD141+(BDCA3) DC. CD1c+ (BDCA-1) cDC express a range of toll-like receptors (TLR), including TLR1, 2, 3, 4, 5, 6, 7, 8, 10. Upon stimulation with TLR ligands, they generate proinflammatory cytokines. CD141+ (thrombomodulin, BDCA-3) constitutes a small population that expresses CLEC9A (DNGR-1).

Plasmacytoid DCs

pDC are present in the bone marrow, blood, and peripheral organs and move into lymphoid organs, respond to viral infection, and produce type I interferons which have antiviral properties. Their response is characterized by three main mechanisms: release of antiviral factors, immediate activation of memory cytotoxic CD8+ T cells through MHC class I, and late activation of CD4+ T cells via MHC class II molecules.[4] pDC are also important for antibody responses by plasma cells and intensify B-cell responses through type I interferons and IL-6 secretion upon viral stimulation.[4] pDC morphology is similar to antibody-producing plasma cells, express endosomal TLR3, 7, 8, 9, respond to viral nucleic acids that have been internalized by the cell, and produce antiviral cytokines, type I interferons in response to viral infections.[5]

Cutaneous (or Langerhans) DCs

Cutaneous DCs have high phagocytic and endocytic capacity and are quite efficient in antigen capture. Two subsets of cutaneous DC are present in the skin: Langerhans cells (LCs) found within the epidermis and dermal/interstitial DCs present in the dermis. LCs express TLR1, 2, 3, 6, and 10. Intersitital DC are further separated into CD1a+ and CD14+ subsets. LCs are very efficient at cross-presenting antigens and prime CD8+ T cells through IL-15, and intersitital CD14+ stimulate humoral immunity and can produce a large set of cytokines upon stimulation with CD40 including IL-1, IL-6, IL-8 IL-10, IL12, granulocyte-macrophage colony-stimulating factor (GM-CSF), MCP, and TCF. CD1c+ and CD1A+ DC and CD141+Clec9A+ DC are found in the skin, lung, intestine, and Langerhans cells and CD14+DCs are found in the skin and vaginal mucosa.[6]

Follicular DCs

One specialized type of DC is follicular DC that displays antigens to B lymphocytes.[5] Follicular DC are found in the germinal centers of lymphoid organs.

DC DEVELOPMENT

DCs differentiate from both myeloid and lymphoid progenitors.[9] In embryogenesis, at about five weeks gestation, hematopoietic stem cells (HSCs) seed the fetal liver and give rise to mature erythroid, lympoid, and myeloid cells. Myeloid cells include granulocytes, monocytes, macrophages, and DCs. HSCs develop through various multipotent progenitor stages into monocyte/macrophage and DC progenitors, which then give rise to a common DC precursor. DCs develop from these bone marrow precursors but can also arise from monocytes in inflammatory conditions.[10]

DC ACTIVATION UPTAKE, PROCESSING, AND PRESENTATION

DCs use several pathways to capture antigens: macropinocytosis, receptor-mediated endocytosis via C-type lectins (mannose receptor, DEC-205, DC-SIGN) or Fc-gamma receptor type I (CD64) and type II (CD32), or phagocytosis. DCs phagocytose apoptotic or necrotic cells, viruses, bacteria and intercellular parasites.[4] MHC class I presentation involves internalized antigens by phagocytosis or receptor-mediated endocytosis, which are degraded by proteosome and enter the endopasmic reticulum and interact with MHC class I molecules. With MHC class II presentation, antigens that are taken up by phagocytosis or endocytosis leads to endosome formation and proteolysis and peptides are loaded onto MHC class II molecules and transported to the surface after maturation, characterized by co-expression of CD86.[4] Blood and lymphoid DC are capable of cross-presentation, which refers to the capability to engulf exogenous antigens with different minor histocompatibility antigens and present them via MHC class I molecules.

DC MATURATION AND IMMUNE STIMULATION

In order to achieve an antigen-specific immune response by the T cell, the DC must present antigen in a mature state. Immature DC are highly phagocytic and sample soluble and cell-associated antigens. An immature DC fails to elicit an immune response but actually induce immune tolerance of these antigens. Maturation of DCs takes place in lymph nodes and occurs by stimulation by pathogen-associated molecular patterns, danger-associated molecular patterns, inflammatory mediators, and CD40L. Mature DC are characterized by expression of costimulatory molecules, such as CD80 and CD86 (which bind to CD28 receptor on T cell), CD40, CD70, or ICOS-L[11] as well as CD11a, CD11c, CD50, CD54, and CD102.[12] A mature DC stains with antibody to CD83 and produces IL-12 which is important for differentiation of Th1 cells.[4] In vitro, after DCs are differentiated from peripheral monocytes (typically using media enriched with GM-CSF and IL-4, discussed later), they are matured using a standard combination of tumor necrosis factor alpha (TNF-α), IL-1β, IL-6, and prostaglandin E2.[13,14] An alternate mixture that includes IFN-α, polyI:C, IL-1β,

TNF, and INF-γ as opposed to the standard combination can produce improved cytotoxic T cells (CTL) response.[14,15] Upon interaction with T cells, DCs undergo terminal maturation provided by interaction with CD40/CD40L, RANK/TRANCE, 4-1BB/41BBL, or OX40/OX40L.

DC REGULATION OF CD8+ CYTOTOXIC T LYMPHOCYTE RESPONSES

Mature DC present antigens via MHC class I to naïve CD8+ T cells. With the proper co-stimulation, CD8+ T cells become activated and, upon interaction with HLA-restricted antigen, respond via release of cytotoxic granzyme and perforin particles to eliminate cells. After interaction with T cells, it is thought that DCs die by apoptosis. Maturation of DCs is very important step in regulation of CD8+ T cell responses.

If antigens are presented by DCs in the immature state, this actually promotes tumor tolerance and Treg cell production.[7,8] Several DC subsets actually induce Treg cells, including dermal/intersitial CD14+ DC, intestinal CD1C+ CD, CD103-CD172a+ DC, IL-3 or TLR activated tonsil pDC, and bacteria-exposed Langerhans cells.[6] While dermal/intersitial CD14+ DC regulate B cell differentiation, Langerhans cells are more efficient in the priming of antigen specific CD8+ T cells and induce proliferation of naïve CD8+ T cells in vitro.[14]

DC-BASED TUMOR VACCINES

For cancer vaccines, a patient's DCs are first extracted and exposed to antigen derived from the patient's cancer cell and then reinfused into the patient with the goal to initiate immune response.[4] DC vaccines are aimed to stimulate T lymphocytes, and

TABLE 8.3 **ADVANTAGES AND DISADVANTAGES OF VARIOUS ANTIGEN SOURCES UTILIZED IN DC VACCINES**

Strategy	Advantages	Disadvantages
Peptide, whole protein	Well tolerated Stable and easy to produce	Usually weak antigens Induces only a restricted repertoire of T cells
Necrotic whole tumor cell lysate	Easy to prepare Mixture of all cellular components Induces polyclonal immune response	Limited amount of vaccine available after preparation Safety concerns
Apoptotic whole tumor cells	Easy to prepare Presents whole repertoire of TAA	Modest T-cell expansion Low frequency of tumor-reactive T cells are detected Limited access to tumor-derived material
Oxidation of whole tumor cells	Stronger tumor-specific immune response Improvement in antigen immunogenicity	Only used in recent early clinical trials
DC-tumor cell fusion	Endogenously synthesized antigens have better access to MHC class I pathway	No clinical studies yet available
Recombinant adenovirus-associated vector	High transfection efficiency More efficient activation of CD8+ cells Higher epitope presentation	DNA insert limited to 7.5 kb in size

NOTE: DC = dentritic cell; TAA = tumor-associated antigens; MHC = major histocompatibility complex.

vaccines aim to disrupt the tolerogenic state of the immune system and direction of an effector T-cell response which would lead to cancer regression.[11]

SOURCES OF DCS FOR CLINICAL USE

DCs make up less than 1% of circulating blood mononuclear cells. Two sources of DC are ex vivo generation of DCs or using native DCs in vivo (Table 8.3).

Ex Vivo

Ex vivo generation of DCs is performed by culturing monocytes or CD34+ progenitor cells obtained from peripheral blood in the presence of GM-CSF and IL-4 or IL-13.[16] Monocytes can be obtained by plastic adherence or immunomagnetic selection of CD14+ cells from peripheral blood. Ex vivo education of DCs would bypass the dysfunction of endogenous DCs that has been observed in cancer patients.[17,18] Once the DCs are obtained, they are cocultured in vitro with the selected tumor antigen, then matured and given back to the patient.[8]

Because humoral immunity is preferentially induced by CD14+ dermal DC, and cellular immunity preferentially induced by Langerhan's cell, the cytokine combinations used to differentiate monocytes into DCs is critical for the elicited T-cell response. Using GM-CSF and IL-15 to develop Langerhans-type DCs may actually produce better cells for cancer vaccines, and several studies have used these as source of DCs.[8,14]

In Vivo

Another method of activation of DCs has been to try and improve the capture of tumor-specific antigens by endogenous DCs in vivo.[8] In vivo DC activation and antigen loading has the benefit of using DCs in their natural environment. Adjuvants used in infectious disease vaccines, including mineral salts, emulsions, and liposomes, can enhance the magnitude of immune response over antigen alone.[19]

SOURCE OF TUMOR ANTIGENS

Common sources of tumor antigens are tumor-derived peptide or protein, RNA from tumor cells, and tumor lysates. When using peptides and protein tumor antigen, escape of induced tumor-specific immune response occurs. This escape can theoretically be overcome by using combination with tumor lysate.[4]

Types of Tumor Lysates

Necrotic Whole Tumor Cell Lysates

One method of preparation of tumor lystaes uses repetitive freeze-thaw cycles to induce cell necrosis. The resultant lysate is a mixture of call cellular components including fragments of destroyed cellular membrane and intracellular organelles, as well as cellular RNA and DNA. Necrotic tumor cells release large amount of heat shock proteins (HSP70 and 90) after necrosis that induces DC maturation,[20] as well as proinflammatory factor HMGB1 which binds to TLR4 on DCs and stimulates processing and presentation of tumor antigens.[21,22] In addition, necrotic cells rapidly degrade their RNA and DNA to purines and uric acid which aids in immune activation.[23] Ovarian cancer lysate pulsed DCs can activate T cells and mediate cytotoxic activity against autologous tumor cells.[24]

Apoptotic Whole Tumor Cells

Another method of preparing tumor cell lysate is irradiating tumor cells to created apoptotic tumor cells. Part of the apoptotic process exposes the phosphatidylserine of the plasma membrane externally. DCs have phosphatidylserine receptors that mediate uptake of apoptotic cells and cross-presentation of tumor antigens.[25] In patients with ovarian cancer, peripheral blood mononuclear cells (PBMC)-derived DCs pulsed with UVB-irradiated autologous ovarian tumor cells and matured with TNF-α has produced modest expansion of tumor-specific T-cell precursors.[26]

Oxidation of Whole Tumor Cells

Proteins that have been oxidized by hypochlorous acid (HOCl) are easily recognized and processed by APCs, which results in improved immunogenicity and activation of antigen-specific T cells.[27] HOCl produces dose-dependent necrotic cell death, and DCs pulsed with oxidized tumor cells were able to take up these cells and cross-present to activate T cells.[28]

STRATEGIES FOR LOADING ANTIGENS

Commonly used strategies for loading antigens are pulsing DCs with peptide or protein, exosomes plus peptides, whole tumor cell lysates, DC-tumor cell fusion, and recombinant adeno-associated viral vectors.

Pulsing DC with Peptide, Full Protein, or Tumor Lysates

Mature DCs can be exposed to tumor antigens for a short period of time in vitro to allow antigen uptake. Durable cytotoxic T-cell responses were shown in vivo in 10 patients with HLA-A2 and Her-2 or MUC1 expressing breast and ovarian cancer using mature autologous DCs pulsed with Her-2 or MUC-1 peptides. There was evidence of epitope spreading, and two patients had stable disease, one lasting eight months.[29] Using full-length endogenous or recombinant proteins or tumor lysates allows for immune response against different epitopes that could be restricted by multiple HLA alleles and allows for MHC class I and class II immune responses. Some recombinant proteins that have been tried include fusion proteins of tumor antigens with mannan or GM-CSF.

Two separate Phase I trials used DCs pulsed with mannan-MUC1 fusion protein[30], and DCs cultured with portions of HER-2/neu protein linked to GM-CSF, called lapuleucel-T,[31] showed T-cell immune response and disease stabilization.

DC-Tumor Cell Fusion

Tumor-associated antigens can also be delivered in vivo using chimeric proteins that incorporate an anti-DC receptor antibody fused to the selected antigen.[14] Fusion of DCs and tumor cells can be achieved through chemical, physical, or biological methods. One advantage of DC-tumor fusion vaccines over DC pulsed with whole tumor lysates is that endogenous antigens have better access to the MHC class I pathway. Cells produced from human ovarian cancer cells fused to DCs has shown T-cell proliferation and activity in vitro but has not yet been shown efficacy in a clinical trial.[32]

RNA/DNA Transfection/Transduction— Recombinant Adeno-Associated Viral Vectors

Tumor antigens can be genetically delivered via transduction of recombinant viruses with RNA or DNA specific for tumor antigen or whole tumor RNA. Recombinant adeno-associated viral (rAAV) vector have a single-stranded DNA genome bordered with inverted repeats which facilitate integration of the viral genome into chromosome 19. The virus is then transformed into a double-stranded, nonintegrated episome.[33] In vitro, Her-2/neu rAAV-transduced DC generated potent stimulation of HLA class I-restricted CTLs.[34]

OPTIMAL ROUTES OF DC ADMINISTRATION

The route of administration of DC-based vaccines has been studied in many different routes including subcutaneously, intravenously, intradermally, intraperitoneally, and intranodally, and the most optimal route has not been established. The intravenous (IV) route appears to be the best administration of antigens for reaching DC subsets residing in blood and lymphoid tissues. But when infusing mature DC, some do not express CD62L, which is the homing receptor required to enter lymph nodes across endothelial venules,[35,36] and intradermal, intraperitoneal, subcutaneous, or intranodal injections may be superior. One study found DC-infused IV accumulated in the spleen and nonlymphoid tissues but not in lymph nodes,[37] yet some preclinical data suggests IV routes are most effective in generating an immune response.[38] Intranodal injections have also been employed to overcome the time and difficulty in DCs actually reaching the secondary lymphoid organs. Typically the dose ranges between 10^5 and 10^9 DC per dose, yet there is considerable variability in number and frequency of doses in clinical trials.

SUMMARY OF THE CURRENT CLINICAL TRIALS FOR PERSONALIZED DC VACCINES IN OVARIAN CANCER

The early studies of DC vaccination immediately faced several difficulties. First was the determination that DCs needed to be matured with additional stimuli for optimal antigen presentation.[3] The next challenge was to determine the best tumor antigen, yet without one specific antigen in ovarian cancer, many studies used tumor lysate. One of the earliest studies to show that vaccination with DCs pulsed with a single tumor antigen may induce immunologic responses in patients with ovarian cancer was in 2000 (Table 8.4). Patients with advanced ovarian and breast cancer were vaccinated with autologous DCs pulsed with HER2/neu or MUC1-derived peptide combinations.[29] Peptide-specific CTLs were detected in the peripheral blood

of 5 out of 10 vaccinated patients using both intracellular IFN-γ immunohistochemistry staining and 51 Chromatin release assays. The main CTL response in vivo was stimulated by the HER2/neu derived E75 and the MUC1-derived M1.2 peptides. Interestingly, in one patient immunized with the HER2/neu peptides, MUC1-specific T lymphocytes were induced after seven vaccinations, suggesting that antigen spreading in vivo may occur after successful immunization with a single tumor antigen.

In another early study of DC vaccination published in 2002, patients with advanced gynecological malignancies were effectively vaccinated with DCs pulsed with keyhole limpet hemocyanin (KLH) to enhance immunity and autologous tumor antigens derived from tumor lysate.[39] Six subjects with ovarian carcinoma and two patients with uterine sarcoma received multiple intracutaneous injections (range 3–23) of antigen pulsed DCs at 10-day or four-week intervals. Three patients showed stable disease lasting 14, 25, and 45 weeks, respectively, and five experienced early tumor progression within the first 14 weeks of beginning therapy. Lymphoproliferative responses to KLH and to tumor lysate were observed in eight patients in this study. Conclusions were made that this treatment was immunologically active and essentially lacking significant adverse events.

Similarly in 2007, Hernando et al. reported a case report of a woman with recurrent ovarian cancer treated with autologous DCs transfected with mRNA encoded folate receptor α.[40] Imaging performed scans three months posttreatment (10 vaccinations at four-week intervals) revealed a partial response with very low toxicity. Homma et al. found elevated levels of antinuclear antibody (ANA) in the sera of patients with cancer who had received immunotherapy with a DC tumor cell fusion vaccine.[41] Twenty-two patients were treated with a vaccine composed of fusion cells created from autologous DCs and tumor cells. Nine out of the 22 vaccinated patients were also treated with recombinant human IL-12.

TABLE 8.4 SUMMARY OF CLINICAL TRIALS

Study	Patients (# pts)	Phase	Treatment (DC pulsed with)	Outcome
Brossart et al., 2000	Advanced breast and ovarian cancer, (10)	I	HER-2/neu- or MUC1-derived peptides	T-cell responses were detected in 5 patients
Hernando et al., 2002	Uterine sarcoma (2), ovarian carcinoma (6)	I	Keyhole limpet haematocyanine and autologous tumor antigens	3 patients with SD lasting 25-45 weeks
Schlienger et al., 2003	Ovarian cancer (10)	I	Autologous tumor lysate with TNF α +TRANCE	DCs vaccine could stimulate MHC class I-restricted T cells capable of secreting IFN-γ in response to autologous tumors
Loveland et al., 2006	Adenocarcinoma expressing MUC 1: ovary (1), fallopian tube (1), lung (1) breast (2), colon (1), esophagus (1), renal cell (3)	I	Mannan-MUC1 fusion protein	T-cell responses in all patients with evidence of tumor stabilization in 2 of the 10 patients
Homma et al., 2006	Ovarian (4), colon (4), gastric (3), breast (3), other (8)	I	DC vaccine of fusion cells composed of autologous DCs and tumor cells (DC/tumor-fusion vaccine)	Elevated serum ANA levels in 3 patients induced by vaccination
Hernando et al., 2007	Ovarian cancer (1)		Dendritic cells engineered with mRNA-encoded folate receptor type alpha	Partial response
Peethambaram et al., 2009	HER-2/neu-expressing tumors: ovarian (4), breast (11), colorectal (3)	I	BA7072, a recombinant fusion antigen consisting of portions of HER-2/neu (Lapuleucel-T)	7 pts with SD, median TTP was 12.8 weeks (observed range 3.9 to 71.9 weeks, including censored patients)
Chu et al., 2012	Ovarian cancer in remission (NED) (11)	I/II	Her2/neu, hTERT, and PADRE peptides	6 stayed NED at 36 months; 3 year OS 90%
Rahma et al., 2012	Recurrent ovarian cancer overexpressing the p53 protein in remission (NED) (21)	II	Arm A: received SC wild-type p53:264-272 peptide admixed with Montanide and GMCSF. Arm B received wild-type p53:264–272 peptide-pulsed DC IV	9/13 pts (69%) in arm A and 5/6 pts (83%) in arm B developed an immunologic response. The median OS was 40.8 and 29.6 months; the median PFS was 4.2 and. 8.7 months for arm A and B, respectively
Chiang et al., 2014	Recurrent ovarian cancer (5)	I	Oxydized autologous whole-tumor lysate	2 SD lasted 36 and 44 months; 1 mixed response

TABLE 8.4 CONTINUED

Study	Patients (# pts)	Phase	Treatment (DC pulsed with)	Outcome
Tanyi et al., 2015	Recurrent ovarian cancer (35)	I/II	Autologous oxidized whole-tumor antigen vaccine in combination with angiogenesis blockade	2 PR, 20 SD
Coosemans et al., 2013	Ovarian carcinosarcoma (1), serous ovarian cancer (1)		Autologous DCs electroporated with mRNA coding for the Wilms' tumor gene 1	Survival of 19 (OCS) and 12 (SOC) months. Increased CD137+ antigen-specific T-cells and IL-10 production post-vaccination
Bapsy et al., 2014	Ovarian cancer (7), other (31)	II	Autologous tumor lysate	Objective response rate by RECIST was 28.9% (11/38) and immune-related response criteria was 42.1% (16/38); median TTP 9 weeks
Kobayashi et al., 2014	Recurrent ovarian cancer (56)	II	MHC class I-restricted mutated WT1 and MUC1 synthetized peptide antigens	71% of the patients developed an immunologic response. The MST from diagnosis was 30.4 months and from the first vaccination was 14.5 months
Mitchel et al., 2014	Ovarian cancer (28)	II	Autologous monocyte-derived DCs incubated with mannosylated mucin 1protein	4 patients showed CA125 response or stabilization (2 patients with major responses, 1 minor response, 1 stabilization) of median duration 10.3 months (5.3–16.3 months)

NOTE: DC = dentritic cell; SD = stable disease; TNF = tumor necrosis factor; TTP = time to disease progression; NED = no evidence of disease; OS = overall survival; PFS = progression-free survival; PR = Partial response; SC = subcutaneously; IV = intravenously; IL = interleukin; RECIST = Response Evaluation Criteria in Solid Tumors; MST = median survival time.

One patient with gastric carcinoma (patient 1, DC tumor cell fusion vaccine alone), one patient with breast cancer (patient 2, DC tumor cell fusion vaccine alone), and one patient with ovarian cancer (patient 3, DC tumor cell fusion vaccine plus recombinant human IL-12) showed significant elevations of serum ANA levels during treatment. Patients 2 and 3 remained in good physical condition during treatment for 24 and 9 months, respectively. Patients with elevated serum levels of ANA had significantly longer treatment periods than those without it. This study concluded that elevated serum levels of ANA after DC tumor cell fusion vaccine are associated with anti-tumor immune response induced by the vaccination.[41]

Peethambaram et al. evaluated the use of lapuleucel T (APC8024) in patients with HER2/neu expressing tumors.[31] Lapuleucel T is an investigational active immunotherapy product consisting of autologous PBMCs, including APCs, which are cultured ex vivo with BA7072, a recombinant fusion antigen consisting of portions of the intracellular and extracellular regions of HER2/neu linked to GMCSF.[31] Eighteen patients with metastatic ovarian, colorectal, and breast cancer whose tumors expressed HER2/neu were enrolled; however, no objective responses were noted and only two patients experienced stable disease lasting >48 weeks. Chu et al., in a Phase I/II trial, evaluated the responses of patients with advanced EOC in remission to vaccination with PBMC-derived DCs loaded with HER2/neu, human telomerase reverse transcriptase, and pan HLADR epitope peptides.[42] In this study, the peptide-loaded DC vaccination elicited only modest immune responses by Enzyme-Linked ImmunoSpot (ELISPOT) assay, although OS of 90% at three years was very promising. Two patients from the enrolled 11 experienced recurrence during vaccination, and nine received all four doses. Unfortunately, three patients recurred at 6, 17, and 26 months, respectively. Six had no evidence of disease at 36 months. The authors concluded that peptide-loaded DC vaccination elicits modest immune responses, but the survival outcome was promising.

A Phase I study assessed the effect of autologous DCs pulsed with mannan-MUC1 fusion protein (MFP) to treat patients with advanced ovarian and renal adenocarcinomas.[30] The DCs were culture ex vivo and were then pulsed with MFP. Patients underwent three cycles of leukapheresis and reinjection at monthly intervals. The DC/MFP vaccine created both a strong T cell IFN-α ELISPOT response to the vaccine and a delayed type hypersensitivity response at the injection site in 8 out of the 10 enrolled patients. Two patients with clearly progressive disease (ovarian and renal carcinoma) at entry were stable after initial therapy and went on to further leukapheresis and DCMFP immunotherapy. The authors concluded that immunization produced T-cell responses in all patients with evidence of tumor stabilization in 2 of the 10 advanced cancer patients treated.

A gynecologic oncology group Phase II trial assessed the immune response to two p53 peptide vaccine approaches: subcutaneous injection and IV-pulsed DCs in high recurrence risk ovarian cancer patients.[38] Twenty-one HLA-A2.1 patients with stage III, IV, or recurrent ovarian cancer overexpressing the p53 protein with no evidence of disease were treated in two cohorts. Arm A received SC wt p53:264–272 peptide admixed with Montanide and GM-CSF. Arm B received wt p53:264–272 peptide-pulsed DCs IV. IL-2 was administered to both cohorts in alternative cycles. Nine out of 13 patients (69%) in the first arm and five out of six patients (83%) in the second arm showed an immunologic response as determined by ELISPOT and tetramer assays. The median OS was 40.8 and 29.6 months for the first and second arm, respectively, with median progression free survival of 4.2 and 8.7 months, respectively.[38]

A recent proposal presented a combination immunotherapy approach to introduce novel therapeutic immunomodulation, which could enable otherwise less effective vaccines to gain clinical efficacy. The authors identified important barriers in the tumor microenvironment: such as the blood-tumor barrier, which prevents homing of effector T cells.[43] They hypothesized that DC vaccine therapy will benefit from adjuvant treatment and a combinatorial approach of a new DC vaccine pulsed with autologous whole tumor oxidized lysate, in combination with antiangiogenesis therapy (bevacizumab) and metronomic cyclophosphamide.[43] Currently only the first cohort of five patients who received the DC vaccine in this trial has been published.[44] Three subjects entered the study with radiographically measurable disease, and two subjects progressed during the trial, whereas one subject showed a mixed response by RECIST criteria at EOS. This patient showed radiographic progression in 13 lesions at EOS (day 86) via CT, however, six weeks later, in the absence of additional therapy, she showed regression or stabilization of 6 of 13 tumor metastatic deposits. Two other patients entered the study with no evidence of disease and these subjects experienced durable progression-free intervals of 36 and 44 months. Both subjects experienced a longer second progression-free survival after vaccine therapy compared with the progression-free survival (PFS) after previous chemotherapy.[44]

As a continuation of this work, Tanyi et al. conducted a pilot clinical trial testing an autologous oxidized whole tumor cell lysate

DC-based vaccine injected intranodally, alone, or in combination with bevacizumab (Bev) with or without low-dose IV cyclophosphamide (Cy) and/or oral aspirin (ASA), in advanced recurrent ovarian cancer patients. Patients were treated every three weeks, until exhaustion of vaccine or progression. The majority of patients were platinum-resistant and heavily pretreated. To date, 35 patients (cohort 1 (vx only; n = 5), 2 (vx+bev; n = 10), 3 (vx+bev+Cy; n = 10), and 4 (vx+Bev+Cy+ASA; n = 10) have received over 392 vaccine doses (Tanyi ASCO). Six patients achieved a partial response or were disease-free at the end of treatment. The median PFS of cohort 1, 2, 3, and 4 were 4, 3.8, 11.1, and 10.1 months, respectively. The median OS of cohorts 1 and 2 were 35.3 and 11.4 months, respectively, while for cohorts 3 and 4 it has not been reached, with median potential follow-up of 19 months. Estimated PFS at six months was 70% for cohorts 3 and 4. Additionally, OS at 20 months was 100% and 90% for cohorts 3 and 4.[45] Coosemans et al. evaluated one patient with ovarian carcinosarcoma (OCS) and one with serous ovarian cancer (SOC) who received four weekly vaccinations of autologous DCs electroporated with mRNA coding for the Wilms' tumor gene 1 (WT1). In an ex vivo antigen restimulation assay of peripheral blood mononuclear cells, both patients showed increasing CD137+ antigen-specific T cells and IL-10 production postvaccination. Moreover, IL-2 production increased (OCS) as well as IFN-γ and TNF-α (SOC). Unfortunately both patients progressed after four vaccines but, after cessation of immunotherapy, they had an extended survival of 19 (OCS) and 12 (SOC) months.[46]

Another Phase II clinical trial of an autologous DC formulation for the management of refractory solid malignant tumors was conducted across six sites in India.[47] A total of 51 patients with refractory cancer (either sex) were recruited. Monocytes obtained by leukapheresis, differentiated into DCs by cytokines and primed with autologous tumor lysate (fresh tissue biopsy or paraffin block).

On the eighth day, mature DCs were analyzed for expression of CD40, CD80, CD83, CD86, DC205, and DC209. The treatment regimen consisted of six doses (IV) over 14 weeks with two posttreatment follow-up visits, six weeks apart. Objective response rate by RECIST was 28.9% (11/38), and immune-related response criteria was 42.1% (16/38).[47] The median time to treatment progression was >9 weeks. Median OS was 397 days.[47]

A retrospective study included 56 recurrent ovarian cancer (ROC) patients who initially received standard chemotherapy followed by DC-based immunotherapy targeting synthesized peptides at two different institutions in Japan.[48] Seventy-one percent of the enrolled patients developed an immunologic response. The median OS from diagnosis was 30.4 months and from the first vaccination was 14.5 months. Albumin levels of ≥4.0 g/dL and lactate dehydrogenase levels of <200 IU/L before vaccination were identified as significant independent factors by multivariate Cox proportional hazard analysis. The median survival time from the first vaccination in patients with albumin levels of ≥4.0 and <4.0 g/dL were 19.9 and 11.6 months, respectively. The corresponding disease control rates were 36% and 15%, respectively. They demonstrated potential clinical effectiveness of DC-based immunotherapy for ROC patients and showed that a good nutritional status might be an important factor for clinical efficacy.[48] Mitchell et al. conducted a Phase II, single-arm study of an autologous DC treatment against mucin 1 in patients with advanced EOC.[49] Mucin 1 antigen, highly expressed by EOC, is a potential target for immunotherapy. This Phase II trial was conducted in patients with EOC with progressive disease who were injected with Cvac, autologous monocyte-derived DCs incubated with mannosylated mucin 1protein intradermally every four weeks for three doses, then every 10 weeks for up to 12 months. All together 28 patients were enrolled, and only four patients showed CA125 response or stabilization (two patients with major responses, one minor response, one stabilization) of median duration 10.3 months (5.3–16.3 months). They concluded that Cvac immunotherapy was well tolerated and some patients showed some clinical activity based on decline or stabilization of CA125 levels.[49]

TREATMENT-RELATED TOXICITIES

DC vaccination is a relatively non-toxic treatment, with very few grade 3 or 4 adverse events reported in the literature; toxicities are summarized in Table 8.5. No deaths related to study therapy have been published. Mitchell et al. reported grade 2 (moderate) adverse events that occurred in more than one patient such as gastrointestinal disorders in nine patients (35%), fatigue in five patients (19%), and anemia in two patients (8%).[49] There were two grade 3 (severe) events (8%), abdominal pain and vomiting. Three patients had

lethargy, one of whom also had influenza-like symptoms.[49] Hernando et al. reported only minor grade 2 adverse events in two patients (25%) such as fatigue, chills, and low-grade fever which did not require any treatment.[39] Five patients (63%) showed mild repeated hypersensitivity skin reaction as an erythema at the injection site, and one patient (13%) developed temporary lymphadenopathy.[39] Loveland reported no clinical toxicity of the vaccine.[30] One patient (10%) developed elevation of antithyroid antibodies up to a maximal titer of 1:400 with no evidence of clinical autoimmune disease, and another had anti–smooth muscle antibodies at 1:80.[30] Homma et al. used DC/tumor-fusion vaccine alone; three patients showed significant elevations of serum ANA levels during treatment, but none of the treated patients showed clinical symptoms suggesting autoimmune disease.[41] In another study evaluating 18 patients with HER-2/neu-expressing tumors treated with

TABLE 8.5 **GRADE 3 AND 4 ADVERSE EVENTS ASSOCIATED WITH DC TREATMENT**

Adverse Event	Percentage of Patients	Grade	Attribution Per Author	Author
Abdominal pain and vomiting	4	3	Related	Mitchell et al., 2014
Vomiting	4	3	Related	
Acquired pyloric stenosis	5	4	Unrelated	Peethambaram et al., 2009
Fecal impaction	5	4	Unrelated	
Hydronephrosis,	5	4	Unrelated	
Urosepsis	5	4	Unrelated	
Worsening glaucoma	9	3	Unrelated	Chu et al., 2002
Fatigue	10	3	Unrelated	Rahma et al., 2012
Athralgia	10	3	Unrelated	
Cardiac arrhythmia	4	3	Unrelated	
Hepatic toxicity	8	4	Unrelated	
Rigors	3	4	Related	Bapsy et al., 2013

NOTE: DC = dentritic cell. Safety events were graded by use of the revised National Cancer Institute Common Terminology Criteria for Adverse Events, version 4.0.

lapuleucel-T, fatigue and rigors were the most commonly reported adverse events, occurring in 66.7% and 44.4% of patients, respectively.[31] The majority of events of fatigue (8 of 12, 66.7%) and rigors (7 of 8, 87.5%) occurred within one day of treatment. Other events that occurred in more than 25% of patients included arthralgia, headache, nausea, and vomiting. Four patients (22%) developed serious adverse events (SAEs) during this study although there were classified as unrelated to the study drug. These SAEs consisted of acquired pyloric stenosis, fecal impaction and hydronephrosis, urosepsis, and disease progression. No patient experienced an adverse event that resulted in an intervention, withdrawal of test drug, dose reduction, or significant additional concomitant medications other than those previously described as SAEs. The only cardiac disorder reported during the study was tachycardia not otherwise specified, which was seen in two patients (11%).[31]

Chu et al. administered a total of 39 vaccines to 11 subjects and all tolerated the vaccines well.[42] No grade 3 or 4 vaccine-related toxicities were reported. The most common study-related toxicities included reactogenicity as indicated by erythema, induration, pruritus, and pain at the site of injection, fever, and fatigue.[42] Only one patient experienced a grade 3 toxicity consisting of worsening of pre-existing glaucoma, deemed to be unrelated to vaccination.[42] In a two-arm study the patients in Arm A received a total of 143 vaccines and all of them experienced grade 1 or grade 2 toxicities.[38] The most common toxicities were erythema or induration at the sites of the vaccination, occurring in 77% of patients. Other common side effects included fatigue and elevated liver enzymes. Grade 3 or 4 toxicities occurred in 11 patients (14% of vaccines) and included fatigue, elevated liver enzymes, and arthralgia. The authors stated that all grade 3 toxicities occurred during the IL-2 cycles, required IL-2 dose reduction, and were attributed to the IL-2 usage and not to the vaccine itself. One patient who experienced grade 3 cardiac arrhythmia after receiving IL-2 with the third vaccine was removed from the study.

Another patient developed grade 4 hepatic toxicity after the fourth vaccine and continued vaccination without IL-2. In Arm B, patients received a total of 68 vaccines. Eighty-five percent experienced grade 1 or 2 toxicities in 44% of vaccines, all of which occurred during IL-2 cycles. Other adverse events included fatigue and increases in liver enzymes. Grade 3 toxicities occurred in five patients (23% of vaccines) and included fatigue, lymphopenia, and increased liver enzymes. All occurred during the IL-2 cycles.[38] In an Indian, open-label, multicenter, non-randomized, single-arm study of DC immunotherapy, adverse events were reported in 29 patients (56.9%).[47] Only one patient developed chills and rigors, which was judged as related to study therapy by the investigator. The SAEs were reported in 21.6% of the patients but not related to the study therapy. All SAEs were attributed to the primary cancer condition and associated metastases and not adjudged related to study therapy.[47] In Kobayashi et al.'s study, all the adverse events were tolerable in all patients.[48] No serious acute allergic reaction such as anaphylaxis was observed. The most common adverse events were injection-site reaction (68%) and fever (32%). Other common adverse events such as arthralgia and elevated liver enzyme levels were not observed. No grade 3–4 toxicity or evidence of autoimmune sequelae was detected.[48]

IMMUNOMODULATORY THERAPIES TO INCREASE CLINICAL EFFICACY

After injecting DC as a vaccine, many more steps in the immune response are required for an anti-tumor effect. One of the reasons we do not see a profound tumor regression in these DC clinical trials may be in part due to immune suppression preventing a full response.

INHIBITION OF REGULATORY T CELLS

If DCs are not properly matured, immune tolerance and/or suppression and Treg cell responses may be induced. Tregs are CD4+ T cells with immunosuppressive effects. Tregs have been associated with poorer outcomes in cancer. Patients with advanced ovarian cancer have been shown to have increased number of Tregs in blood and tumor microenvironment.[50,51] In a DC vaccine trial in melanoma, Treg were higher in patients with progressive disease, which suggests that Tregs may suppress anti-tumor immune responses in vaccinated patients.[52] Techniques to inhibit or reduce numbers of Tregs include cyclophosphamide and treatment with an anti-CD25 monoclonal antibody. A single-arm study with low-dose "metronomic" cyclophosphamide given orally was shown to decrease Tregs in patients with advanced cancer.[53] A randomized study of DC vaccine with or without cyclophosphamide showed that a single intravenous dose of cyclophosphamide had a nonsignificant improvement in survival but no associated effect on the number of circulating Treg.[42] In a clinical DC vaccine study in melanoma which depleted Tregs using a monoclonal antibody did not improve the efficacy of the vaccine.[54]

CHECKPOINT INHIBITORS

Negative costimulatory molecules such as cytotoxic T lymphocyte-associated antigen 4 (CTLA-4) and programmed death 1 (PD-1) have profound inhibitory effects on effector T-cell responses. These proteins are present on the T-cell surface and are referred to as immune checkpoint proteins. CTLA-4 is a receptor on T-cell surface and blocks immune response by inhibiting T-cell activation. Its effect occurs in secondary lymphoid tissues. An anti-CTLA-4 antibody has been approved in melanoma, and an anti-PD-1 antibody has been approved in melanoma and lung cancer. PD-1 is also a T-cell receptor that interacts with PD-1 ligands (such as PD-L1 or PD-L2) present on APC or parenchymal cells in peripheral tissues and is thought to have dual roles in immunological tolerance: induction and maintenance of peripheral tolerance.

PD-1 knockout mice have spontaneous autoimmune diseases.[55] In ovarian cancer, higher PD-L1 expression is associated with poorer prognosis,[56] and PD-1 inhibitors are currently being studied in ovarian cancer. Combination therapy with DC vaccine immunotherapy as well as checkpoint inhibitors are promising areas to be explored as blocking the negative effects of CTLA-4 and PD-1 may make DC vaccines more effective. In preclinical models in mice, silencing PD-L1 and PD-L2 in DC vaccine augmented T-cell expansion with ex vivo primed T cells.[57]

ENHANCEMENT OF T CELL CO-STIMULATION

DC can activate many immune cells, including antibody or natural killer cell responses, but the most important of their ability is to stimulate naïve T cells, specifically CD8+ cytotoxic T cells which actually kill tumor targets. For complete activation, T cells require two signals; the first is antigen-specific and the second is a co-stimulatory signal. Co-stimulatory molecules include CD28, ICOS, and 41BB. Co-stimulation allows for proliferation, differentiation, and persistence of T cells and can lead to anergy or immune tolerance without proper co-stimulation. Some work has been done to investigate the role of T-cell co-stimulation in context of a DC vaccine. One vaccine strategy was to use patient-derived tumor cells fused with autologous DCs. This study showed dramatic expansion in T cells co-cultured with DC/tumor fusion cells followed by anti-CD3/CD28-coated plates, as opposed to either agent alone or in the reverse order.[58]

Th1/Th2 Responses

CD4+ T cells on stimulation produce two major phenotypes of helper T cell, Th1 and Th2, and the cytokines they produce will either stimulate or inhibit cytotoxic T cell response. Lymphoid-DC subset induces Th1 cytokines (IFN-γ, IL-2), while myeloid DCs produce more Th2 cytokines (IL-10 and IL-4).[4] It is also hypothesized that polyanhydride microparticles are internalized by DCs and possess intrinsic adjuvant properties. g-poly-glutamic acid causes DC stimulation by TLR2 and TLR4 receptors producing IL-10 secreting memory T cells and the release of IL-12 causing enhanced Th1 response.[59]

TECHNIQUES OF IMMUNE RESPONSE ASSESSMENT

Immune response assessment is an important part of the evaluation of Phase I and II vaccine studies and is often used as an initial endpoint which is typically correlated with clinical outcome. The immune response is often measured by cytokine production (most commonly using ELISPOT for IFN-γ), T cell functionality, and delayed type-hypersensitivity (DTH) responses.

CYTOKINE PRODUCTION

T cells produce specific cytokines in response to antigen stimulation. The classic CD8 cytotoxic T cell produces IFN-γ which is identified in individual T cells by an ELISPOT assay.[60,61] ELISPOT is a modification of traditional enzyme-linked immunosorbent assay (ELISA) immunoassay, in which PBMC are plated on 96 well plate coated with anti-IFN-γ monoclonal antibodies(or other cytokine of interest) with or without the antigen of interest. Spot forming cells are then determined by a video image analyzer.

T CELL FUNCTIONALITY

Cytotoxic T lymphocyte (CTL) assays measure cytotoxicity classically by 51Cr release. Flow cytometry-based measurement of T cells induced caspase-3 or annexin-V activation through detection of

fluorescence. *T-cell proliferation assays* aim to measure the overall number and function of the entire T-cell population in aggregate. The most frequently applied form of the above assay is the radionuclide method. In this in vitro method for assessing antigen-specific T-cell proliferation in the assessment of T-cell clonal expansion, the T cells are incubated with antigens in the presence of a radiolabeled nucleotide. The cell proliferation degree can be speculated by the amount of 3H labeled TDR (tritiated thymidine). An activated T cell phenotype can also be shown by the expression of CD69 or granzyme B by flow cytometry. *Multimer assay* and *T cell receptor (TCR) analysis* are two methods to detect antigen specific responses. With multimer analysis, the binding of MHC-peptide complexes to T cells is detected by flow cytometry. With TCR analysis, clonal expansion of antigen-specific T cell can be detected by flow cytometry using antibodies against TCR Vβ epitopes, or alternatively polymerase chain reaction (PCR)-based techniques can be used when only small numbers of T cells are available.

Delayed Type-Hypersensitivity

DTH response has been used in clinical trials to show response to specific vaccination. This technique is similar to the idea in purified protein derivative (PPD) testing for tuberculosis exposure. After vaccination, the antigen of interest or tumor cell lysate is applied intradermally to patient's forearm to assess local inflammatory response after 48 hours.

Clinical Response

Clinical efficacy can be more difficult to show in Phase I and II clinical trials, but it is arguably the outcome of interest. Clinical efficacy can be shown by a decrease in tumor size or increased time to progression. RECIST

(Response Evaluation Criteria in Solid Tumors), originally published in 2000 with revised guidelines in version 1.1 in 2009,[62] has traditionally been used to evaluated response to chemotherapy. Tumor response to immunotherapy can be quite different using the iRECIST guidelines that were published in 2009.[63] Overall survival is the gold standard, yet this outcome can take many years, so laboratory end points showing immune correlates of clinical efficacy are important.

LIMITATION OF CURRENT DC VACCINE STRATEGIES IN OVARIAN CANCER

In a study looking at 56 patients with recurrent ovarian cancer who received DC pulsed with WT1 peptide, 71% of the evaluable patients showed an immunologic response as described by an increase in frequency of WT1-specific CTL.[48] Unfortunately this was not associated with an increase in median survival time. While there have been effective anti-tumor responses in animal models, human clinical trials have limited results such as these.

To improve immunogenicity of DC vaccines, some authors have administered adjuvants such as GM-CSF, IL-2, IL-15, and KLH. A Phase I trial in melanoma showed that a DC vaccine derived from monocytes generated more antigen-specific effector memory T cells when supplemented with IL-15.[53] In addition to adding adjuvants, possibly the source of DCs may be limiting the clinical effect. Most studies use monocytes obtained from peripheral apheresis as the source of DC, yet research suggests that Langerhans-type cells may actually serve as better vaccines.[64]

CONCLUSION AND FUTURE DIRECTIONS

Since the first clinical trials in ovarian cancer in 1999, clinical trials with DC vaccines have shown safety and immunologic response, yet the best clinical outcomes have been disease stabilization and rare partial responses. Future directions will be combinatorial techniques with chemotherapy and adjuvant agents, either biologic adjuvants such as cytokines or synthetic adjuvants such as polymeric nanoparticles. These early studies have shaped our understanding of immune system interactions and will guide future trials.

REFERENCES

1. Zhang L, et al. (2003) Intratumoral T cells, recurrence, and survival in epithelial ovarian cancer. *The New England Journal of Medicine* 348(3):203–13.
2. Nestle FO, et al. (1998) Vaccination of melanoma patients with peptide- or tumor lysate-pulsed dendritic cells. *Nature Medicine* 4(3):328–32.
3. Morse MA, et al. (1999) A phase I study of active immunotherapy with carcinoembryonic antigen peptide (CAP-1)-pulsed, autologous human cultured dendritic cells in patients with metastatic malignancies expressing carcinoembryonic antigen. *Clinical Cancer Research* 5(6):1331–38.
4. Mody N, Dubey S, Sharma R, Agrawal U, & Vyas SP (2015) Dendritic cell-based vaccine research against cancer. *Expert Review of Clinical Immunology* 11(2):213–32.
5. Abbas AK, Lichtman AH, & Pillai S (2015) *Cellular and molecular immunology* 8th ed. Philadelphia, PA: Elsevier.
6. Durand M, & Segura E (2015) The known unknowns of the human dendritic cell network. *Frontiers in Immunology* 6:129.
7. Steinman RM, Turley S, Mellman I, & Inaba K (2000) The induction of tolerance by dendritic cells that have captured apoptotic cells. *The Journal of Experimental Medicine* 191(3):411–16.
8. Tanyi JL, & Chu CS (2012) Dendritic cell-based tumor vaccinations in epithelial ovarian cancer: a systematic review. *Immunotherapy* 4(10):995–1009.
9. Hargadon KM (2013) Tumor-altered dendritic cell function: implications for anti-tumor immunity. *Frontiers in Immunology* 4:192.
10. De Kleer I, Willems F, Lambrecht B, & Goriely S (2014) Ontogeny of myeloid cells. *Frontiers in Immunology* 5:423.
11. Pizzurro GA, & Barrio MM (2015) Dendritic cell-based vaccine efficacy: aiming for hot spots. *Frontiers in Immunology* 6:91.
12. Brossart P (2002) Dendritic cells in vaccination therapies of malignant diseases. *Transfusion and Apheresis Science* 27(2):183–86.
13. Jonuleit H, et al. (1997) Pro-inflammatory cytokines and prostaglandins induce maturation

of potent immunostimulatory dendritic cells under fetal calf serum-free conditions. *European Journal of Immunology* 27(12):3135–42.

14. Palucka K, Ueno H, Zurawski G, Fay J, & Banchereau J (2010) Building on dendritic cell subsets to improve cancer vaccines. *Current Opinion in Immunology* 22(2):258–63.

15. Mailliard RB, et al. (2004) Alpha-type-1 polarized dendritic cells: a novel immunization tool with optimized CTL-inducing activity. *Cancer Research* 64(17):5934–37.

16. Alters SE, Gadea JR, Holm B, Lebkowski J, & Philip R (1999) IL-13 can substitute for IL-4 in the generation of dendritic cells for the induction of cytotoxic T lymphocytes and gene therapy. *Journal of Immunotherapy* 22(3):229–36.

17. Kalinski P, et al. (2011) Dendritic cells in cancer immunotherapy: vaccines or autologous transplants? *Immunologic Research* 50(2–3):235–47.

18. Pinzon-Charry A, Maxwell T, & Lopez JA (2005) Dendritic cell dysfunction in cancer: a mechanism for immunosuppression. *Immunology and Cell Biology* 83(5):451–61.

19. Dubensky TW Jr, & Reed SG (2010) Adjuvants for cancer vaccines. *Seminars in Immunology* 22(3):155–61.

20. Somersan S, et al. (2001) Primary tumor tissue lysates are enriched in heat shock proteins and induce the maturation of human dendritic cells. *Journal of Immunology* 167(9):4844–52.

21. Scaffidi P, Misteli T, & Bianchi ME (2002) Release of chromatin protein HMGB1 by necrotic cells triggers inflammation. *Nature* 418(6894):191–95.

22. Apetoh L, et al. (2007) Toll-like receptor 4-dependent contribution of the immune system to anticancer chemotherapy and radiotherapy. *Nature Medicine* 13(9):1050–59.

23. Hu DE, Moore AM, Thomsen LL, & Brindle KM (2004) Uric acid promotes tumor immune rejection. *Cancer Research* 64(15):5059–62.

24. Zhao X, Wei YQ, & Peng ZL (2001) Induction of T cell responses against autologous ovarian tumors with whole tumor cell lysate-pulsed dendritic cells. *Immunological Investigations* 30(1):33–45.

25. Larsson M, Fonteneau JF, & Bhardwaj N (2001) Dendritic cells resurrect antigens from dead cells. *Trends in Immunology* 22(3):141–48.

26. Schlienger K, et al. (2003) TRANCE- and CD40 ligand-matured dendritic cells reveal MHC class I-restricted T cells specific for autologous tumor in late-stage ovarian cancer patients. *Clinical Cancer Research* 9(4):1517–27.

27. Allison ME & Fearon DT (2000) Enhanced immunogenicity of aldehyde-bearing antigens: a possible link between innate and adaptive immunity. *European Journal of Immunology* 30(10):2881–87.

28. Chiang CL, et al. (2008) Oxidation of ovarian epithelial cancer cells by hypochlorous acid enhances immunogenicity and stimulates T cells that recognize autologous primary tumor. *Clinical Cancer Research* 14(15):4898–907.

29. Brossart P, et al. (2000) Induction of cytotoxic T-lymphocyte responses in vivo after vaccinations with peptide-pulsed dendritic cells. *Blood* 96(9):3102–108.

30. Loveland BE, et al. (2006) Mannan-MUC1-pulsed dendritic cell immunotherapy: a phase I trial in patients with adenocarcinoma. *Clinical Cancer Research* 12(3 Pt 1):869–77.

31. Peethambaram PP, et al. (2009) A phase I trial of immunotherapy with lapuleucel-T (APC8024) in patients with refractory metastatic tumors that express HER-2/neu. *Clinical Cancer Research* 15(18):5937–44.

32. Gong J, et al. (2000) Fusions of human ovarian carcinoma cells with autologous or allogeneic dendritic cells induce antitumor immunity. *Journal of Immunology* 165(3):1705–11.

33. Bohenzky RA, LeFebvre RB, & Berns KI (1988) Sequence and symmetry requirements within the internal palindromic sequences of the adeno-associated virus terminal repeat. *Virology* 166(2):316–27.

34. Yu Y, et al. (2008) rAAV/Her-2/neu loading of dendritic cells for a potent cellular-mediated MHC class I restricted immune response against ovarian cancer. *Viral Immunology* 21(4):435–42.

35. von Bergwelt-Baildon M, et al. (2006) CD40-activated B cells express full lymph node homing triad and induce T-cell chemotaxis: potential as cellular adjuvants. *Blood* 107(7):2786–89.

36. Miyasaka M, & Tanaka T (2004) Lymphocyte trafficking across high endothelial venules: dogmas and enigmas. *Nature Reviews. Immunology* 4(5):360–70.

37. Robert C, et al. (2003) Gene therapy to target dendritic cells from blood to lymph nodes. *Gene Therapy* 10(17):1479–86.

38. Rahma OE, et al. (2012) A gynecologic oncology group phase II trial of two p53 peptide vaccine approaches: subcutaneous injection and intravenous pulsed dendritic cells in high recurrence risk ovarian cancer patients. *Cancer Immunology, Immunotherapy: CII* 61(3):373–84.

39. Hernando JJ, et al. (2002) Vaccination with autologous tumour antigen-pulsed dendritic cells in advanced gynaecological malignancies: clinical and immunological evaluation of a phase I trial. *Cancer Immunology, Immunotherapy: CII* 51(1):45–52.

40. Hernando JJ, et al. (2007) Vaccination with dendritic cells transfected with mRNA-encoded folate-receptor-alpha for relapsed metastatic ovarian cancer. *The Lancet Oncology* 8(5):451–54.

41. Homma S, Sagawa Y, Ito M, Ohno T, & Toda G (2006) Cancer immunotherapy using dendritic/tumour-fusion vaccine induces elevation of serum anti-nuclear antibody with better clinical responses. *Clinical and Experimental Immunology* 144(1):41–47.

42. Chu CS, et al. (2012) Phase I/II randomized trial of dendritic cell vaccination with or without cyclophosphamide for consolidation therapy of advanced

ovarian cancer in first or second remission. *Cancer Immunology, Immunotherapy: CII* 61(5):629–41.

43. Kandalaft LE, et al. (2013) A phase I vaccine trial using dendritic cells pulsed with autologous oxidized lysate for recurrent ovarian cancer. *Journal of Translational Medicine* 11:149.

44. Chiang CL, et al. (2013) A dendritic cell vaccine pulsed with autologous hypochlorous acid-oxidized ovarian cancer lysate primes effective broad antitumor immunity: from bench to bedside. *Clinical Cancer Research* 19(17):4801–15.

45. Tanyi JL KL, Ophir E, Bobisse S, Genolet R, Zsiros E, Torigian DA, Mick R, Harari A, & Coukos G (2015) Autologous oxidized whole-tumor antigen vaccine in combination with angiogenesis blockade to elicit antitumor immune response in ovarian cancer. *Journal of Clinical Oncology* 33(15 Suppl.):5519.

46. Coosemans A, et al. (2013) Immunological response after WT1 mRNA-loaded dendritic cell immunotherapy in ovarian carcinoma and carcinosarcoma. *Anticancer Research* 33(9):3855–59.

47. Bapsy PP, et al. (2014) Open-label, multi-center, non-randomized, single-arm study to evaluate the safety and efficacy of dendritic cell immunotherapy in patients with refractory solid malignancies, on supportive care. *Cytotherapy* 16(2):234–44.

48. Kobayashi M, et al. (2014) The feasibility and clinical effects of dendritic cell-based immunotherapy targeting synthesized peptides for recurrent ovarian cancer. *Journal of Ovarian Research* 7:48.

49. Mitchell PL, et al. (2014) A phase 2, single-arm study of an autologous dendritic cell treatment against mucin 1 in patients with advanced epithelial ovarian cancer. *Journal for Immunotherapy of Cancer* 2:16.

50. Woo EY, et al. (2001) Regulatory CD4(+)CD25(+) T cells in tumors from patients with early-stage non-small cell lung cancer and late-stage ovarian cancer. *Cancer Research* 61(12):4766–72.

51. Shah CA, et al. (2008) Intratumoral T cells, tumor-associated macrophages, and regulatory T cells: association with p53 mutations, circulating tumor DNA and survival in women with ovarian cancer. *Gynecologic Oncology* 109(2):215–19.

52. Bjoern J, Brimnes MK, Andersen MH, Thor Straten P, & Svane IM (2011) Changes in peripheral blood level of regulatory T cells in patients with malignant melanoma during treatment with dendritic cell vaccination and low-dose IL-2. *Scandinavian Journal of Immunology* 73(3):222–33.

53. Ghiringhelli F, et al. (2007) Metronomic cyclophosphamide regimen selectively depletes CD4+CD25+ regulatory T cells and restores T and NK effector functions in end stage cancer patients. *Cancer Immunology, Immunotherapy: CII* 56(5):641–48.

54. Jacobs JF, et al. (2010) Dendritic cell vaccination in combination with anti-CD25 monoclonal antibody treatment: a phase I/II study in metastatic melanoma patients. *Clinical Cancer Research* 16(20):5067–78.

55. Okazaki T & Honjo T (2006) The PD-1-PD-L pathway in immunological tolerance. *Trends in Immunology* 27(4):195–201.

56. Hamanishi J, et al. (2007) Programmed cell death 1 ligand 1 and tumor-infiltrating CD8+ T lymphocytes are prognostic factors of human ovarian cancer. *Proceedings of the National Academy of Sciences of the United States of America* 104(9):3360–65.

57. van der Waart AB, et al. (2015) siRNA silencing of PD-1 ligands on dendritic cell vaccines boosts the expansion of minor histocompatibility antigen-specific CD8(+) T cells in NOD/SCID/IL2Rg(null) mice. *Cancer Immunology, Immunotherapy: CII* 64(5):645–54.

58. Rosenblatt J, et al. (2010) Generation of tumor-specific T lymphocytes using dendritic cell/tumor fusions and anti-CD3/CD28. *Journal of Immunotherapy* 33(2):155–66.

59. Broos S, et al. (2010) Immunomodulatory nanoparticles as adjuvants and allergen-delivery system to human dendritic cells: Implications for specific immunotherapy. *Vaccine* 28(31):5075–85.

60. Czerkinsky C, et al. (1988) Reverse ELISPOT assay for clonal analysis of cytokine production. I. Enumeration of gamma-interferon-secreting cells. *Journal of Immunological Methods* 110(1):29–36.

61. Schmittel A, Keilholz U, Thiel E, & Scheibenbogen C (2000) Quantification of tumor-specific T lymphocytes with the ELISPOT assay. *Journal of Immunotherapy* 23(3):289–95.

62. Eisenhauer EA, et al. (2009) New response evaluation criteria in solid tumours: revised RECIST guideline (version 1.1). *European Journal of Cancer* 45(2):228–47.

63. Wolchok JD, et al. (2009) Guidelines for the evaluation of immune therapy activity in solid tumors: immune-related response criteria. *Clinical Cancer Research* 15(23):7412–20.

64. Mantia-Smaldone GM & Chu CS (2013) A review of dendritic cell therapy for cancer: progress and challenges. *BioDrugs: Clinical Immunotherapeutics, Biopharmaceuticals and Gene Therapy* 27(5):453–68.

9.

HEAT SHOCK PROTEIN VACCINE THERAPY FOR OVARIAN CANCER

Hiroyuki Abe, Amane Sasada, Shigeki Tabata, and Minako Abe

BACKGROUND

Ovarian cancer occurs with a lifetime incidence of approximately 1 in 58 women and is the fifth leading cause of death by cancer in women.[1] Despite advances in chemotherapy and surgery, ovarian cancer has a poor prognosis and is the leading cause of death from gynecological malignancies. For all types of ovarian cancer, the five-year relative survival rate is 45%. If ovarian cancer is found at stages IA and IB, the five-year relative survival rate is 94% and 92%, respectively. However, due to a mostly asymptomatic early stage and lack of early diagnostic tools, only 15% of all ovarian cancers are found at stage I. Sixty-seven percent of patients are diagnosed at stage III and IV, with resultant low survival rates.[2] The list shown in Table 9.1 is the five-year survival rate for the different types of ovarian cancer. The most recent FIGO staging system was published in January of 2014, and so statistics for survival based on this staging are not yet available.

Because of low survival rates from ovarian cancer, innovative and effective therapeutic modalities are urgently needed. Many studies have reported that the immune system plays a critical role in disease progression and overall survival. Numbers of tumor-infiltrating T cells correlate with improved progression-free survival (PFS). On the other hand, presence of regulatory T cells (Treg) and expression of T cell inhibitory molecules such as programmed death (PD)-1 are correlated with poor prognosis. Therefore, cell-based immunotherapy will become a promising novel option to the conventional treatments of ovarian cancer. Herein, we review several key issues and discuss the molecular targeting cellular immunotherapies in ovarian cancer.

FUNCTION OF HEAT SHOCK PROTEIN IN OVARIAN CANCER

Heat shock proteins (HSP) are group of proteins induced by heat shock or stress. HSPs are present in all cells in all forms of life and in a variety of intracellular locations, such as the cytosol, nuclei, endoplasmic reticulum, and mitochondria. HSPs can be classified into 10 families by their molecular size, which consists of one to eight closely related proteins (see Table 9.2).[3]

Expression of HSPs is induced in response to a wide variety of physiological and environmental stressors. HSPs normally constitute up to 5% of the total intracellular proteins. However, under stress their levels can rise to 15% or more.[3] These proteins play an essential role as molecular chaperones by assisting the correct folding of misfolded proteins, and preventing their aggregation.

TABLE 9.1 RELATIVE FIVE-YEAR SURVIVAL RATE FOR DIFFERENT TYPES OF OVARIAN CANCER BY STAGE

Stage	Invasive Epithelial Ovarian Cancer	Ovarian Stromal Tumors	Germ Cell Tumors of Ovary	Fallopian Tube Carcinoma
I	90%	95%	93%	87%
IA	94%			
IB	92%			
IC	85%			
II	70%	78%	94%	86%
IIA	78%			
IIB	73%			
III	39%	65%	87%	52%
IIIA	59%			
IIIB	52%			
IIIC	39%			
IV	17%	35%	69%	40%

NOTE: National Cancer Institute, SEER Database; based on patients diagnosed from 2004 to 2010.

TABLE 9.2 THE MAIN FAMILIES OF HSPS[a]

HSP Family	Members	Intracellular Location
Small HSPs	HSP10, GROES, HSP16, α-crystallin, HSP20, HSP25, HSP26, HSP27	Cytosol
HSP40	HSP40, DNAJ, SIS1	Cytosol
HSP47	HSP47	Endoplasmic reticulum
Calreticulin	Calreticulin, calnexin	Endoplasmic reticulum
HSP60	HSP60, HSP65, GROEL	Cytosol and mitochondria
HSP70[b]	HSP72, HSC70 (HSP73), HSP110/SSE, DNAK SSC1, SSQ1, ECM10 GRP78 (BiP), GRP170	Cytosol Mitochondria Endoplasmic reticulum
HSP90	HSC84, HSP86, HTPG Gp96 (GRP94, HSP108, endoplasmin)	Cytosol Endoplasmic reticulum
HSP100	HSP104, HSP110[c] CLP proteins HSP78	Cytosol Cytosol Mitochondria

NOTE: HSP = heat shock protein.

[a] The list is not all-inclusive. [b] Co-chaperones HIP (p48), HOP (p60), BAG-1, RAP46. [c] Distinct from the HSP70 member with the same name.

Modified from Srivastava P. Roles of heat-shock proteins in innate and adaptive immunity. *Nat Rev Immunol*. 2002 Mar;2(3):185–94.

HSPs have a dual function depending on their intracellular or extracellular location.[4] Intracellular HSPs have a protective function, through direct interactions with various components of the tightly regulated programmed cell death machinery. In contrast to these, extracellularly located or membrane-bound HSPs mediate immunological functions. They can elicit an immune response modulated either by the adaptive or innate immune system. Most patients with advanced ovarian cancer respond well to initial chemotherapy; however, within two years chemoresistance and recurrence follows. In order to explain this phenomenon, considerable attention has been paid to the important role of HSPs in carcinogenesis processes and their participation in developing resistance to anticancer treatments.[5] It was demonstrated that the levels of circulating HSPs and antibodies could be useful biomarkers for prognosis factors and susceptibility to treatment.[6,7] Presence of antibodies reactive to tumor-associated antigens (TAAs) can be shown in the circulation already in early stages of cancer development including ovarian cancer and much earlier than circulating antigens.[8-11] Some HSPs were identified as TAAs recognized by antibodies present in serum of patients with ovarian cancer,[11] and HSP27, heat shock protein 70 (HSP70), HSP90 expression in tumor tissues was positively correlated to clinical stage of disease (FIGO).[12] Recent studies show usefulness of assessment of anti-HSP60/65 antibody levels as a "diagnostic marker" especially in early clinical stages of ovarian cancer, when lack of specific markers in serum and lack of clinical symptoms often delay diagnosis.[13] Presently, the molecular nature of HSPs transport has not yet been identified. However, it can be hypothesized that after binding of HSP70 to phosphatidylserine, a flip-flop mechanism similar to that shown for annexin might facilitate the transport of HSP70 from inside the cell to the outer surface membrane of cell.[14] An alternative vesicular pathway bypassing the endoplasmic reticulum (ER)-Golgi route has been hypothesized for HSP70.[15] Schmitt

and his group[14] demonstrated an active release of HSP70 in concert with Bag-4 from viable human colon and pancreatic carcinoma cell in detergent-soluble lipid vesicles, which was recently identified as "exosome."[16] HSP70 originating from tumors was found to facilitate receptor-mediated endocytosis.[17] After uptake a HSP-peptide complexes into antigen presenting cells (APCs), processing and presentation of HSP-chaperoned peptides on major histocompatibility complex (MHC) class I, then, a CD8+ cytotoxic T lymphocyte response is initiated.[18]

ROLE OF EXOSOME IN HSP TRANSPORT

Exosomes are cell-derived vesicles that are secreted by all cell types and are also present in many body fluids such as blood, urine, cerebrospinal fluid, breast milk, saliva, bronchoalveolar lavage fluid, ascitic fluid, and amniotic fluid.[19] HSPs localized on the surface of exosomes, secreted by normal and tumor cells, could be key players in intercellular cross-talk, particularly during the course of different diseases, such as cancer. Exosomal HSP offers significant opportunities for clinical applications, including their use as potential novel biomarkers for the diagnosis or prognoses of different diseases or for therapeutic application and drug delivery.[20] Importantly extracellular HSP70 exert immunomodulatory effects and play a key role in the immune response to cancer cells.[21] Microvesicles containing HSP70 on their surface activate macrophages,[22] or natural killer (NK) cells[23] and play an important role in the regulation of vascular homeostasis.[16] Therefore, HSPs found on the surface of exosomes might be key players in intercellular cross-talk. Elsner and his associates demonstrated that HSP70-positive exosome releases by tumor cells increase the NK cell activity against cell targets, resulting in reduced tumor growth.[24] Another interesting observation is that treatment with the histone deacetylase inhibitor (MS-275) increased the expression of HSP70. Exosome modification by MS-275 can significantly increase the cytotoxicity of NK cells and the proliferation of peripheral blood mononuclear cells (PBMCs), determining a reduction in tumor growth.[24-26] Most HSP-based immunotherapeutic approaches against cancer exploit their carrier function for immunogenic peptides.[27,28]

HSP70 and GP96 peptide complexes purified from patient-derived tumors were used as a vaccine to treat and prevent cancer. In contrast, HSP preparations derived from normal tissues did not induce an anticancer immune response. These results indicated that the immunogenicity in this approach is dependent on the tumor-specific peptides chaperoned by HSPs. Besides their chaperone activity, HSP-peptide complexes are internalized into antigen-presenting cells by receptor-mediated endocytosis, then they traffic into cellular compartments where the chaperoned peptides are released, processed, and represented on MHC class I molecules[14] as well as class II molecules (see Figure 9.1).

HSP70-PEPTIDES COMPLEX VACCINE FOR CLINICAL USE

For molecular chaperone function, HSP70 family members are equipped with two major functional domains, including a carboxy-terminal region that binds peptides and denatured proteins and an N-terminal ATPase domain that controls the opening and closing of the peptide binding domain.[29] These two domains play important roles in functions of HSP70 in tumor immunity, mediating the acquisition of cellular antigens and their delivery to immune effector cells.[30,31] Weng and his group developed an enhanced molecular chaperone-based vaccine through rapid isolation of HSP70 peptide complexes after the fusion of tumor and dendritic cells (HSP70 PC-F).[32] Preclinical studies show HSP70 extracted from fusions of dendritic cell (DC) and tumor cells possess superior properties such as stimulation of DC maturation and T cell-mediated antitumor immunity[33-35] and therefore constitutes a formation of chaperone protein-based tumor vaccine for clinical use. Belli and his group[36] reported the usefulness of autologous tumor

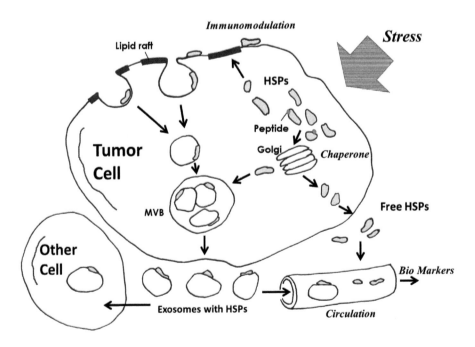

Figure 9.1 HSPs and exosomes. MVB= multivesicular body. Modified from Campanella C, Bavisotto CC, Gammazza AM, et al. Exosomal heat shock proteins as new players in tumour cell-to-cell communication. *J Circ Biomark*. 2014, 3: 4.

derived HSP gp96-peptide complexes in 42 patients with surgically resected metastatic melanoma. No treatment-related toxicity was observed. Out of 28 patients with measurable disease, two had a complete remission response (CR) and three had stable disease (SD) at the end of follow up. Duration of CR was 599+ and 703+ days; whereas SD lasted for 153, 191, and 272 days, respectively.[36] It was also shown that HSP gp96 vaccination after resection of colorectal liver metastasis was safe and elicits a significant increase in CD8+ T cell response against colon cancer (see Figure 9.2).[37]

DEVELOPMENT OF DC VACCINE FOR OVARIAN CANCER

The standard treatment of advanced stage epithelial ovarian cancer is optimal debulking surgery as feasible plus chemotherapy with a platinum plus a taxane agent. If this front-line approach fails, as it is too often the case, several Food and Drug Administration–approved agents are available for salvage therapy. Because there is no second-line therapy for advanced-stage epithelial ovarian cancer,

immunotherapy is theoretically the next step in treating ovarian cancer. Immunotherapy based on DC-based vaccine pulsed with ovarian tumor antigens leads to produce specific T-cell responses, which has potential as an alternative treatment to prevent disease recurrence or progression after the first-line therapy for ovarian cancer. As far as antigens, the hepsin 48-84 peptide was widely used as an ovarian tumor antigen for T-cell stimulation.[38] Hepsin is a serine protease that is highly overexpressed by ovarian cancer and is associated with invasion and metastasis.[39] The hepsin 48-84 sequence is "QEPLYPVQVS SADARLMVFDKTEGTWRLLCSSRSNAR." DCs loaded with hepsin 48-84 peptide efficiently stimulated CD4+ T cell responses from ovarian cancer patients or healthy adults.[38] However, tumor-associated immunosuppression through recruitment and expression of CD4+ Treg remains a significant barrier to effective treatment. Cannon and his group's approach, based on DC vaccination and designed to drive a tumor antigen-specific Th17 T cell response, holds the potential to be of clinical benefit for patients with ovarian cancer.[38] For this approach, several recent

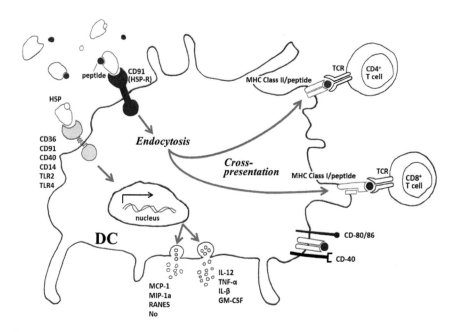

Figure 9.2 The HSP-DC interaction integrates adaptive and innate immune events. Modified from Srivastava P. Roles of heat-shock proteins in innate and adaptive immunity. *Nat Rev Immunol.* 2002; 2(3): 185-94, p. 188.

studies have indicated that regulation of the p38 and ERK/MAPK signal transduction pathway in DCs plays a central role in the direction of T-cell differentiation.

Inhibition of MEK1/2 and ERK/MAPK signaling promotes interleukin (IL)-12 production and Th1 T cell responses. On the other hand, inhibition of p38 MAPK increases signal transduction through ERK1/2 and blocks IL-12 production.[40] Treatment of DCs with pharmacological inhibitors of p38 signaling may confer benefit for patients with ovarian cancer.

Recently, Prima Bio Med (Sydney, Australia) developed CVac. CVac is an autologous DC vaccine that targets the abnormal forms of MUC1 found on tumor cells. Gray and his group have recently completed a Phase II clinical trial of CVac in ovarian cancer. The trial, known as CAN-003, is an open label Phase II study evaluating CVac as compared to the standard of care (SOC). PFS was not improved in first-line patients by CVac treatment as compared to SOC. In second-line patients, however, CVac demonstrated a significant improvement in PFS. The median PFS for SOC was 4.94 months, while the median PFS for CVac was not reached but is greater than 12.91 months. They concluded that CVac treatment was safe and showed a significant improvement in PFS in 20 second-line epithelial ovarian cancer patients.[41] On the other hand, Sabbatini and his group demonstrated that NY-ESO-1 overlapped long peptide (OLP) vaccine was safe and rapidly induced consistent integrated immune responses (antibody, CD8+ and CD4+) in nearly all vaccinated advanced ovarian cancer patients, when given with Poly-ICLC + Montanide adjuvants.[42] This work suggests the possibility of using OLPs as tumor associated antigen in DC-based vaccines.

DEVELOPMENT OF MULTIPEPTIDE DC-BASED VACCINE LOADED HSP70-PC

DCs can take up a diverse array of antigens and present them to T cells as peptides bound to both MHC class I and II products. Relative to other APCs, DCs are adept at stimulating naïve T cells. DCs also control the quality of the T-cell response, driving naïve lymphocytes into distinct classes of effectors. These antigen-specific, adaptive responses are critical for resistance to tumors. Controversially, DCs can also generate Treg that suppress activated T cells, a function of likely importance in autoimmunity and transplant rejection.[43] Current immunotherapy strategies include monoclonal antibodies against tumor cells or immune-regulatory molecules (checkpoint blockade), cell-based therapies such as adoptive transfer of ex vivo-activated T cells, and NK cells and cancer vaccines.[44]

Herein we discuss the clinical basis for DC-based vaccine and activated NK cells with the supportive use of immune checkpoint inhibitor anti-PD-1 antibody.

STRATEGIES USING DC-BASED VACCINE PULSED WITH HSP70-PC

Because of burst function, DCs can conduct all of the elements of the immune orchestra, and they are therefore a fundamental target and tool for vaccines.[45] TAAs are a key factor implicated in the design of DC vaccine strategies. If a patient's own cancer cells are available for lysate, this will be used for the production of an individual DC-based vaccine which is utilized for the optimally matched tumor surface antigen. In most instances, however, a patient's own cancer cells are not available; then artificial cancer antigens are utilized for the production of a DC-based vaccine. A pilot project by the National Cancer Institute reported on the prioritization of cancer antigens to develop a well-vetted, priority-ranked list of cancer vaccine target antigens based on predefined and preweighted objective criteria.[46]

Tumor-Associated Antigens

Among these antigens, frequently used artificial tumor antigens are listed in Table 9.3.

TABLE 9.3 FREQUENTLY USED TUMOR
ANTIGENS

HLA-A2 or HLA-A24 Restricted		Nonrestricted	
Short Epitope Peptide		Short Epitope Peptide	Overlapped Long Peptide or Protein
WT1	MAGE1, MAGE3	MUC1	WT1
NY-ESO-1	HER2	CA125	NY-ESO-1
MUC1	Gp100	PSA	MUC1
CEA	PSMA	NY-ESO-2	MAGE-A3
Survivin	SART1, SART3		hTERT
EBVBMLF1	MART1		Survivin
Melan-A	HPV16-E7		HPV16-E6
			HPV16-E7
			Lysate

Some of these are restricted by HLA-A1 or HLA-A24, so that an HLA study is needed to select and match the TAAs to DCs. Recently, new therapy strategies that focus on multipeptides use of TAAs have been suggested as additional options to currently available treatments, due to their fewer adverse events and better tolerability. The establishment and maintenance of immune cell therapy for cancer relies on special TAAs, such as WT1, MUC1, and hTERT, which have become primary targets for cancer vaccines.[47] Synthetic OLPs representing the entire sequence of immunogenic proteins are efficiently activated both CD4+ and CD8+ T cells irrespective of HLA typing of the patient, after intracellular processing by DCs.[42,48]

Therefore vaccination is an effective medical procedure in clinical oncology, based on the induction of long-lasting immunologic memory and characterized by mechanisms endowed with high destruction potential and specificity. These functions will elicit a persistent immune memory that can eliminate residual cancer cells and protect against relapses. As described, DCs internalize the OLPs, process them, and display them with MHC class I and II molecules. Thereafter DC-based vaccine is injected intradermally; DCs migrate into corresponding lymph nodes, where they present the antigens to naïve T lymphocytes. Helper T cell (CD4+) recognize their cognate antigens on MHC class II molecules, whereas CD8+ T cells (cytotoxic T lymphocytes [CTLs]) recognize the peptide-MHC class I molecule complex on the cell surface of DCs. Adapting a single peptide for the development of vaccines is not an optimal approach. It has been shown that after complete objective response to NY-ESO-1 peptide vaccine, a NY-ESO-1 negative tumor later recurred showing that single-target immunization approaches can result in the development of immune escape tumor variants.[49] Since MHC expression levels vary with tumor type (e.g., primary tumors vs. metastatic lesions and stages), it is difficult to eradicate cancer by the administration of the DC vaccine alone. So it is rational to use NK cells together with the cancer vaccine, which we call "hybrid immunotherapy." CTLs activated by DC-based vaccine target MHC expressing cancer cells, whereas NK cells attack cancer cells that do not express MHC molecules.

Role of HSP70 as a Chaperone

HSP70 are involved in binding short epitope peptides as well as OLPs and presenting them to the immune system. It is known that HSP70 interacts with DCs through common HSP receptor CD91;[50] this leads to internalization of the HSP70-peptide, which complies into a non-acidic endosomal compartment, followed by a transfer of the complexes (HSP70-PC), or of the peptide alone, to the cytosol.[27,51] The peptides are processed by the proteasomes and are transported into ER through the transporters that are associated with antigen processing. The peptides are then loaded onto MHC class I molecules and presented by the DC to CD8[+] T cells. Recent evidence indicates that a relatively small proportion of the HSP-PC that are internalized through the CD91 receptor enters an acidic compartment, where the peptide is loaded onto the MHC class II molecules, leading to stimulation of CD4[+] T cells.[3,52] The representation of HSP-chaperoned peptides by DCs has also been shown in the human system.[53]

Preparation of DCs

Preparations of DCs are as follows: PBMC-rich fraction is obtained usually by leukapheresis using COM TEC (Fresenius Kabi, Hamburg, Germany). However, recently we developed a new method for production of enough numbers of DCs from a small amount of PBMCs obtained by 25ml of blood sampling (see Figure 9.3). PBMCs were isolated from heparinized peripheral blood by Ficoll-Hypaque gradient density centrifugation.[54] These PBMCs are placed into 100mm plastic tissue culture plates (Becton Dickinson Labware, Franklin Lakes, NJ) in AIM-V medium (Gibco, Gaithersburg, MD). Following 30-minute incubation at 37deg C, non-adherent cells are removed and adherent cells are cultured in AIM-V medium containing granulocyte-macrophage colony stimulating factor (500ng/ml, Primmune Inc., Kobe, Japan) and IL-4 (250ng/ml, R&D Systems Inc., Minneapolis, MN), to generate immature DCs.[55] The population of adherent cells remaining in the wells is composed of 95.6 +/- 3.3% CD14[+] cells. After 5 days of cultures, the immature DCs are stimulated with OK-432 (10 μ/mL) and prostaglandin E2 (50ng/mL, Daiichi Fine Chemical Co., Ltd., Toyama, Japan) for 24 hours to induce differentiation. Then WT1, MUC1, and other OLP or proteins after mixing with HSP70 are pulsed onto the DCs in the same culture media and incubated for 24 hours. The concentrations usually used are shown in Table 9.4.

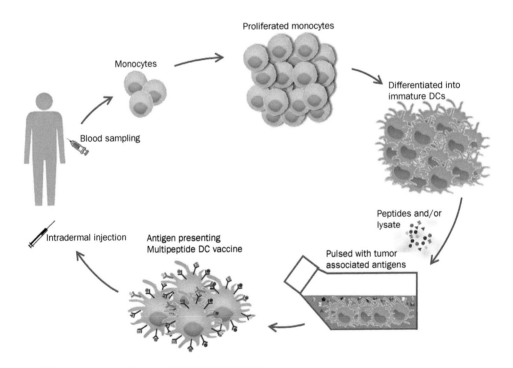

Proliferated monocytes

Monocytes

Differentiated into immature DCs

Blood sampling

Peptides and/or lysate

Intradermal injection   Antigen presenting Multipeptide DC vaccine

Pulsed with tumor associated antigens

Figure 9.3 Clinical application of multipeptide DC-based vaccine.

TABLE 9.4 CONCENTRATIONS OF PEPTIDE USING DENDRITIC CELL VACCINE

HSP70	5 μg/mL each peptide
WT1 (OLP)	1 μg/mL each peptide
MUC1, long peptide (30-mer)	20 μg/mL each peptide
NY-ESO-1 (OLP)	1 μg/mL each peptide
MAGE-A3 (OLP)	1 μg/mL each peptide
hTERT (OLP)	560 μg/mL each peptide
PHV16-E6, E7 (OLP)	20 μg/mL each peptide
CA125 protein	500 μg/mL each peptide
CEA	20 μg/mL each peptide
HER2	20 μg/mL each peptide
gp100	25 μg/mL each peptide
Survivin (OLP)	30 μg/mL each peptide
Autologous tumor lysates	50 μg/mL each peptide

NOTE: OLP = overlapped long peptide.

To prepare the autologous tumor lysates, tumor masses were obtained by surgical resection exclusion and are homogenized. Aliquots of isolated tumor cells are then lysed by 10 cycles of repeated freeze in liquid nitrogen and thaw in a 37°C water bath. The lysed cells are centrifuged at 14,000G for five minutes and supernatants are passed through a 0.22 μm filter (Millipore Corporation, Bedford, MA). Protein concentrations in the resultant cell-free lysates are determined using DC protein assay kits (Bio-Rad Laboratories, Hercules, CA). Aliquots (500μg/tube) are then cryopreserved at −135°C until use.[56]

Surface molecules are determined using flow cytometry. The cells defined as mature DCs are CD14, HLA-DR+, HLA-ABC+, CD83+, CD86+, CD40+, and CCR7+. Vaccine quality control and fluorescence-activated cell sorting (FACS) analysis are as follows: all vaccines are subjected to quality control evaluation, which involves assessing the total number of live DCs, monocyte-derived DC characteristics, and percentage of viable cells. For vaccines to be deemed "adequate" >1×10^7 viable DCs are required. Usually, fresh DC vaccines are injected intradermally to the patients within four hours. If needed, cryopreservation of DC vaccines is performed. The frozen DC cells are allowed to thaw quickly in a 37°C water bath and are retrieved from the cryopreservation tube by rinsing with 0.02% albumin-containing FACS buffer cell Wash™ (Bioscience, San Hose, CA). The FACS analysis is performed for cell surface antigen detection. FITC-labeled anti-human CD14, CD40, CD80, HLA-A, B, C, PE-labeled anti-human CD11C, CD83, CD197 (CCR7+), HLA-DR, and the FACS Calibur flow cytometer were used from DC Biosciences (Franklin Lakes, NJ).

Role of Natural Killer Cell in Hybrid Immunotherapy

NK cells are present in the peripheral blood and number approximately 10% to 15% in the lymphocyte fraction. NK cells are the most important innate immune cell because of their ability to directly kill target cells as well as produce immunoregulatory cytokines. NK cells are defined by the surface expression of CD56, a neural cell adhesion molecule that lacks the T cell antigen CD3.[57] The function of NK cells are direct cytotoxic activity against virus-infected cells and tumor cells.[58] There are two distinct subsets of human NK cells based on the density of surface CD56 expression. Approximately 90% of human NK cells are CD 56^dim and have high-density expression of CD16; others are CD56^bright and CD16^dim/neg. The CD56^bright and CD56^dim NK cell subsets show an important difference in cytotoxic potential, capacity for cytokine production, and response to cytokine activation (see Table 9.5).[59,60]

NK cells can mediate antibody-dependent cellular cytotoxicity (ADCC) through membrane FcγRIII (CD16) expressed on the majority of NK cells. CD56^dim NK cells are more cytotoxic against

TABLE 9.5 FUNCTIONAL DIFFERENCES IN NK CELL SUBSETS

	CD56[bright]	CD56[dim]
NK receptors		
FcγRIII (CD16)	-/+	+ + +
KIR	-/+	+ + +
CD94/NKG2	+	-/+
Cytokine receptors		
IL-2Rαβγ	+ +	-
IL-2Rβγ	+ +	+ +
CCR7	+ +	-
Adhesion molecules	+ +	-/+
Effector functions		
ADCC	-/+	+ + +
Natural cytotoxicity	-/+	+ + +
Cytokine production	+ + +	-/+

NOTE: NK = natural killer; KIR=killer immunoglobulin-like receptor; IL=interleukin; ADCC=antibody-dependent cellular cytotoxicity.

Reprinted with permission from Farag SS, VanDeusen JB, Fehniger TA, Caligiuri MA. Biology and clinical impact of human natural killer cells. *Int J Hematol.* 2003;78(1):7–17.

NK-sensitive targets than CD56[bright] NK cells and respond to IL-2 with increased cytotoxicity. It is of clinical importance to know that CD56[bright] cells, after activation with IL-2, can exhibit similar or enhanced cytotoxicity against NK targets compared with CD56[dim] cells.[61-63] In addition, more than 95% of all CD56[dim] NK cells express CD16 (FcγRIII) and are capable of ADCC. On the other hand, 50% to 70% of CD56[bright] NK cells lack expression of CD16 or have only low-density expression of CD16 and therefore function minimally in ADCC.

It is well known that MHC class I molecules are critical for the inhibition of NK cell-mediated lysis of normal autologous cells.[64,65]

NK cells selectively lyse autologous cell that have lost MHC class I self-expression.[66]

In humans, two families of paired inhibitory and activating NK receptors have been identified, killer immunoglobulin-like receptor (KIR) family and the heterodimeric CD94/NKG2 C-type lectin family. In this text, these receptors are not discussed in order to simplify the clinical application of NK cell therapy. Although the activating KIR and CD95/NKG2 receptors are important in mediating NK cytotoxicity, natural cytotoxicity receptors and the homodimeric NKG 2D receptors may be important in mediating cytotoxicity against abnormal, MHC class I-deficient, or class I-negative targets. This biological information will result in the clinical application of NK cell-based therapies for cancer. As shown in Table 9.6, the incidence of MHC class I deficient or negative cancer cells are different in primary cancer or metastatic lesions. Because of the heterogeneity of cancer cells, it is insufficient to kill all cancer cells by CTLs, which are activated by a DC-based antigen targeted vaccine; it is necessary to also utilize NK cells to avoid immune escape of the MHC class I deficient cancer cells (Table 9.6).

Role of Immune Checkpoint Inhibitor

Disappointing results that we sometimes encounter with DC-based vaccine therapy are likely due to inherent tumor-induced immune suppression and enhanced immunologic tolerance. As pointed out by Postow,[67] current research directed toward understanding the mechanisms of immunologic tolerance has led to the development of promising therapeutic immune regulatory antibodies that inhibit immunologic checkpoints such as CTLA-4 blocking antibodies and anti-PD-1 or anti-PD-1 ligand (PD-L1) antibodies. Immunotherapeutic modalities, aimed at manipulating these immunologic checkpoints, are now proving indispensable in the field of cancer immunotherapy. Among them, PD-1 is the most interesting inhibitory receptor

TABLE 9.6 INCIDENCE OF MHC CLASS I DEFICIENT OR NEGATIVE CANCER CELLS

Tumor	Primary Cancer (%)	Metastatic Lesions (%)
Melanoma	16	58
Colon cancer	32	72
Osteosarcoma	52	88
Lung cancer	38	
Breast cancer	81	
Pancreatic cancer	76	
Prostate cancer	74	
Ovarian cancer	37	
Uterine cervical cancer	90	

NOTE: MHC = major histocompatibility complex.

Reprinted with permission from Abe H, Akiyama S, Okamoto M. Clinical Cancer Immunotherapy: Molecular Targeting Immunotherapy. *J Integ Med.* 2008;1(1):38–46.

and promising therapeutic target. PD-1 is expressed on T cells, B cells, and myeloid cells after activation,[68] and its ligands PD-1 and PD-L1 are expressed on APCs, tumor cells, and other cells found in the inflammatory microenvironment.[69] Interaction between PD-L1 and PD-1 appears to contribute to tumor-induced immune suppression through multiple immunosuppressive pathways, including induction T-cell death and enhancement of resistance of tumor cells to T-cell mediated apoptosis.[70,71] High levels of PD-L1 correlate with poor clinical outcomes in a variety of tumors including pancreatic,[72] ovarian,[73] renal,[74] urothelial,[75] gastric,[76] head and neck,[77] and melanoma.[78] Results from the trials of the several PD-1 inhibitory antibodies suggest these antibodies are well tolerated and can result in disease response in patients with solid tumors. A Phase II trial of 21 patients with treatment refractory metastatic non-small cell lung cancer, renal cell carcinoma, melanoma, or prostate cancer shows treatment with MDX1106 (later BMS-936558, Bristol-Myers Squibb, Princeton, NJ) demonstrated efficacy in patients with renal cell carcinoma and melanoma without serious toxicity.[79,80] Recently, Hamanishi and his associates reported the first trial for clinical application of anti-PD-1-antibody (nivolumab) in patients with platinum-resistant ovarian cancer at the 2014 ASCO annual meeting. Fifteen patients were treated with nivolumab (1mg/kg n = 10, 3mg/kg n = 5) and evaluated. Nivolumab at 1mg/kg was well tolerated and has encouraging clinical efficacy; a 3mg/kg cohort is now under investigation.[81] In addition to immune regulatory antibodies directly targeting PD-1, an alternative strategy has involved targeting PD-L1.[67] Research involving a preclinical murine model of leukemia has shown that an anti-PD-L1 antibody resulted in decreased tumor burden and prolonged survival.[82] Thus, PD-1 inhibitory antibodies and/or PD-L1 inhibitory antibodies will be an ideal tool in combination therapy with a DC-based vaccine (see Figure 9.4).

Role of Hyperthermia in DC-Vaccine Therapy

Hyperthermia is widely used to enhance the efficacy of chemotherapy or radiation in patients with inoperable cancer.[83] It has been given much attention for the cellular response to heat stress with respect to the immune system in cancer. The anti-tumor immune response can be markedly enhanced by treatment with hyperthermia particularly in the fever range.[84] Immunological effects of mild hyperthermia are twofold. One is the effect on dendritic and other immune cells.[85] The other is the effect on tumor cells. Protein or peptides derived from cancer which are chaperoned by heat shock protein (HSP) are possible sources of antigens, transferred to antigen-presenting cells for priming CD8+ T-cell responses.[86] Human tumor-derived HSP70 peptide complexes (HSP70-PC) have the immunogenic potential to instruct DCs and cross-present endogenously expressed, nonmutated, tumor antigenic peptides. The

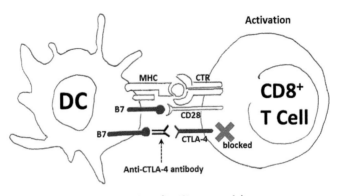

Anti-CTLA-4 (Ipilimumab)

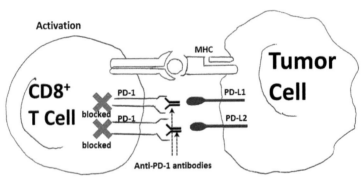

Anti-PD-1 (Nivolumab)

Figure 9.4 Block of immune inhibitory signal by antibodies.

cross-presentation of a shared human tumor antigen together with its exquisite efficacy is an important new aspect for HSP70-based immunotherapy in clinical anticancer vaccination strategies and suggests a potential extension of HSP70-based vaccination protocols from a patient-individual treatment modality to its use in an allogeneic setting.[30] Other studies support various clinical uses of hyperthermia as part of an immunotherapeutic strategy in treating cancer.[84,87]

The mechanisms by which a tumor cell can escape CTL is critical for the design and modification for effective vaccine strategies against cancer. These mechanisms fall into four broad categories: (a) inadequate antigen presentation by tumor cells resulting in their poor sensitivity to lysis by CTL, (b) inhibitory signals provided by the tumor microenvironment, (c) inability of TAA-specific CTL to localize at a tumor site, and (d) inability of the tumor microenvironment to sustain T-cell function in vivo.[88] Therefore, adequate antigen expression by tumor cells is of crucial importance. Many research papers show the possible augmentation of MHC class I antigen presentation via HSP expression by hyperthermia. It has been demonstrated that the cell surface presentation of MHC class I antigen is increased in tandem with increased HSP70.[89] It is clear that mild hyperthermia enhances both the expression of TAA on the surface of tumors and also increased presentation of TAA chaperoned by HSP on the DC. These findings are encouraging for the usage of hyperthermia at the time of DC-based vaccination.

CLINICAL APPLICATION OF DC-BASED VACCINE LOADED HSP70-PC

DC-based HSP70-PC vaccines are applicable to any patient with any type of cancer, because the vaccines are customized to fit the patient as well as the cancer itself. The patient's evaluation for inclusion to this DC-based vaccine include a medical history and physical examination, performance status (PS) evaluation, serum albumin, hemoglobin, white blood cell and platelet count, blood urea nitrogen (BUN), creatinine, alkaline phosphatase, LDH, AST, ALT, bilirubin, HbA1c, tumor markers, and HLA. As image markers, computed tomography (CT) scans, magnetic resonance imaging, positron emission tomography (PET), PET-CT, as well as ultrasound studies are indicated. To be eligible to DC-based vaccine therapy, patients are required to have an ECOG PS of ≤3. They are also required to have adequate hematologic and hepatorenal functions as determined by the following parameters:

WBC counts of ≥2,500/μL, platelet counts of ≥80,000/μL, hemoglobin value of ≥9.0g/dL, BUN<50mg/dL, serum bilirubin level <5.0mg/dL, and AST level<500IU/L

Our immunological treatment is performed in a stepwise fashion. First, the autologous DC-based vaccine (>1×10⁷ cells) is administered intradermally at 14-day intervals, for a total of five to six times. In most of cases one to five KE doses of OK-432 (Chugai Pharmaceutical Co., Ltd., Tokyo, a streptococcus immunological adjuvant) is administered together with the DC vaccine. Second, NK cells (>1×10⁹ cells) are simultaneously injected intravenously in most patients after DC vaccine injection at 14-day intervals. Third, as combination therapy, following NK cell administration, escalating doses (0.1~1mg/kg) of anti-PD-1 antibody OPDIVO (nivolumab) are administered by intravenous drip infusion. Clinical response is evaluated according to the Response Evaluation Criteria in Solid Tumors version 1.0 as follows: complete remission (CR), partial remission (PR), stable disease (SD), and progressive disease (PD). Adverse events are evaluated by grading the toxicity according to the National Cancer Institute Common Terminology Criteria for Adverse Events (CTCAE) version 4.0. Our experience with previous series of studies was that patients with advanced cancer such as breast, lung, pancreatic, and colorectal cancer that were refractory to standard therapy were treated with DC-based vaccine.[90] The most important factor for prolonged survival was good PS before entry into DC-based vaccine treatment. Patients in the better PS group had a significantly longer survival time compared to those in the poorer group. The overall survival based on our risk score was significantly better for patients with clinical response of CR, PR, and SD compared to those with a response of PD group. Therapy was well tolerated during treatment and for three months after the final treatment. None of the patients experienced adverse events of grade 3 or higher during the treatment period. Grade 1 to 2 fevers and grade 1 injection site reactions, consisting of erythema, induration, and tenderness lasting one to five days after injection occurred in most patients and did not result in any dosage modifications or delayed treatments. No signs of autoimmune disease (arthritis, rash, colitis, etc.) were observed either during or after therapy. Included are the results of our retrospective study of the DC-based vaccine in ovarian cancer treated in our clinic. All patients had prior surgical resection with chemotherapy, then were noted to have peritoneal dissemination or recurrence of tumors. Twelve patients with stage IV or IIIc ovarian cancer were entered in this study. Ages ranged between 15 years old and 79 years old with a mean of 57.9 years (see Table 9.7).

Among these patients, the longest survival at this study point (as of May 31, 2015) is 1,329 days after the first injection of DC-based vaccine. Kaplan-Meier plots of overall survival of this group are shown in Figure 9.5. As discussed, the factor for

Case	Age	Stage	Pathology	PS	Prev.Chemo	IX	Peptide	Survival (days)
1	60	IV	Carcinosarcoma	1	TC	DC+NK	W, M, C	201
2	56	IV	Unknown	0	Unknown	DC	W, M, C	420
3	57	IV	Mucinous	2	TC	DC	W, M, C	120
4	56	IV	Clear cell	2	TC	DC+NK	W, M, C, CEA	120
5	56	IV	Clear cell	0	TC	DC	W, M, C	1,329 alive (PS:0)
6	41	IV	Mucinous	1	TC	DC	W, M, C	210
7	65	IV	Unknown	0	TC	DC	W, M, C	760 alive (PS:0)
8	77	IV	Adenocarcinoma	1	TC	DC+NK	W, M, C, Survivin	180
9	79	IIIc	Serous	1	TC	DC+NK	W, M	507 alive (PS:0)
10	59	IV	Unknown	2	TC	DC	W, M, C	263
11	15	IV	Yolk sac tumor	1	ETP+ CBDCA	DC+NK +PD-1	W, M, C, NY, hT	100 alive (PS:1)
12	74	IIIc	Serous	1	DC	DC+NK	W, M, C, NY, hT	87 alive (PS:1)

NOTE: TC = paclitaxel and carboplatin; DC = decetaxel and carboplatin; IX = immunotherapy; DC = dendritic cell-based vaccine; NK = activated natural killer cell; PD-1 = anti PD-1 antibodies; W = WT1; M = MUC1; C = CA125; NY = NY-ESO-1; hT = hTERT; PS = The Eastern Cooperative Oncology Group (ECOG) Scale of Performance Status. PS:0 = Fully active, able to carry on all pre-disease performance without restriction; PS:1 = Restricted in physically strenuous activity but ambulatory and able to carry out work of a light or sedentary nature, e.g., light house work, office work; PS:2 = Ambulatory and capable of all selfcare but unable to carry out any work activities; up and about more than 50% of waking hours.

prolonged survival is good PS (0 or 1) before entry into DC vaccine treatment. Severe adverse events of more than grade 2 were not observed, assessing the toxicity analysis by CTCAE. After DC-based vaccine injection, survival time was markedly prolonged. As severe side effects of more than grade 2 were not observed, it was strongly suggested that the DC-based vaccine pulsed with HSP-PC especially in combination with immune checkpoint inhibitors was safe and effective in patients with end-stage ovarian cancer refractory to standard treatment.

DISCUSSION AND CONCLUSION

DC-based vaccine immunotherapy has been a focus of promising strategies for cancer treatment. Currently the scope of cancer immunotherapy is limited because most targeted antigens are restricted to a subset of patients. However, long synthetic peptides of 25 to 50 mer have the advantage of potentially inducing broad immunity with both CD8[+] T-cell and CD4[+] T-cell responses against multiple epitopes.[91] It has been reported that vaccination of subjects suffering from recurrent ovarian cancer with long peptides covering p53 led to the expansion of p53-specific CD4[+] T cells in blood and tumors.[92] Application of HSP70 as chaperones of antigenic peptides may have a direct bearing on the DCs, and HSP70-PCs are taken by DCs' CD91 receptor through endocytosis. Molecular target DC-based vaccines evoke the power of each patient's immune system to help prevent recurrence and increase the long-term survival rate. If the patient's resected tumor is available,

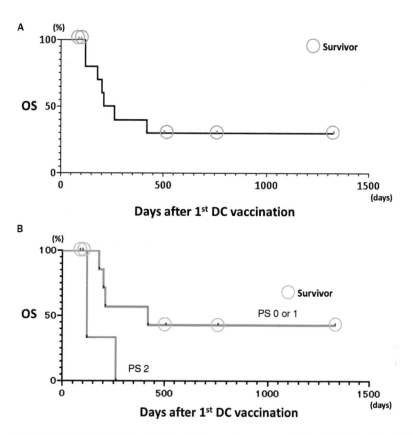

Figure 9.5 (A) Kaplan-Meier plots of overall survival of end-stage ovarian cancer patients after DC vaccine. (B) Kaplan-Meier plots of overall survival of end-stage ovarian cancer patients after DC vaccine according to performance status.

lysate is used as a molecular antigen. Using this lysate, the vaccine induces an immune response against cancerous cells and creates immunologic memory. Because it is derived from the individual patient's tumor cells, this vaccine is a true targeted and personalized cancer therapy. When a patient's own tumor cells are not available, integrating several candidates of peptides such as WT1, MUC1, CEA, CA125, NY-ESO-1, hTERT, Her2, and so on can be used for the design of an anti-tumor vaccine which is restricted to the patient's HLA typing. A multicancer clinical study of 60 advanced-cancer patients who were previously treated with conventional therapy followed by mulitpeptide immunotherapy or no therapy showed that patients undergoing immunotherapy had significantly higher PFS rates. Especially patients with peptide-specific CTL responses confirmed by ELISpot assay had better overall survival rates.[93] Moreover, Hazama and his associates[94] reported that patient survival significantly improved when three or more peptides were used. It is rational to pulse multiple peptides on DCs for a better response to the DC vaccine. Among these antigens, it is known that WT1 and MUC1 are the most important antigens expressed and are also present in cancer stem cells. Cancer stem cells form new tumors and may not be eliminated by chemotherapy or radiation. This has changed the perspective with regard to new approaches for treating cancer. Cancer stem cells are slow-dividing and inherently chemotherapy resistant. Eradication of these cancer stem cells may be necessary for the long-term success in cancer treatment. Using this strategy, a DC-based vaccine pulsed with WT1 and MUC1 and other specific antigens would possibly eliminate cancer stem cells in some patients.

Hyperthermia is often used to activate the immune system. There is evidence that when DCs take up HSPs together with the peptide they chaperone, the accompanying peptides are delivered into the antigen-processing pathways, leading to peptide presentation by MHC molecules. When DCs travel to the lymph nodes, T cells recognize the antigenic peptides and are specifically activated against cancer cells bearing these peptides.

The challenge for next-generation vaccines is to resolve the discrepancy between the immune and clinical efficacy measured by the rate of cancer rejection.[44] CD4+ T cells regulate CD8+ T cell immunity in both the priming and the effector phases. Thereby, Treg cells can inhibit the effector functions of CD8+ T cells but also prevent tumor rejection. However, Treg cells also play a critical role during the priming by promoting the selection of high-avidity CD8+ cells.[95] Although they mostly help tumor rejection, Th1 cells might contribute to tumor escape via secretion of interferon-gamma (IFN-γ) that triggers expression of PD-L1 in tissues, thus providing an off signal to effector CD8+ T cells.[96] IL-17 can synergize with IFN-γ to induce tumor cells to secrete CXCL9 and CXCL10, which attract cytotoxic CD8+ T cells.[97] This knowledge can be applied to the design of next-generation vaccines for directing the differentiation of antigen-specific CD4+ T cell to the desired phenotype and function.[44] Once elicited, CD8+ T cell must confront numerous barriers, including (a) intrinsic regulators, such as CD28-CTLA-4, PD-1-PD-L1, and ILTs,[98] and extrinsic regulators such as Treg cells[99] or myeloid-derived suppressor cells (MDSCs);[100] (b) a corrupted tumor microenvironment with pro-tumor inflammation;[101,102] (c) antigen loss and immune evasion of tumor targets;[102] and (d) tissue-specific alterations, such as fatty cells in breast cancer or desmofibrosis in pancreatic cancer stroma (see Box 9.1). Defining strategies for bypassing these obstacles is the object of intense studies to improve the clinical efficacy of vaccination via DCs. A logical approach to addressing

these issues is the combination of DC-based vaccine candidates and agents that target different pathways.[44] For example, checkpoint inhibitors such as antagonists to CTLA-4 or PD-1 might offset inhibitor signals.[103] The combination of GVAX and CTLA-4 antibody (ipilimumab) has shown to be safe,[104] and preclinical models show increased effector CD8+ T cells and enhanced tumor-antigen-directed CTL function.[105]

Given the wide interest for targeted vaccine intervention in treating miscellaneous cancers, our previous findings may help in guiding and designing future trials and the development of novel cancer treatment strategies. As Palucka and Banchereau stated, the considerable progress made in the understanding of the biology of DCs and effector and Treg cells has opened avenues for the development of new vaccine strategies. At present, we are proposing new combination therapy protocols for supporting hybrid immunotherapy (DC-based vaccine with NK cells), which include (a) low dose

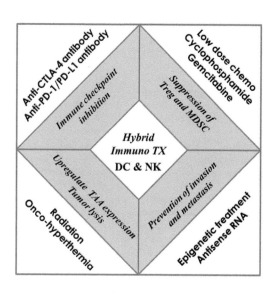

Figure 9.6 Combination therapy in the era of new immunological treatment.

of cyclophosphamide or gemcitabine against Treg or MDSC, (b) use of anti PD-1/PD-L1 antibodies or anti CTLA-4 antibodies as immune checkpoint inhibitors, (c) onco-hyperthermia or radiation therapy to enhance antigen display on the tumor cell surface, and (d) antisense RNA as epigenetic therapy. Novel protocols will be tailored to individual-specific mutations[106] and immune alterations (see Figure 9.6). As more is elucidated, we can look forward with optimism that immunotherapy will play a key role in the future of effective cancer treatments and eradication.

REFERENCES

1. Liu B, Nash J, Runowicz C, Swede H, Stevens R, Li Z. Ovarian cancer immunotherapy: opportunities, progress and challenges. *J Hematol Oncol.* 2013;3:7. doi:10.1186/1756-8722-3-7
2. Howlader N, Noone AM, Krapcho M, et al. SEER Cancer Statistics Review, 1975–2012. Bethesda, MD: National Cancer Institute, April 2015. http://seer.cancer.gov/csr/1975_2012/
3. Srivastava P. Roles of heat-shock proteins in innate and adaptive immunity. *Nat Rev Immunol.* 2002;2(3):185–94.
4. Schmitt E, Gehrmann M, Brunet M, Multhoff G, Garrido C. Intracellular and extracellular functions of heat shock proteins: repercussions in cancer therapy. *J Leukoc Biol.* 2007;81(1):15–27.
5. Cohen M, Dromard M, Petignat P. Heat shock proteins in ovarian cancer: a potential target for therapy. *Gynecol Oncol.* 2010;119(1):164–66. doi:10.1016/j.ygyno.2010.05.027
6. Ciocca DR, Calderwood SK. Heat shock proteins in cancer: diagnostic, prognostic, predictive, and treatment implications. *Cell Stress Chaperones.* 2005;10(2):86–103.
7. Wu T, Tanguay RM. Antibodies against heat shock proteins in environmental stresses and diseases: friend or foe? *Cell Stress Chaperones.* 2006;11(1):1–12. doi:10.1379/CSC-155R.1
8. Korneeva I, Bongiovanni AM, Girotra M, Caputo TA, Witkin SS. IgA antibodies to the 27-kDa heat-shock protein in the genital tracts of women with gynecologic cancers. *Int J Cancer.* 2000;87(6):824–28.
9. Anderson KS, LaBaer J. The sentinel within: exploiting the immune system for cancer biomarkers. *J Proteome Res.* 2005;4(4):1123–33.
10. Nesterova M, Johnson C, Cheadle C, Cho-Chung YS. Autoantibody biomarker opens a new gateway for cancer diagnosis. *Biochim Biophys Acta.* 2006;1762(4):398–403.
11. Luborsky JL, Barua A, Shatavi SV, Kebede T, Abramowicz J, Rotmensch J. Anti-tumor antibodies in ovarian cancer. *Am J Reprod Immunol.* 2005;54(2):55–62.
12. Elpek GO, Karaveli S, Şimşek T, Keles N, Aksoy NH. Expression of heat-shock proteins hsp27, hsp70 and hsp90 in malignant epithelial tumour of the ovaries. *APMIS.* 2003;111(4):523–30.
13. Bodzek P, Partyka R, Damasiewicz-Bodzek A. Antibodies against Hsp60 and HSP65 in the sera of women with ovarian cancer. *J Ovarian Res.* 2014;7:30. doi:10.1186/1757-2215-7-30
14. Schmitt E, Gehrmann M, Brunet M, Multhoff G, Garrido C. Intracellular and extracellular functions of heat shock proteins: repercussions in cancer therapy. *J Leukoc Biol.* 2007;81(1):15–27.

15. Broquet AH, Thomas G, Masliah J, Trugnan G, Bachelet M. Expression of the molecular chaperone Hsp70 in detergent-resistant microdomains correlates with its membrane delivery and release. *J Biol Chem.* 2003;278(24):21601–606.

16. Lancaster GI, Febbraio MA. Exosome-dependent trafficking of HSP70: a novel secretory pathway for cellular stress proteins. *J Biol Chem.* 2005;280(24):23349–55.

17. Becker T, Hartl FU, Wieland F. CD40, an extracellular receptor for binding and uptake of Hsp70-peptide complexes. *J Cell Biol.* 2002;158(7):1277–85.

18. Singh-Jasuja H, Toes RE, Spee P, et al. Cross-presentation of glycoprotein 96-associated antigens on major histocompatibility complex class I molecules requires receptor-mediated endocytosis. *J Exp Med.* 2000;191(11):1965–74.

19. Vlassov AV, Magdaleno S, Setterquist R, Conrad R. Exosomes: current knowledge of their composition, biological functions, and diagnostic and therapeutic potentials. *Biochim Biophys Acta.* 2012;1820(7):940–48. doi:10.1016/j.bbagen.2012.03.017

20. Campanella C, Bavisotto CC, Gammazza AM, et al. Exosomal heat shock proteins as new players in tumour cell-to-cell communication. *J Circ Biomark.* 2014, 3:4. doi:10.5772/58721

21. Bausero MA, Gastpar R, Multhoff G, Asea A. Alternative mechanism by which IFN-gamma enhances tumor recognition: active release of heat shock protein 72. *J Immunol.* 2005;175(5):2900–12.

22. Vega VL, Rodríguez-Silva M, Frey T, et al. Hsp70 translocates into the plasma membrane after stress and is released into the extracellular environment in a membrane-associated form that activates macrophages. *J Immunol.* 2008;180(6):4299–307.

23. Gastpar R, Gehrmann M, Bausero MA, et al. Heat shock protein 70 surface-positive tumor exosomes stimulate migratory and cytolytic activity of natural killer cells. *Cancer Res.* 2005;65(12):5238–47.

24. Elsner L, Muppala V, Gehrmann M, et al. The heat shock protein HSP70 promotes mouse NK cell activity against tumors that express inducible NKG2D ligands. *J Immunol.* 2007;179(8):5523–33.

25. Radons J, Multhoff G. Immunostimulatory functions of membrane-bound and exported heat shock protein 70. *Exerc Immunol Rev.* 2005;11:17–33.

26. Xiao W, Dong W, Zhang C, et al. Effects of the epigenetic drug MS-275 on the release and function of exosome-related immune molecules in hepatocellular carcinoma cells. *Eur J Med Res.* 2013;18:61. doi:10.1186/2047-783X-18-61

27. Suto R, Srivastava PK. A mechanism for the specific immunogenicity of heat shock protein-chaperoned peptides. *Science.* 1995;269(5230):1585–88.

28. Janetzki S, Palla D, Rosenhauer V, Lochs H, Lewis JJ, Srivastava PK. Immunization of cancer patients with autologous cancer-derived heat shock protein gp96 preparations: a pilot study. *Int J Cancer.* 2000;88(2):232–38.

29. Bukau B, Horwich AL. The Hsp70 and Hsp60 chaperone machines. *Cell.* 1998;92(3):351–66.

30. Noessner E, Gastpar R, Milani V, et al. Tumor-derived heat shock protein 70 peptide complexes are cross-presented by human dendritic cells. *J Immunol.* 2002;169(10):5424–32.

31. Srivastava PK, Amato RJ. Heat shock proteins: the "Swiss Army Knife" vaccines against cancers and infectious agents. *Vaccine.* 2001;19(17–19):2590–97.

32. Weng D, Calderwood SK, Gong J. Preparation of a heat-shock protein 70-based vaccine from DC-tumor fusion cells. *Methods Mol Biol.* 2011;787:255–65. doi:10.1007/978-1-61779-295-3_19

33. Koido S, Ohana M, Liu C, et al. Dendritic cells fused with human cancer cells: morphology, antigen expression, and T cell stimulation. *Clin Immunol.* 2004;113(3):261–69.

34. Wang J, Saffold S, Cao X, Krauss J, Chen W. Eliciting T cell immunity against poorly immunogenic tumors by immunization with dendritic cell-tumor fusion vaccines. *J Immunol.* 1998;161(10):5516–24.

35. Enomoto Y, Bharti A, Khaleque AA, et al. Enhanced immunogenicity of heat shock protein 70 peptide complexes from dendritic cell-tumor fusion cells. *J Immunol.* 2006;177(9):5946–55.

36. Belli F, Testori A, Rivoltini L, et al. Vaccination of metastatic melanoma patients with autologous tumor-derived heat shock protein gp96-peptide complexes: clinical and immunologic findings. *J Clin Oncol.* 2002;20(20):4169–80.

37. Mazzaferro V, Coppa J, Carrabba MG, et al. Vaccination with autologous tumor-derived heat-shock protein gp96 after liver resection for metastatic colorectal cancer. *Clin Cancer Res.* 2003;9(9):3235–45.

38. Cannon MJ, Goyne HE, Stone PJ, et al. Modulation of p38 MAPK signaling enhances dendritic cell activation of human CD4+ Th17 responses to ovarian tumor antigen. *Cancer Immunol Immunother.* 2013;62(5):839–49. doi:10.1007/s00262-013-1391-0

39. Tanimoto H, Yan Y, Clarke J, et al. Hepsin, a cell surface serine protease identified in hepatoma cells, is overexpressed in ovarian cancer. *Cancer Res.* 1997;57(14):2884–87.

40. Jackson AM, Mulcahy LA, Zhu XW, O'Donnell D, Patel PM. Tumour-mediated disruption of dendritic cell function: inhibiting the MEK1/2-p44/42 axis restores IL-12 production and Th1-generation. *Int J Cancer.* 2008;123(3):623–32. doi:10.1002/ijc.23530

41. Gray HJ, Gargosky SE, CAN-003 Study Team. Progression-free survival in ovarian cancer patients in second remission with mucin-1 autologous dendritic cell therapy. *J Clin Oncol.* 2014;32(5 Suppl.): Abstract 5504.

42. Sabbatini P, Tsuji T, Ferran L, et al. Phase I trial of overlapping long peptides from a tumor self-antigen and poly-ICLC shows rapid induction of integrated immune response in ovarian cancer patients. *Clin*

Cancer Res. 2012;18(23):6497–508. doi:10.1158/1078-0432.CCR-12-2189

43. Mellman I, Steinman RM. Dendritic cells: specialized and regulated antigen processing machines. *Cell.* 2001;106(3):255–58.

44. Palucka K, Banchereau J. Dendritic-cell-based therapeutic cancer vaccines. *Immunity* 2013:39(1):38–48. doi:10.1016/j.immuni.2013.07.004

45. Banchereau J, Palucka AK. Dendritic cells as therapeutic vaccines against cancer. *Nat Rev Immunol.* 2005;5(4):296–306.

46. Cheever MA, Allison JP, Ferris AS, et al. The prioritization of cancer antigens: a National Cancer Institute pilot project for the acceleration of translational research. *Clin Cancer Res.* 2009;15(17):5323–37. doi:10.1158/1078-0432.CCR-09-0737

47. Akiyama S, Abe H. Successful treatment by hybrid immune therapy and high dose vitamin C therapy against hepatocellular carcinoma. *Int J Integ Med.* 2011;3:147–51.

48. Melief CJ, van der Burg SH. Immunotherapy of established (pre)malignant disease by synthetic long peptide vaccines. *Nat Rev Cancer.* 2008;8(5):351–60. doi:10.1038/nrc2373

49. Odunsi K, Qian F, Matsuzaki J, et al. Vaccination with an NY-ESO-1 peptide of HLA class I/II specificities induces integrated humoral and T cell responses in ovarian cancer. *Proc Natl Acad Sci U S A.* 2007;104(31):12837–42.

50. Binder RJ, Han DK, Srivastava PK. CD91: a receptor for heat shock protein gp96. *Nat Immunol.* 2000;1(2):151–55.

51. Basu S, Binder RJ, Ramalingam T, Srivastava PK. CD91 is a common receptor for heat shock proteins gp96, hsp90, hsp70, and calreticulin. *Immunity.* 2001;14(3):303–13.

52. Matsutake T, Srivastava PK. CD91 is involved in MHC class II presentation of gp96-chaperoned peptides. *Cell Stress Chaperones.* 2000;5:378.

53. Castelli C, Ciupitu AM, Rini F, et al. Human heat shock protein 70 peptide complexes specifically activate antimelanoma T cells. *Cancer Res.* 2001;61(1):222–27.

54. Böyum A. Isolation of mononuclear cells and granulocytes from human blood. Isolation of mononuclear cells by one centrifugation, and of granulocytes by combining centrifugation and sedimentation at 1 g. *Scand J Clin Lab Invest Suppl.* 1968;97:77–89.

55. Okamoto M, Furuichi S, Nishioka Y, et al. Expression of toll-like receptor 4 on dendritic cells is significant for anticancer effect of dendritic cell-based immunotherapy in combination with an active component of OK-432, a streptococcal preparation. *Cancer Res.* 2004;64(15):5461–70.

56. Nagayama H, Sato K, Morishita M, et al. Results of a phase I clinical study using autologous tumour lysate-pulsed monocyte-derived mature dendritic cell vaccinations for stage IV malignant melanoma

patients combined with low dose interleukin-2. *Melanoma Res.* 2003;13(5):521–30.

57. Melder RJ, Whiteside TL, Vujanovic NL, Hiserodt JC, Herberman RB. A new approach to generating antitumor effectors for adoptive immunotherapy using human adherent lymphokine-activated killer cells. *Cancer Res.* 1988;48(12):3461–69.

58. Farag SS, VanDeusen JB, Fehniger TA, Caligiuri MA. Biology and clinical impact of human natural killer cells. *Int J Hematol.* 2003;78(1):7–17.

59. Nagler A, Lanier LL, Cwirla S, Phillips JH. Comparative studies of human FcRIII-positive and negative natural killer cells. *J Immunol.* 1989;143(10):3183–891.

60. Miller JS, Oelkers S, Verfaillie C, McGlave P. Role of monocytes in the expansion of human activated natural killer cells. *Blood.* 1992;80(9):2221–29.

61. Baume DM, Caligiuri MA, Manley TJ, Daley JF, Ritz J. Differential expression of CD8 alpha and CD8 beta associated with MHC-restricted and non-MHC-restricted cytolytic effector cells. *Cell Immunol.* 1990;131(2):352-65.

62. Rabinowich H, Pricop L, Herberman RB, Whiteside TL. Expression and function of CD7 molecule on human natural killer cells. *J Immunol.* 1994;152(2):517–26.

63. Lee DM, Patel DD, Pendergast AM, Haynes BF. Functional association of CD7 with phosphatidylinositol 3-kinase: interaction via a YEDM motif. *Int Immunol.* 1996;8(8):1195–203.

64. Keever CA, Pekle K, Gazzola MV, Collins NH, Gillio A. NK and LAK activities from human marrow progenitors. I. The effects of interleukin-2 and interleukin-1. *Cell Immunol.* 1990;126(1):211–26.

65. Trinchieri G, Matsumoto-Kobayashi M, Clark SC, Seehra J, London L, Perussia B. Response of resting human peripheral blood natural killer cells to interleukin 2. *J Exp Med.* 1984;160(4):1147–69.

66. Baume DM, Robertson MJ, Levine H, Manley TJ, Schow PW, Ritz J. Differential responses to interleukin 2 define functionally distinct subsets of human natural killer cells. *Eur J Immunol.* 1992;22(1):1–6.

67. Postow M, Callahan MK, Wolchok JD. Beyond cancer vaccines: a reason for future optimism with immunomodulatory therapy. *Cancer J.* 2011;17(5):372–78. doi:10.1097/PPO.0b013e31823261db

68. Freeman GJ, Long AJ, Iwai Y, Bourque K, et al. Engagement of the PD-1 immunoinhibitory receptor by a novel B7 family member leads to negative regulation of lymphocyte activation. *J Exp Med.* 2000;192(7):1027–34.

69. Hirano F, Kaneko K, Tamura H, et al. Blockade of B7-H1 and PD-1 by monoclonal antibodies potentiates cancer therapeutic immunity. *Cancer Res.* 2005;65(3):1089–96.

70. Dong H, Strome SE, Salomao DR, et al. Tumor-associated B7-H1 promotes T-cell apoptosis: a

potential mechanism of immune evasion. *Nat Med.* 2002;8(8):793–800.

71. Azuma T, Yao S, Zhu G, Flies AS, Flies SJ, Chen L. B7-H1 is a ubiquitous antiapoptotic receptor on cancer cells. *Blood.* 2008;111(7):3635–43. doi:10.1182/blood-2007-11-123141

72. Nomi T, Sho M, Akahori T, et al. Clinical significance and therapeutic potential of the programmed death-1 ligand/programmed death-1 pathway in human pancreatic cancer. *Clin Cancer Res.* 2007;13(7):2151–57.

73. Hamanishi J, Mandai M, Iwasaki M, et al. Programmed cell death 1 ligand 1 and tumor-infiltrating CD8+ T lymphocytes are prognostic factors of human ovarian cancer. *Proc Natl Acad Sci U S A.* 2007;104(9):3360–65.

74. Thompson RH, Kuntz SM, Leibovich BC, et al. Tumor B7-H1 is associated with poor prognosis in renal cell carcinoma patients with long-term follow-up. *Cancer Res.* 2006;66(7):3381–85.

75. Nakanishi J, Wada Y, Matsumoto K, Azuma M, Kikuchi K, Ueda S. Overexpression of B7-H1 (PD-L1) significantly associates with tumor grade and postoperative prognosis in human urothelial cancers. *Cancer Immunol Immunother.* 2007;56(8):1173–82.

76. Wu C, Zhu Y, Jiang J, Zhao J, Zhang XG, Xu N. Immunohistochemical localization of programmed death-1 ligand-1 (PD-L1) in gastric carcinoma and its clinical significance. *Acta Histochem.* 2006;108(1):19–24.

77. Hsu MC, Hsiao JR, Chang KC, et al. Increase of programmed death-1-expressing intratumoral CD8 T cells predicts a poor prognosis for nasopharyngeal carcinoma. *Mod Pathol.* 2010;23(10):1393–403. doi:10.1038/modpathol.2010.130

78. Hino R, Kabashima K, Kato Y, et al. Tumor cell expression of programmed cell death-1 ligand 1 is a prognostic factor for malignant melanoma. *Cancer.* 2010;116(7):1757–66. doi:10.1002/cncr.24899

79. Brahmer JR, Topalian SL, Powderly J, et al. Phase II experience with MDX-1106 (Ono-4538), an anti-PD-1 monoclonal antibody, in patients with selected refractory or relapsed malignancies. *J Clin Oncol.* 2009;27(15 Suppl.):Abstract 3018.

80. Brahmer JR, Topalian S, Wollner I, et al. Safety and activity of MDX-1106 (ONO-4538), an anti-PD-1 monoclonal antibody, in patients with selected refractory or relapsed malignancies. *J Clin Oncol.* 2008;26(15 Suppl. 3006).

81. Hamanishi J, Mandai M, Ikeda T, et al. Efficacy and safety of anti-PD-1 antibody (Nivolumab: BMS-936558, ONO-4538) in patients with platinum-resistant ovarian cancer. *J Clin Oncol.* 2014;32(5 Suppl.):Abstract 5511.

82. Zhang L, Gajewski TF, Kline J. PD-1/PD-L1 interactions inhibit antitumor immune responses in a murine acute myeloid leukemia model. *Blood.* 2009;114(8):1545–52. doi:10.1182/blood-2009-03-206672

83. Feyerabend T, Wiedemann GJ, Jäger B, Vesely H, Mahlmann B, Richter E. Local hyperthermia, radiation, and chemotherapy in recurrent breast cancer is feasible and effective except for inflammatory disease. *Int J Radiat Oncol Biol Phys.* 2001;49(5):1317–25.

84. Calderwood SK, Theriault JR, Gong J. How is the immune response affected by hyperthermia and heat shock proteins? *Int J Hyperthermia.* 2005;21(8):713–16.

85. Srivastava P. Interaction of heat shock proteins with peptides and antigen presenting cells: chaperoning of the innate and adaptive immune responses. *Annu Rev Immunol.* 2002;20:395–425.

86. Binder RJ, Srivastava PK. Peptides chaperoned by heat-shock proteins are a necessary and sufficient source of antigen in the cross-priming of CD8+ T cells. *Nat Immunol.* 2005;6(6):593–99.

87. Ostberg JR, Repasky EA. Emerging evidence indicates that physiologically relevant thermal stress regulates dendritic cell function. *Cancer Immunol Immunother.* 2006;55(3):292–98.

88. Marincola FM, Jaffee EM, Hicklin DJ, Ferrone S. Escape of human solid tumors from T-cell recognition: molecular mechanisms and functional significance. *Adv Immunol.* 2000;74:181–273.

89. Ito A, Shinkai M, Honda H, Wakabayashi T, Yoshida J, Kobayashi T. Augmentation of MHC class I antigen presentation via heat shock protein expression by hyperthermia. *Cancer Immunol Immunother.* 2001;50(10):515–22.

90. Abe H, Shimamoto T, Akiyama S, Abe M. Targeted cancer therapy by dendritic cell vaccine. In: Rangel L, ed. *Cancer Treatment—Conventional and Innovative Approaches.* Rijeka, Croatia: InTech; 2013:249–317.

91. Quakkelaar ED, Melief CJ. Experience with synthetic vaccines for cancer and persistent virus infections in nonhuman primates and patients. *Adv Immunol.* 2012;114:77–106. doi:10.1016/B978-0-12-396548-6.00004-4

92. Leffers N, Lambeck AJ, Gooden MJ, et al. Immunization with a P53 synthetic long peptide vaccine induces P53-specific immune responses in ovarian cancer patients, a phase II trial. *Int J Cancer.* 2009;125(9):2104–13. doi:10.1002/ijc.24597

93. Kono K, Iinuma H, Akutsu Y, et al. Multicenter, phase II clinical trial of cancer vaccination for advanced esophageal cancer with three peptides derived from novel cancer-testis antigens. *J Transl Med.* 2012;10:141. doi:10.1186/1479-5876-10-141

94. Hazama S, Oka M, Yoshida K, et al. Phase I clinical trial of cancer vaccine with five novel epitope peptides for patients with metastatic colorectal cancer (mCRC). *J Clin Oncol.* 2011;29(Suppl.):Abstract 2510.

95. Pace L, Tempez A, Arnold-Schrauf C, et al. Regulatory T cells increase the avidity of primary CD8+ T cell responses and promote memory. *Science.* 2012;338(6106):532–36. doi:10.1126/science.1227049

96. Sharpe AH, Wherry EJ, Ahmed R, Freeman GJ. The function of programmed cell death 1 and its ligands in regulating autoimmunity and infection. *Nat Immunol.* 2007;8(3):239–45.

97. Wei S, Zhao E, Kryczek I, Zou W. Th17 cells have stem cell-like features and promote long-term immunity. *Oncoimmunology.* 2012;1(4):516–19.

98. Pardoll DM. The blockade of immune checkpoints in cancer immunotherapy. *Nat Rev Cancer.* 2012;12(4):252–64. doi:10.1038/nrc3239

99. Fehérvari Z, Sakaguchi S. CD4+ Tregs and immune control. *J Clin Invest.* 2004;114(9):1209–17.

100. Gabrilovich DI, Nagaraj S. Myeloid-derived suppressor cells as regulators of the immune system. *Nat Rev Immunol.* 2009;9(3):162–74. doi:10.1038/nri2506

101. Coussens LM, Zitvogel L, Palucka AK. Neutralizing tumor-promoting chronic inflammation: a magic bullet? *Science.* 2013;339(6117):286–91. doi:10.1126/science.1232227

102. Klebanoff CA, Acquavella N, Yu Z, Restifo NP. Therapeutic cancer vaccines: are we there yet? *Immunol Rev.* 2011;239(1):27–44. doi:10.1111/j.1600-065X.2010.00979.x

103. Chen DS, Mellman I. Oncology meets immunology: the cancer-immunity cycle. *Immunity.* 2013;39(1):1–10. doi:10.1016/j.immuni.2013.07.012

104. van den Eertwegh AJ, Versluis J, van den Berg HP, et al. Combined immunotherapy with granulocyte-macrophage colony-stimulating factor-transduced allogeneic prostate cancer cells and ipilimumab in patients with metastatic castration-resistant prostate cancer: a phase 1 dose-escalation trial. *Lancet Oncol.* 2012;13(5):509–17. doi:10.1016/S1470-2045(12)70007-4

105. Wada S, Jackson CM, Yoshimura K, et al. Sequencing CTLA-4 blockade with cell-based immunotherapy for prostate cancer. *J Transl Med.* 2013;11:89. doi:10.1186/1479-5876-11-89

106. Schreiber H, Rowley JD, Rowley DA. Targeting mutations predictably. *Blood.* 2011;118(4):830–31. doi:10.1182/blood-2011-06-357541

10.

PD-1/PDL-1 INHIBITORS AS IMMUNOTHERAPY FOR OVARIAN CANCER

Scott Moerdler and Xingxing Zang

BACKGROUND

Programmed death 1 (PD-1) is a member of the B7-CD28 immunoglobulin (Ig) superfamily. It encodes a 55 kDa type I transmembrane monomeric glycoprotein that is expressed on activated T and B lymphocytes, natural killer (NK) cells as well as myeloid cells.[1-5] Unlike other members of the B7-CD28 family, PD-1 is a monomeric glycoprotein lacking an extracellular cysteine which prohibits covalent dimers.[6] Its extracellular region contains a single Ig-like variable IgV domain,[7] while its cytoplasmic region consists of an immunoreceptor tyrosine-based inhibitory motif (ITIM).[7,8] The ligands for PD-1 include PD-L1 (aka B7-H1 and CD274) and PD-L2 (aka B7-DC and CD273).[9,10] PD-L1 expression is seen in normal tissues such as the heart, pancreas, placenta, vascular endothelium, liver, lung, and skin.[9,10] Additionally, CD80 (B7-1) can act as receptor for PD-L1 and induces inhibitory T-cell signals when bound.[11-13] PD-L2 also has a second receptor, repulsive guidance molecule b, which functions in respiratory immunity.[14]

PD-1 is structurally similar to another member of the B7 family, cytotoxic T lymphocytes-associated antigen 4 (CLTA-4), which binds B7-1 and B7-2 and is involved in maintenance of T-cell homeostasis. PD-1 ligation, like CLTA-4, is involved in inhibition of lymphocyte proliferation.[9] In another similarity with CLTA-4, PD-1 is also expressed on regulatory T cells (Tregs) and helps to enhance and sustain their proliferation.[15] Since PD-1 is expressed not only on activated T cells but also B cells and NK cells, blockade will lead to augmented effector T-cell activity in both the periphery as well as tumor microenvironment, increased NK cell activity in tumor or tissues, and increased antibody production.[16,17]

Unlike its name, PD-1 does not directly cause cell death. Rather, when bound to its ligands PD-1 inhibits T-cell signaling and cytokine production, as well as limits effector T-cell proliferation and increases their susceptibility to apoptosis.[18] The role of PD-1 was initially evaluated by Nishimura et al. with deficient mice who were found to have consistently mild splenomegaly secondary to proliferation of lymphoid and myeloid cells, selected augmentation in IgG3 antibody response to type 2 T-independent antigen, as well as increased in vitro response to anti-IgM stimulation. All this suggested that PD-1 plays a negative regulatory role in the immune response.[19] PD-1 engagement with its ligands directly inhibits TCR signaling via the Zap-70 and Ras pathways.[20-23] Binding also has downstream effects on the PI3K pathway. Specifically, the cytoplasmic immunoreceptor tyrosine-based inhibitory motif (ITIM) and immunoreceptor tyrosine-based switch motif (ITSM) have been shown to act as negative regulators of tyrosine kinase-based signaling pathways of immunological receptors. Phosphorylation of the ITIM and ITSM leads to recruitment of tyrosine phosphatases such as SHP-1 and SHP-2.[19-22,24] These phosphatases lead to inactivation of PI3K/AKT and MAPK signaling pathways, therefore blocking cell-cycle progression in immune cells,[21,23] impairing proliferation, blunting cytokine production, and increasing apoptosis.[25]

Additionally, PD-1 limits the effector activity of T cells in peripheral tissues to prevent excessive inflammatory damage in the setting of infection and works to limit autoimmunity by inducing T-cell exhaustion. These effects of PD-1 were described in PD-1 deficient mice who developed various autoimmune syndromes depending on the strain of mouse.[19,26] T-cell exhaustion was demonstrated in viral infection models,[27-29] where high PD-1 expression was correlated with increased viremia due to the dysfunctional proliferation and cytokine secretion of T cells,[30] which lead to an ineffective immune response. This early research showed that deficiency of PD-1 leads to dysfunction of peripheral self-tolerance at the T-cell level, which has since been shown to occur via inhibition of TCR, lymphocyte proliferation, and cytokine secretion.[9]

PD-1/PD-L1 IN CANCER

Based on these initial findings, the role of PD-1/PD-L1 has been extensively studied in cancer immunology (Figure 10.1). PD-1 was initially found on many of the tumor infiltrating lymphocytes (TILs) in the tumor microenvironments of various types of cancer including melanoma[30] and prostate.[31] The ligands for PD-1 can be upregulated on the tumor cell surface of many different cancers[10] as well as tumor-associated macrophages (TAMs), myeloid derived suppressor cells,

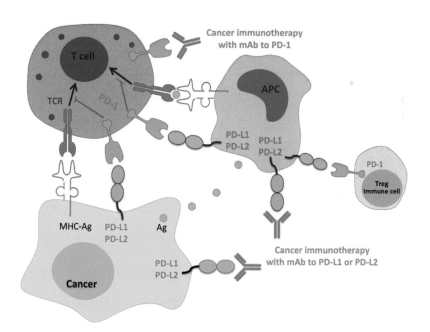

Figure 10.1 Anti- PD-1 receptor and anti-PD-L1/L2 antibodies as cancer immunotherapy. Antigen-presenting cells present antigens (Ag) released from cancer cells to T cells within the tumor microenvironment. Cancer cells can also present Ag directly to activated T cells through the use of the MHC. Upon T-cell activation, PD-1 receptors are expressed on T cells. Engagement with its ligands, PD-L1 and PD-L2 on APCs and PD-L1 on cancer cells, leads to inhibited immune responses. Blockade of the PD-1/PD-L1/PD-L2 pathway can enhance anti-tumor immunity.

dendritic cells (DCs), T cells and B cells.[32] Certain solid tumors have been shown to express PD-L1, including melanoma, lung, ovarian, breast, glioblastoma, esophagus, the gastrointestinal tract, and squamous cell carcinoma of head and neck.[33-36] Meanwhile, PD-L2 is more commonly found to have increased expression on B cell lymphomas like primary mediastinal B cell lymphoma, follicular lymphoma, and Hodgkin lymphoma.[37]

Iwai et al. first observed that PD-1 engagement with its ligand PD-L1 lead to inhibited anti-tumor cytolytic activity of CD8+ T-cells.[38] Furthermore, they showed that deficient mice were unable to mount an immune response, which leads to tumor growth and metastatic suppression.[38,39] Two different mechanisms have been described in which tumor cells use PD-1 and its ligands to evade the human immune system, known as the innate and adaptive immune resistance. Innate immune resistance relies on constitutive signaling of the upregulated PD-L1 expression on tumor cells independent of inflammatory or cytokine signals in tumor microenvironment.[16] This signaling is conducted through the AKT and STAT3 pathways. This has been exhibited in glioblastomas which demonstrate increased expression in the setting of PTEN deletion, suggesting involvement of PIK3-AKT pathway.[40] Another model has been shown with constitutive anaplastic lymphoma kinase signaling in lymphoma and lung cancer due to signal transduction and activation of STAT3.[41] Amplification of JAK2 and 9p24.1 copy number variation has been seen in classical Hodgkin lymphoma and mediastinal large B cell lymphoma.[42] There have been some reports of MAPK signaling pathway controlling PD-L1 expression in anaplastic large cell lymphoma and Hodgkin lymphoma; however, Atefi et al. did not identify this association or other mutations in PI3K/AKT pathways either.[43]

Normally, certain cytokines, such as interferon-gamma (IFN-γ), are secreted in the setting of inflammation leading to PD-L1 expression as a negative feedback cycle to dampen the activity of PD-1+ T-cells. Tumors have been found to hijack this normal host negative feedback system which is physiologically used to prevent autoimmunity and protect peripheral tissue damage from inflammation by using similar mechanisms to protect itself from antitumor immune response. This is part of the adaptive immune response. PD-L1 is not automatically expressed, rather it is induced in response to inflammatory signals such as interferons, mainly IFN-γ, in the microenvironment. Taube et al. demonstrated that IFN-γ was only seen in setting of PD-L1+ but not in PD-L1-/- tumors, and more specifically it was seen at the junction of TILs and the PD-L1+ tumors. This suggests that TILs produce inflammatory and cytokine factors which upregulate PD-L1 expression likely as a negative feedback mechanism; however, this also inadvertently leads to decreased anti-tumor immunity.[44] Other cytokines that have been suggested to be involved in this process include interleukin (IL)-2, IL-6, IL-7, IL-10, IL-15, IL-32γ, and common γ-chain cytokines,[45-47] with the different cytokines inducing upregulation on distinct cell types. Additionally, hypoxia has been shown to induce PD-L1 expression via the hypoxia-inducible factor 1 alpha pathway.[48]

PD-L1 PROGNOSTIC VALUE IN CANCERS

PD-L1 expression has varying prognostic values in different solid tumors. High expression is associated with improved survival in melanoma,[49] merkel cell,[50] breast,[51] and cervical carcinomas[52] as opposed to a poor prognosis seen in non-small cell lung cancer (NSCLC),[33,53] renal cancers,[54-58] esophageal.[59] gastric,[60] and bladder cancer.[61] In an effort to predict response to PD-1/PD-L1 blockade, Teng et al. revised a prior classification system[44] of the tumor microenvironment depending on TIL presence and PD-L1 expression in melanoma and suggested a treatment stratification based on this framework (Figure 10.2).[62] TILs alone

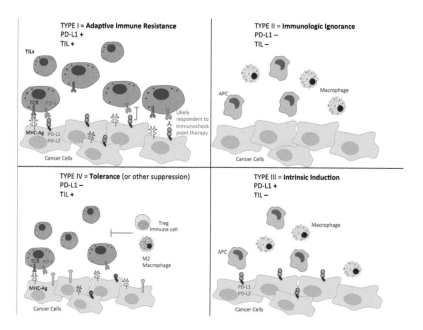

Figure 10.2 Tumor classification framework using presence of TILs and expression of PD-L1. Adapted from Teng MW, et al., Classifying cancers based on T-cell infiltration and PD-L1. *Cancer Res.* 2015. 75(11): 2139-45.

have been investigated as independent prognostic factors. In some studies, presence of TILs in patients with colorectal, ovarian, pancreatic, esophageal, and small-cell lung carcinoma were associated with a better prognosis,[63–67] as opposed to TILs in patients with renal cell carcinoma, who were associated with a poor prognosis.[68] Type 1 was classified as tumors exhibiting adaptive immune resistance with presence of TILs diving PD-L1 expression. These tumors are suggested to be the type most likely to respond to immune checkpoint inhibitor therapy as they already have TILs present in the microenvironment which have been inactivated by the PD-L1+ tumor cells. Therefore the use of checkpoint inhibitors would be able to reactivate those TILs which are already present and allow them to attack the tumor cells. Type 2 is represented by the absence of TILs and no PD-L1 expression, indicating an immunologic resistance. These tumors have been shown to have poor prognosis in melanoma[62] and are unlikely to have a response to immunocheckpoint blockade in the setting of the absence of TILs. However, combination therapy which could attract effector T-cells into the tumor might be successful as the anti-PD-1/PD-L1 therapy could then act on those newly present TILs. Some combination therapy to be considered in conjunction with an PD-1/PD-L1 inhibitor in these situations can include the use of vaccines to increase immunogenicity and recruit TILs, induction of type I IFN response, or CLTA-4 inhibitors.[62] Type 3 includes intrinsic induction with lack of TILs but +PD-L1 expression via oncogenic signaling. These tumors are unlikely to have a response, highlighting that presence of PD-L1 alone cannot predict response to anti-PD-1/PD-L1 therapy as without the presence of inactivated TILs to reactivate, inhibition of PD-1/PD-L1 will not have an anti-tumor response. Therefore, these types of tumors also require enlisting lymphocytes in order to have clinical benefit. Type 4 exhibits presence of TILs but lack of PD-L1 expression leading to immune tolerance, which suggests a possible role of other suppressors driving tolerance. Therefore other immune checkpoint inhibitors might be successful in this situation.

However, this treatment stratification framework is not perfect, as some studies have shown that there is a role for anti-PD-1/L1 therapy even in the setting of PD-L1 negative tumors.[62,69-72] Additionally, immunohistochemistry protocols are not standardized, therefore presence or absence of PD-1/PD-L1 is based on different stains and the analysis is somewhat subjective with different studies using different cutoffs[73] and antibodies used in the various studies and a degree of intratumoral heterogeneity suggesting possible sampling bias. Despite these limitations and the fact that this framework was based on melanoma, this can help us better understand the tumor microenvironment and rationale for the use of anti-PD-1/PD-L1 therapies and combination therapies in ovarian cancer.[18]

PD-1/PLD1 IN OVARIAN CANCER

As already discussed, the tumor microenvironment is not the same in all cancers, with different immune cells present and differing proteins or cytokines and therefore varying actions which leads to distinct responses to therapy and prognoses. The tumor microenvironment in ovarian cancer has been shown to contain TILs which recognize tumor antigens and have cytolytic activity.[74-76] Initially, the presence of CD3+ TILs in ovarian cancer were demonstrated to have a significantly improved median progression free survival (22.4 vs. 5.8 months, $p < 0.001$) and overall survival (50.3 vs. 18.0 months, $p < 0.0001$) compared to tumors without presence of TILs.[64]Subsequent studies indicated that the types of T cells present and the ratio of regulator versus effector T cells impact outcomes.[77,78] For example, an increase in intraepithelial CD8+ TILs and a high CD8 T cell to Treg cell ratio was associated with improved survival,[79] while an increased proportion of CD4+CD25+FoxP3+ Tregs and NK cells was shown to be a poor prognostic factor.[80,81] Tregs have been shown to curb CD4 and CD8 activity as well as activate the

immunosuppressive effect of macrophages, which would add to this decreased survival.[82-84] Tumors are often found to have high levels of infiltrating Tregs, which likely help dampen effector response leading to tumor immune escape; PD-1 blockade likely enhances anti-tumor effect by depleting Treg population in the tumor microenvironment. Some investigators are examining the effect of depleting FoxP3+ Tregs on anti-tumor response.[85-89]

Different cancers are not only classified differently based on these criteria due to the varying immune infiltrative cells in their respective tumor microenvironments, but they also as a result have diverse prognoses and response to immunotherapy. Immune responses differ not only based on the overall type or cancer, but they have been seen to change based on histologic subtype within certain cancers. For example, when analyzing by stage some studies showed that advanced stage epithelial ovarian cancer (EOC) with presence of Tregs were associated with increased survival[90] as opposed to the studies which use heterogeneous populations including different ovarian cancer subtypes. Similarly, when analyzing by histologic subtype, high-grade serous cancer, the most common and fatal form of EOC, is associated with favorable TIL response, and presence of Tregs were found to be associated with increased survival as opposed to other subtypes.[79,91-94] The authors theorize that this increase in survival seen with Treg presence might be indicative of a stronger CD8 response which overshadows the suppressive effects of Tregs,[92] but more research is needed to better understand these differences. Some proposed reasons for these inconsistencies in survival include varying study methodology, specifically in the use of various antibodies or markers and their subjective scoring criteria, and analyzing subtypes separately as opposed to grouping them all in one.[92,94] Another reason for further investigation and detailing of the specific types of infiltrative cells and their locations in the microenvironment is that these elements might be able help direct future therapy.[94] This thinking is extrapolated from the ovarian cancer mouse model findings in which certain chemotherapies were found to lead to activation of these specific cells but other treatments did not elicit an immune response in those infiltrative cells.[95,96]

Other criteria which alter prognosis include surgical outcome, effect of neoadjuvant chemotherapy, and TIL differentiation.[93] While surgical outcomes are an independent prognostic indicator of ovarian cancer, they have been seen to be related to presence of TILs. Specifically, the presence of TILs has been suggested to control disease burden allowing for suboptimal debulking and cytotoxic therapy whereas those without TILs present required maximal surgery to maintain outcomes.[94] However, these distinctions still require further investigation and validation. Wouters et al. have complemented these findings, explaining that surgical outcomes in ovarian cancer can negate the prognostic value of TILs, as incomplete resection outweighed presence of positive prognostic CD8+ TILs.[93] In terms of TIL differentiation, the authors found that patients with tumors infiltrated by less differentiated CD8+ TILs, measured by CD27 expression, had better outcomes in those with maximal cytoreductive surgery, possibly indicating an activated tumor-reactive environment.[93] As a result, these different factors including prior treatment regimens, surgical outcome, and the type or location of TILs all must be evaluated together when thinking about patient prognosis and future treatment plans.

In addition to TILs, other antigen presenting cells are of interest as they too play a role in the PD-1/PD-L1 pathway, specifically macrophages. Macrophages in ovarian cancer have been described to be differentiated to an M2 phenotype, consisting of IL-10 and TGF-b expression, which is believed to lead to tumor progression likely due to IL-10's effect of inducing PD-L1.[84,92,97-99] Additionally, macrophages have been known to produce CCL22, which attracts Tregs into the tumor microenvironment.[83] Webb et al. demonstrated

that PD-L1 was seen to be upregulated on TAMs as compared to tumor cells, and all the tumors that had PD-L1 expression also had associated TAMs.[91] One possible explanation for increased expression of PD-L1 on TAMs is that while they scour the tumor microenvironment they ingest large amounts of proteins and antigen loads which they subsequently present, making them recognizable by T cells. In such a setting, PD-L1 upregulation allows for a means of self-defense and protection from T-cell mediated killing. In that study, PD-L1+ TAMs were not only noted to be present but also found to have positive association of PD-L1+ TAMs as a marker of favorable prognosis.[91] However, immunohistochemical staining has been inconsistent in different studies with some demonstrating significant tumor staining and others showing staining limited to TAMs.[91,100,101]

Another immune cell involved in the PD-1/PD-L1 axis are DCs, which have been shown to constitute up to 40% of the tumor microenvironment.[102,103] DCs have the ability to shift their immune response depending on the cytokines in the microenvironment and have been shown develop the ability to express PD-1 as ovarian cancer progresses.[104] When expressing PD-1, NF-kB activity of DCs is inhibited, therefore affecting downstream activities such as suppressing its co-stimulatory function and cytokine production.[104]

PD-L1 AS PROGNOSTIC FACTOR IN OVARIAN CANCER

In early studies of PD-L1 in cancer Hamanishi demonstrated that PD-L1 was associated with a poor prognosis in EOC, with a five-year survival rate of 52.6% in patient with high expression of PD-L1 versus 80.2% in those with low expression ($p = 0.016$).[69] This data goes along with the thought that PD-1-PD-L1 engagement would render these local T cells ineffective, which leads to tumor survival and the poor prognosis seen here. Subsequently, other studies have also explored the prognostic indication of PD-L1 expression including

Maine et al., who demonstrated that PD-L1+ monocytes in the ascites and blood of patients with malignant ovarian cancer were more common than those with benign or borderline disease.[105] However, more recently, some studies have found the opposite with improved prognosis associated with PD-L1 expression. Darb-Esfahani investigated PD-1/PD-L1 expression on cancer cells where CD3+, PD-1+, PD-L1+, and TIL densities were all positive prognostic factors. One theory to explain this improved prognosis is that the increased PD-L1 expression is a result of a compensatory upregulation in the setting of the adaptive immune reaction's attempt at combating the tumor with cytokines which have induced marker expression.[106] Similarly, Webb et al demonstrated a positive association between PD-L1 and TIL presence in HGSC. They theorized that these contradictory studies were due to differences in staining antibody protocols, the histologic subtypes evaluated in each study, and the degree prior surgical debulking in the representative studies.[91] Another distinction between these studies is the innate differences in varying histological subtypes of EOC, as Kobel et al. reported that various subtypes have significant molecular, immunological, and clinical differences and therefore have varying associations of biomarkers with outcomes.[107] Though this study did not specifically look at PD-1/PDL1 as a biomarker, their hypothesis can be extrapolated to the PD-1/PD-L1 axis in ovarian cancer subtypes and might explain why some studies had opposing findings.[69,91,105,106,108] PD-L1 expression status on tumor cells alone is not enough to use as a marker of prognosis or response to immunotherapy; instead, PD-L1 expression might be an indicator of a setting in which immunotherapy will be of use since PD-L1 is likely suppressing Tregs and other immunosuppressive cells.[18]

IMMUNOTHERAPY

Durable objective responses and improved overall survivals with PD-1 inhibitors have been documented in 19% to 44% of patients with multiple tumor types including melanoma, NSCLC, and renal cancers.[109-117] Based on these studies two PD-1 inhibitors, Nivolimab and Pembrolizumab, both IgG4 monoclonal antibodies, were granted Food and Drug Administration (FDA) approval for these cancers and with continued trials in other cancer types will likely gain approval in the near future. However, not all cancers have exhibited responses to anti-PD-1/PD-L1 therapy, including prostate and colorectal cancer, and even within those cancers which have shown response, not every patient has experienced benefit.[109]

In their Phase I study of humanized IgG1 monoclonal antibody to PD-1 in hematologic malignancies, Berger et al. found the antibody to be safe and well tolerated. They also observed clinical benefit in 33% of patients, one with complete remission (CR).[118] A subsequent Phase I study of anti-PD-1 in solid tumors, including melanoma, NSCLC, prostate, renal, and colorectal cancers was carried out. In this study the observed cumulative response rates were 18% in NSCLC, 28% in melanoma, and 27% in renal cell. Durable responses were seen in 20 out of 31 patients, and responses were noted at one year or more.[119] In 2012 Brahmer et al. investigated the use of Nivolumab, which was FDA approved for treatment of melanoma, NSCLC, renal cell carcinoma, and Hodgkin lymphoma. This was a multicenter Phase I trial of anti-PD-L1 therapy in advanced solid tumors. Seventeen patients with ovarian cancer were enrolled, and the investigators observed one partial remission (PR) and three patients with stable disease, with a disease control rate of 23.5%.[115] More recently, Hamanishi et al. published the results of their single-center Phase II trial using Nivolimab in 20 patients with platinum-resistant, recurrent, or advanced ovarian cancer with a history of at least two chemotherapy regimens including platinum and taxane agents. Patients were treated with either 1mg/kg or 3mg/kg of Nivolumab every two weeks until disease progression was identified or up to

48 weeks maximum. Their primary endpoint was best overall response which was assessed by RECIST 1.1 criteria. They observed grade 3 or 4 treatment-related adverse events in eight patients (20%) and serious events in two patients (one with disorientation and gait abnormality in the setting of a month of fevers; the other developed fever and deep vein thrombosis). The best overall response rate was 15% with a disease control rate of 45%. A complete response was observed in two patients in the 2mg/kg group, and prolonged stable disease was noted in four patients.[108] These response rates were similar to those of patients treated with routine chemotherapy[120,121] in patients with platinum-resistant tumors; however, the durable anti-tumor response seen has been clinically encouraging in this pretreated population.[18] Hamanishi et al. also evaluated expression levels of PD-L1, which were not significantly correlated with objective response. Sixteen of the patients' tumors (80%) were classified as having high expression of PD-L1, but only two of those patients with high expression showed objective response, and one of the patients with low levels of expression showed a response to therapy.

Pembrolizumab, another anti-PD-1 humanized IgG4 monoclonal antibody, has been FDA approved for treatment of melanoma and NSCLC. In the non-randomized multicohort Phase Ib (KEYNOTE-028, NCT02054806) trial of Pembrolizumab in patients with solid tumors, 26 patients with ovarian cancer enrolled. Using 10mg/kg of Pembrolizumab every two weeks, best overall response rate was assessed using RECIST 1.1 criteria. The objective response rate observed was 11.5% with one CR, two PR, and 23% stable disease with a durable response.[18,122]

Avelumab was the first anti-PD-L1 therapy to be evaluated. It is a humanized selective IgG1 monoclonal antibody to PD-L1 (which does not affect PD-L2-PD-1 interaction). In a Phase Ib study 124 recurrent or refractory ovarian cancer patients were treated with 10mg/kg every two weeks until progression or toxicity. Twelve patients were

observed to have PR with an objective response rate (ORR) 9.7%. While 55 patients reported to have stable disease burden and the disease control rate was 54%, the ORR in PD-L1+ tumors was 12.3% and in PD-L1- ORR was 5.9%. They did not demonstrate statistically significant difference between PFS or OS based on PD-L1 expression status.[18,72]

Of these published studies using anti-PD-1/PD-L1 as immunotherapy, they were all in patients with platinum-resistant ovarian cancer, the ORR at best was 15% and a few had durable long-lasting disease control. While these results were encouraging, the hope is to continue improving outcomes. Therefore, the next step in many upcoming trials is using these agents as combination therapy, first with standard chemotherapy and then with other immunotherapies.

Standard treatments like chemotherapy or radiation leads to apoptosis and subsequent dispersal of antigens which can affect other tissues or tumors in the body.[123] Recently presented preclinical models showed that standard chemotherapy with platinum and taxanes increased expression of PD-L1 therefore adding to chemoresistance.[124,125] Similarly, Mesnage showed that both TIL and PD-L1 expression were augmented after standard neoadjuvant chemotherapy in patients with EOC.[126] Bohm et al. also documented the effect of neoadjuvant chemotherapy with platinum therapy in boosting the immune response.[127] However, this stimulation of the immune response has not been shown to alter outcomes.[49] Other chemotherapies aside from platinums and taxanes are also involved in augmenting anti-tumor response. Mantia-Smaldone et al. evaluated the use of pegylated liposomal doxorubicin (PLD) in patients with BRCA mutated cancers which lead to a heightened immune response with increased TIL recruitment and vulnerability to T-cell cytotoxicity.[128] Therefore, Bohm and others suggest the incorporation of immunotherapy to harness this enhanced immune response and further improve disease control. Current trials are evaluating these combinations. For example, combination therapy of platinum chemotherapy with anti-PD-L1 immuno-therapy in vivo has been shown to control and reduce tumor burden.[124,125,129] And given that BRCA mutated tumors are deficient in homologous recombination and rely on the imperfect poly (ADP-ribose) polymerase (PARP) mediated pathway for double-stranded break repair,[130,131] further research is needed on the combination of PD-1/PD-L1 immunotherapy with PARP inhibitors.

Other therapies aside from standard che-motherapy are being used for combination therapies. Vascular endothelial growth factor (VEGF) inhibitors which affect angiogenesis play a role in ovarian cancers,[64] affecting the T-cell immune response, and inversely cor-relate with TIL infiltration.[64,80] Durvalumab, an Fc optimized IgG1 monoclonal antibody to PD-L1 which has been FDA approved for urothelial bladder cancer, is being used in combination with VEGF inhibitors. In an on-going Phase I/II trial, Durvalumab is being studied in combination with Olaparib (PARP inhibitor) or Cediranib (VEGFR inhib-itor). Recently presented results showed one partial response in nine evaluable ovarian cancer patients lasting over six months with Durvalumab/Olaparib and one PR in five evaluable ovarian cancer patients treated with Durvalumab/Cediranib.[18,132] Some trials are currently exploring the combination of immune-checkpoint blockers such as anti-CLTA-4 therapy Ipilimumab with Nivolumab based on its promising results in melanoma.[113]

The results of these combination therapies are promising and encouraging, leading to many more trials which are ongoing and further research into other related possible pathways. Table 10.1 highlights the open clin-ical trials as of January 2017 using PD-1 and PD-L1 inhibitors. Another active agent being studied is the use of DNA methyltransferase inhibitors. Studies have shown that solid tumors treated with DNA methyltransferase inhibitors exhibit upregulation in genes in-volved in the interferon pathway.[133,134] More recent studies have gone on to show that pre-treatment with a DNA methyltransferase in-hibitor can sensitize melanoma to immune

checkpoint inhibitors like anti-CLTA-4.[135] Given these findings and Wrangle et al., who showed that treatment with Azacytidine led to upregulation of PD-L1, future work should include trials using PD-1/PD-L1 inhibitors in combination with DNA methyltransferase inhibitors.[136]

GENETIC VARIABILITY AND NEOANTIGENS

As therapy evolves, and more combinations are being studied, we need further de-tailed subclassifications based on tumor subtypes. While there are some classifica-tion frameworks such as the one suggested by Teng et al., which was described earlier, more recent research suggests adding a mo-lecular layer to include certain mutations. Genetic variability and mutational load has also been suggested to play a role in PD-1/PD-L1 expression. Recent research (budczies)[136a] has suggested that PD-L1 copy number variation correlates with mRNA ex-pression and with poor prognosis in many cancers including ovarian cancer. T cells rec-ognize foreign peptide epitopes presented on major histocompatibility complexes, pro-viding the initial signal for T cell activation. These epitopes can either be non-mutated proteins from the tissue, for which there is incomplete tolerance, or mutated peptides which are novel compared to the human genome, called neoantigens.[137] There is evi-dence suggesting that increased mutational load leads to increases in neoantigens in the tumor microenvironment which recruits TILs and leads to increased response to PD-1/PD-L1 therapies,[119,138] and with low genetic alterations there have been decreased re-sponse to immunotherapy.[109] However, there are a limited number of mutant epitopes to which T cells react, possibly due to immune editing or ineffective priming and tolerance of the T cells.[138] Based on this, current re-search includes the use of vaccination with neoantigen peptides in an attempt to increase the breadth of T cell reactivity and hopefully

TABLE 10.1 ONGOING CLINICAL TRIALS USING ANTI-PD-1/PD-L1 THERAPIES[a]

NCT	Immunotherapeutic Agent	Combination Therapy	Phase	Population	Trial
NCT02728830	Pembrolizumab		Early I	Gynecologic cancers	A Study of Pembrolizumab on the Tumoral Immunoprofile of Gynecologic Cancers
NCT02856425	Pembrolizumab	Nintedanib (tyrosine kinase inhibitor)	I	Advanced solid tumors	Trial of Pembrolizumab and Nintedanib
NCT02526017	Nivolumab	FPA008 (anti-CSF1R)	I	Advanced solid tumors	Study of FPA008 in Combination with Nivolumab in Patients with Selected Advanced Cancers
NCT02475213	Pembrolizumab	Enoblituzumab (anti-B7-H3)	I	Refractory cancers	Safety Study of Enoblituzumab (MGA271) in Combination with Pembrolizumab in Refractory Cancer
NCT02606305	Pembrolizumab	IMGN853 (folate receptor alpha targeting antibody-drug conjugate)	I	Folate receptor alpha positive advanced epithelial ovarian cancer	Study of IMGN853 in Combination with Bevacizumab, Carboplatin, PLD, or Pembrolizumab in Adults with FRa + Adv. EOC, Primary Peritoneal, Fallopian Tube, or Endometrial Cancer
NCT02298959	Pembrolizumab	Ziv-Aflibercept	I	Advanced solid tumors	Pembrolizumab and Ziv-aflibercept in Treating Patients with Advanced Solid Tumors
NCT02346955	Pembrolizumab	CM-24 (MK-6018)	I	Advanced or recurrent malignancies	Study of CM-24 (MK-6018) Alone and in Combination with Pembrolizumab (MK-3475) in Participants with Selected Advanced or Recurrent Malignancies (MK-6018-001)
NCT02009449	Pembrolizumab	AM0010	I	Advanced solid tumors	A Phase I Study of AM0010 in Patients with Advanced Solid Tumors
NCT02737787	Nivolumab	WT1 Vaccine	I	Recurrent ovarian cancer	A Study of WT1 Vaccine and Nivolumab for Recurrent Ovarian Cancer

(continued)

TABLE 10.1 CONTINUED

NCT	Immunotherapeutic Agent	Combination Therapy	Phase	Population	Trial
NCT02955251	Nivolumab	ABBV-428	I	Advanced solid tumors	A Study Evaluating Safety and Pharmacokinetics, and the Recommended Phase 2 Dose (RPTD) of ABBV-428 in Participants with Advanced Solid Tumors
NCT02812875	CA-170 (targets PD-L1/PD-L2 and V-domain Ig suppressor of T cell activation (VISTA) immune checkpoints)		I	Advanced solid tumors or lymphomas	A Study of CA-170 (Oral PD-L1, PD-L2 and VISTA Checkpoint Antagonist) in Patients with Advanced Tumors and Lymphomas
NCT01772004	Avelumab		I	Advanced solid tumor	Avelumab in Metastatic or Locally Advanced Solid Tumors (JAVELIN Solid Tumor)
NCT02914470	Atezolizumab	Carboplatin, Cyclophosphamide	I	Advanced breast cancer and gynecologic cancer	Carboplatin-Cyclophosphamide Combined with Atezolizumab
NCT01975831	MEDI4736	Tremelimumab (anti-CTLA-4)	I	Advanced solid tumor	A Phase I Study to Evaluate MEDI4736 in Combination with Tremelimumab
NCT02471846	Atezolizumab	GDC-0919 (anti-IDO)	I	Locally advanced or metastatic solid tumors	A Study of GDC-0919 and Atezolizumab Combination Treatment in Participants with Locally Advanced or Metastatic Solid Tumors
NCT02943317	Avelumab	Defactinib (FAK inhibitor)	I	Ovarian cancer	Study to Investigate the Safety, Pharmacokinetics, Pharmacodynamics, and Preliminary Clinical Activity of Defactinib in Combination with Avelumab in Epithelial Ovarian Cancer
NCT03029598	Pembrolizumab	Carboplatin	I/II	Platinum-resistant ovarian, fallopian tube, and primary peritoneal cancer	Pembrolizumab and Carboplatin in Treating Patients with Relapsed or Refractory Ovarian, Fallopian Tube, or Primary Peritoneal Cancer

NCT Number	Drug	Combination Agent	Phase	Indication	Study Title
NCT02335918	Nivolumab	Varlilumab (anti-CD27)	I/II	Advanced refractory solid tumors	A Dose Escalation and Cohort Expansion Study of Anti-CD27 (Varlilumab) and Anti-PD-1 (Nivolumab) in Advanced Refractory Solid Tumors
NCT02961101	anti-PD-1 antibody	Decitabine	I/II	Relapsed or refractory malignancies	Anti-PD-1 Antibody in Combination with Low-Dose Decitabine in Relapsed or Refractory Malignancies
NCT02452424	Pembrolizumab	PLX3397 (CSF1 receptor blockade)	I/II	Advanced melanoma and other solid tumors	A Combination Clinical Study of PLX3397 and Pembrolizumab to Treat Advanced Melanoma and Other Solid Tumors
NCT02657889	Pembrolizumab	Niraparib (PARP inhibitor)	I/II	Triple-negative breast cancer or ovarian cancer	Study of Niraparib in Combination with Pembrolizumab (MK-3475) in Patients with Triple-Negative Breast Cancer or Ovarian Cancer
NCT02452424	Pembrolizumab	PLX3397 (CSF1R inhibitor)	I/II	Solid tumors	A Combination Clinical Study of PLX3397 and Pembrolizumab to Treat Advanced Melanoma and Other Solid Tumors
NCT02331251	Pembrolizumab	Liposomal Doxorubicin	I/II	Advanced cancers	Study of Pembrolizumab Plus Chemotherapy in Patients with Advanced Cancer (PembroPlus)
NCT02178722	Pembrolizumab	Epacadostat	I/II	Solid tumors	A Phase I/II Study Exploring the Safety, Tolerability, and Efficacy of Pembrolizumab (MK-3475) in Combination With Epacadostat (INCB024360) in Subjects with Selected Cancers (INCB 24360-202 / MK-3475-037 / KEYNOTE-037 / ECHO-202)

(continued)

TABLE 10.1 CONTINUED

NCT	Immunotherapeutic Agent	Combination Therapy	Phase	Population	Trial
NCT02327078	Nivolumab	Epacadostat	I/II	Advanced cancers	A Study of the Safety, Tolerability, and Efficacy of Epacadostat Administered in Combination with Nivolumab in Select Advanced Cancers (ECHO-204)
NCT02341625	Nivolumab	BMS-986148 (anti-mesothelin antibody-drug conjugate)	I/II	Advanced solid tumors	A Study of BMS-986148 in Patients with Select Advanced Solid Tumors
NCT01928394	Nivolumab	Ipilimumab, Cobimetinib	I/II	Advanced or metastatic solid tumors	A Study of Nivolumab by Itself or Nivolumab Combined with Ipilimumab in Patients with Advanced or Metastatic Solid Tumors
NCT02484404	Durvalumab	Olaparib (PARP-inhibitor), Cediranib (anti-VEGF)	I/II	Advanced solid tumor	Phase I/II Study of the Anti-Programmed Death Ligand-1 Antibody MEDI4736 in Combination with Olaparib and/or Cediranib for Advanced Solid Tumors and Advanced or Recurrent Ovarian, Triple Negative Breast, Lung, Prostate and Colorectal Cancers
NCT02431559	Durvalumab	Pegylated Liposomal Doxorubicin	I/II	Recurrent, platinum-resistant ovarian cancer	A Phase I/II Study of Motolimod (VTX-2337) and MEDI4736 in Subjects with Recurrent, Platinum-Resistant Ovarian Cancer for Whom Pegylated Liposomal Doxorubicin (PLD) is Indicated
NCT02915523	Avelumab	Entinostat (histone deacetylase inhibitor)	I/II	Advanced epithelial ovarian cancer	Phase Ib/II Study of Avelumab with or without Entinostat in Patients with Advanced Epithelial Ovarian Cancer
NCT02963831	Durvalumab	ONCOS-102	I/II	Advanced peritoneal malignancies	A Phase I/II Study to Investigate the Safety, Biologic and Anti-Tumor Activity of ONCOS-102 in Combination with Durvalumab in Subjects with Advanced Peritoneal Malignancies

NCT Number	Drug	Intervention	Phase	Condition	Title
NCT02734004	Durvalumab	Olaparib	I/II	Advanced solid tumor	A Phase I/II Study of MEDI4736 in Combination with Olaparib in Patients with Advanced Solid Tumors.
NCT02726997	Durvalumab	Carboplatin, Paclitaxel	I/II	Ovarian cancer	Matched Paired Pharmacodynamics and Feasibility Study of Durvalumab in Combination with Chemotherapy in Frontline Ovarian Cancer
NCT02953457	Durvalumab	Olaparib, Tremelimumab	I/II	Recurrent or refractory ovarian cancer with BRAC1/2 mutation	Olaparib, Durvalumab, and Tremelimumab in Treating Patients with Recurrent or Refractory Ovarian, Fallopian Tube, or Primary Peritoneal Cancer with BRCA1 or BRAC2 Mutation
NCT02766582	Pembrolizumab	Carboplatin, Paclitaxel	II	Stage III/IV epithelial ovarian cancer	Phase II: Pembrolizumab/Carboplatin/Taxol in Epithelial Ovary Cancer
NCT02608684	Pembrolizumab	Gemcitabine, Cisplatin	II	Recurrent platinum-resistant ovarian cancer	A Study of Pembrolizumab with Standard Treatment in Patients with Recurrent Platinum-Resistant Ovarian Cancer
NCT03029403	Pembrolizumab	DPX-Survivac Vaccine, Cyclophosphamide	II	Advanced ovarian, primary peritoneal, or fallopian tube cancer	Phase II Study of Pembrolizumab, DPX-Survivac Vaccine and Cyclophosphamide in Advanced Ovarian, Primary Peritoneal, or Fallopian Tube Cancer
NCT02834975	Pembrolizumab	Carboplatin, Paclitaxel	II	Advanced stage epithelial ovarian cancer	Pembrolizumab, Paclitaxel, and Carboplatin in Patients with Advanced Stage Epithelial Ovarian Cancer (EOC).
NCT02644369	Pembrolizumab		II	Advanced solid tumors	Study of the Effects of Pembrolizumab in Patients with Advanced Solid Tumors
NCT02834013	Nivolumab	Iplilimumab	II	Rare tumors	Nivolumab and Ipilimumab in Treating Patients with Rare Tumors

(continued)

TABLE 10.1 CONTINUED

NCT	Immunotherapeutic Agent	Combination Therapy	Phase	Population	Trial
NCT01174121	Pembrolizumab	Young TIL, Aldesleukin (recombinant IL2), Cyclophosphamide, Fludarabine	II	Metastatic cancers	Immunotherapy Using Tumor Infiltrating Lymphocytes for Patients with Metastatic Cancer
NCT02923934	Nivolumab	Ipilimumab	II	Rare cancers	A Phase II Trial of Ipilimumab and Nivolumab for the Treatment of Rare Cancers
NCT02873962	Nivolumab	Bevacizumab	II	Relapsed ovarian cancers	A Phase II Study Of Nivolumab/ Bevacizumab
NCT03012620	Pembrolizumab		II	Rare cancers	Secured Access to Pembrolizumab for Adult Patients with Selected Rare Cancer Types
NCT02520154	Pembrolizumab	Carboplatin, Paclitaxel	II	Ovarian cancer	Pembrolizumab in Combination with Chemotherapy in Frontline Ovarian Cancer
NCT02440425	Pembrolizumab	Paclitaxel	II	Platinum-resistant ovarian cancer	Dose Dense Paclitaxel with Pembrolizumab (MK-3475) in Platinum-Resistant Ovarian Cancer
NCT02900560	Pembrolizumab	CC-486 (oral azacitidine)	II	Platinum-resistant ovarian cancer	Study of Pembrolizumab with or without CC-486 in Patients With Platinum-resistant Ovarian Cancer
NCT02901899	Pembrolizumab	Gemcitabine	II	Platinum-resistant ovarian cancer	Guadecitabine and Pembrolizumab in Treating Patients with Recurrent Ovarian, Primary Peritoneal, or Fallopian Tube Cancer
NCT02865811	Pembrolizumab	Pegylated Liposomal Doxorubicin	II	Recurrent platinum ovarian cancer	Pembrolizumab Combined with PLD for Recurrent Platinum Resistant Ovarian, Fallopian Tube, or Peritoneal Cancer
NCT02853318	Pembrolizumab	Bevacizumab, Cyclophosphamide	II	Recurrent epithelial ovarian cancer	Pembrolizumab, Bevacizumab, and Cyclophosphamide in Treating Patients with Recurrent Ovarian, Fallopian Tube, or Primary Peritoneal Cancer

NCT Number	Agent	Intervention	Phase	Condition	Title
NCT02669914	Durvalumab		II	Patients with brain metastasis from epithelial-derived tumors	MEDI4736 (Durvalumab) in Patients with Brain Metastasis From Epithelial-Derived Tumors
NCT02764333	Durvalumab	TPIV200 (anti-Folate Receptor Vaccine)	II	Platinum-resistant ovarian cancer	TPIV200/huFR-1 (A Multi-Epitope Anti-Folate Receptor Vaccine) Plus Anti-PD-L1 MEDI4736 (Durvalumab) in Patients with Platinum-Resistant Ovarian Cancer
NCT02659384	Atezolizumab	Bevacizumab, Acetylsalicylic acid	II	Recurrent platinum-resistant ovarian, fallopian tube, or primary peritoneal adenocarcinoma	Anti-Programmed Cell Death-1 Ligand 1 (aPDL-1) Antibody Atezolizumab, Bevacizumab, and Acetylsalicylic Acid in Recurrent Platinum Resistant Ovarian Cancer
NCT03026062	Durvalumab	Tremelimumab	II	Malignant neoplasm of female genital organ	Durvalumab and Tremelimumab in Combo Versus Sequential
NCT02811497	Durvalumab	Azacitidine	II	Advanced solid tumor	Study of Azacitidine and Durvalumab in Advanced Solid Tumors
NCT02839707	Atezolizumab	Bevacizumab, Pegylated Liposomal Doxorubicin Hydrochloride	II/III	Recurrent ovarian cancer	Pegylated Liposomal Doxorubicin Hydrochloride with Atezolizumab and/or Bevacizumab in Treating Patients with Recurrent Ovarian, Fallopian Tube, or Primary Peritoneal Cancer
NCT02891824	Atezolizumab	Bevacizumab, platinum chemotherapy	III	Late Relapse ovarian cancer treated with chemotherapy+bevacizumab	ATALANTE: Atezolizumab vs Placebo Phase III Study in Late Relapse Ovarian Cancer Treated with Chemotherapy+Bevacizumab
NCT02580058	Avelumab	Pegylated Liposomal Doxorubicin	III	Resistant/recurrent ovarian cancer	A Study Of Avelumab Alone or in Combination with Pegylated Liposomal Doxorubicin Versus Pegylated Liposomal Doxorubicin Alone in Patients with Platinum Resistant/Refractory Ovarian Cancer (JAVELIN Ovarian 200)
NCT02718417	Avelumab	Carboplatin, Paclitaxel	III	Ovarian cancer	Avelumab in Previously Untreated Patients with Epithelial Ovarian Cancer (JAVELIN OVARIAN 100)

[a] Based on clinicaltrials.gov, January 2017.

improve immunogenicity against the endogenous tumor. In the setting of this heightened immunogenicity and neoantigen load from these vaccines, enhancement of neoantigen-specific reactive T cells can recognize the tumors epitopes, and therefore combination therapy with immunotherapy may be synergistic.[137] A variety of tumors with microsatellite instability or mismatch repair mutations, specifically those with POLD, POLE, or MYH mutations, have been shown to be strongly associated with improved clinical response to anti-PD-1 therapy, likely due to their subsequent increase in neoantigen load.[139] Mutational load has been shown to be a positive prognostic value in melanoma and bladder cancer[140] as well as a predictor of sensitivity to PD-1 immunotherapy in NSCLC.[141] Additionally, based on their analysis of multiple solid tumor types, Danilova et al. showed that PD-L1 expression was independent from BRAF, PTEN, and NRAS mutations; their group therefore suggest these as other future mutational targets which might be able to serve as biomarkers. They also highlight other targetable mutations such as LAG-3, IDO, ICOS, and Tim-3, to name a few, some of which are already part of ongoing clinical trials. Despite all this, the mutational landscape is constantly changing from diagnosis, as a result of treatment, and at time of relapse, leaving the field with more research to be done to continue to understand these pathways.

Data on genetic variability previously documented in other cancers[142,143] may be able to be extrapolated to ovarian cancer. Up to 29% of ovarian cancers have somatic mismatch repair mutations,[144] and in those without mismatch repair mutations the likely abnormality is copy number alteration.[18,145] One such gene being studied is BRCA mutations, which are known to have increased mutational load due to changes in homologous recombination repair.[146] With increased number of mutations comes genetic variability, which is suggested to lead to development of tumor-specific neoantigens. These neoantigens lead to increased mobilization

of TILs which then stimulates upregulation of immunocheckpoints like PD-1/PD-L1. In their preliminary work Strickland et al. observed an improved survival associated with tumors with higher neoantigen load as a result of their DNA repair mutations, suggesting that BRCA mutational status may be more sensitive to PD-1/PD-L1 immunotherapy.[101,147] More specifically, tumors with BRCA mutations contained higher CD8+ TILs, indicating they likely have higher sensitivity to checkpoint inhibitors.[148] However, according to recently presented data, there were no responses seen in the BRCA mutation group treated with Avelumab,[72] though we continue to wait for further results and research.

Another pathway under investigation includes PI3K/Akt/mTOR mutational status. Recent studies have shown that the PI3K/Akt/mTOR pathway is often altered in clear cell carcinoma (CCC),[149] and preclinical data from NSCLC suggest that mutations in this pathway has been correlated with increased PD-L1 expression in tumor cells,[150] which is the suspected reason why CCC patients showed benefit with Nivolumab.[49] While these are some of the relevant mutations, more are being discovered, and in the future we will likely need panels of markers to assess expression levels,[123] which taken together can guide combination therapies specific to that patient.

FUTURE WORK

We still require reliable or validated predictive biomarkers to guide patient-directed therapy and as a predictor or indicator of response. Without standardized protocols, we cannot definitively develop appropriate markers. For example, when evaluating the prognostic value of TILs, some studies qualify all CD3+ cells as TILs as opposed to other studies which specifically target CD8+ cytotoxic T-cells. Furthermore, as discussed previously, not every patient with an otherwise responsive tumor type will actually have benefit, and the contrary is true too: some patients with generally unresponsive cancers might show some response depending on the presence of certain factors. PD-L1 expression on tumor cells has not proven to be a reliable marker of response to immunotherapy as it is inconsistent when comparing different tumor subtypes. Specifically, Hamanishi reported 88% of tumors analyzed as expressing PD-L1[69] whereas Webb et al. and Gottlieb et al. only showed a small portion with expression (13.2% and 8.2%, respectively), and both detected simultaneous PD-L1+ TILs or TAMs.[91,100] Gottlieb et al. explains this discrepancy due to TAMs admixing with tumor cells and given their histologic characteristics they are easily confused for tumor cells.[100] Therefore in their study they distinguish tumor cells from macrophages with concurrent CD68 staining. If one was able to reliably differentiate between tumors cells and macrophages, PD-L1 expression on TAMs could be another area to investigate and validate as a possible prognostic marker. In their cohort of 51 patients, Qu et al. showed that PD-L1+ CD68 macrophages in tumor tissue as well as in peripheral blood were elevated compared to healthy controls and patients with benign ovarian cysts.[151] Similarly, Maine et al. showed comparable results of PD-L1 expression on monocytes in ascites and peripheral blood. Some preliminary studies, which still require validation, are looking into the role of postchemotherapy TILs and PD-L1 expression as predictors of immunotherapy benefit to be used for treatment stratification.[126] And future trials will hopefully evaluate PD-L1 expression both on tumor cells but also on specific immune infiltrates in the tumor microenvironment. Abiko et al. have been evaluating both tumors as well as other related cells. They investigated the relationship of PD-L1+ tumors and the resulting cytology of peritoneal ascites with preclinical models of PD-L1 inhibition associated with reduced peritoneal tumor growth and improved survival. Based on their results, they suggested future evaluation of primary tumor PD-L1 expression as a marker of response but also the possibility of PD-L1 status in ascites.[152]

Additionally, checkpoint expression and immune infiltrates are a moving target. Spatial and temporal heterogeneity in ovarian cancers are a problem, and therefore the current genomic scene cannot be used as a prognostic biomarker.[153] For example, clinically this is seen with tumor sampling, as one might miss focal expression or infiltrates at the edge of the tumor.[18] Recognizing its influence and accounting for this heterogeneity in future studies can help better understand outcomes in immunotherapy.[148]

REFERENCES

1. Ishida, Y., et al., Induced expression of PD-1, a novel member of the immunoglobulin gene superfamily, upon programmed cell death. *EMBO J*, 1992. 11(11): 3887–95.
2. Agata, Y., et al., Expression of the PD-1 antigen on the surface of stimulated mouse T and B lymphocytes. *Int Immunol*, 1996. 8(5):765–72.
3. Vibhakar, R., et al., Activation-induced expression of human programmed death-1 gene in T-lymphocytes. *Exp Cell Res*, 1997. 232(1):25–28.
4. Terme, M., et al., IL-18 induces PD-1-dependent immunosuppression in cancer. *Cancer Res*, 2011. 71(16):5393–99.
5. Liu, Y., et al., B7-H1 on myeloid-derived suppressor cells in immune suppression by a mouse model of ovarian cancer. *Clin Immunol*, 2008. 129(3):471–81.
6. Zhang, X., et al., Structural and functional analysis of the costimulatory receptor programmed death-1. *Immunity*, 2004. 20(3):337–47.
7. Shinohara, T., et al., Structure and chromosomal localization of the human PD-1 gene (PDCD1). *Genomics*, 1994. 23(3):704–706.
8. Finger, L.R., et al., The human PD-1 gene: complete cDNA, genomic organization, and developmentally regulated expression in B cell progenitors. *Gene*, 1997. 197(1–2):177–87.
9. Freeman, G.J., et al., Engagement of the PD-1 immunoinhibitory receptor by a novel B7 family member leads to negative regulation of lymphocyte activation. *J Exp Med*, 2000. 192(7):1027–34.
10. Dong, H., et al., B7-H1, a third member of the B7 family, co-stimulates T-cell proliferation and interleukin-10 secretion. *Nat Med*, 1999. 5(12):1365–69.
11. Butte, M.J., et al., Programmed death-1 ligand 1 interacts specifically with the B7-1 costimulatory molecule to inhibit T cell responses. *Immunity*, 2007. 27(1):111–22.

12. Paterson, A.M., et al., The programmed death-1 ligand 1:B7-1 pathway restrains diabetogenic effector T cells in vivo. *J Immunol*, 2011. 187(3):1097–105.

13. Park, J.J., et al., B7-H1/CD80 interaction is required for the induction and maintenance of peripheral T-cell tolerance. *Blood*, 2010. 116(8):1291–98.

14. Xiao, Y., et al., RGMb is a novel binding partner for PD-L2 and its engagement with PD-L2 promotes respiratory tolerance. *J Exp Med*, 2014. 211(5):943–59.

15. Francisco, L.M., et al., PD-L1 regulates the development, maintenance, and function of induced regulatory T cells. *J Exp Med*, 2009. 206(13):3015–29.

16. Pardoll, D.M., The blockade of immune checkpoints in cancer immunotherapy. *Nat Rev Cancer*, 2012. 12(4):252–64.

17. Velu, V., et al., Enhancing SIV-specific immunity in vivo by PD-1 blockade. *Nature*, 2009. 458(7235):206–10.

18. Gaillard, S.L., A.A. Secord, and B. Monk, The role of immune checkpoint inhibition in the treatment of ovarian cancer. *Gynecol Oncol Res Pract*, 2016. 3:11.

19. Nishimura, H., et al., Immunological studies on PD-1 deficient mice: implication of PD-1 as a negative regulator for B cell responses. *Int Immunol*, 1998. 10(10):1563–72.

20. Yokosuka, T., et al., Programmed cell death 1 forms negative costimulatory microclusters that directly inhibit T cell receptor signaling by recruiting phosphatase SHP2. *J Exp Med*, 2012. 209(6):1201–17.

21. Parry, R.V., et al., CTLA-4 and PD-1 receptors inhibit T-cell activation by distinct mechanisms. *Mol Cell Biol*, 2005. 25(21):9543–53.

22. Sheppard, K.A., et al., PD-1 inhibits T-cell receptor induced phosphorylation of the ZAP70/CD3zeta signalosome and downstream signaling to PKCtheta. *FEBS Lett*, 2004. 574(1-3):37–41.

23. Patsoukis, N., et al., Selective effects of PD-1 on Akt and Ras pathways regulate molecular components of the cell cycle and inhibit T cell proliferation. *Sci Signal*, 2012. 5(230):ra46.

24. Chemnitz, J.M., et al., SHP-1 and SHP-2 associate with immunoreceptor tyrosine-based switch motif of programmed death 1 upon primary human T cell stimulation, but only receptor ligation prevents T cell activation. *J Immunol*, 2004. 173(2):945–54.

25. Riley, J.L., PD-1 signaling in primary T cells. *Immunol Rev*, 2009. 229(1):114–25.

26. Nishimura, H., et al., Development of lupus-like autoimmune diseases by disruption of the PD-1 gene encoding an ITIM motif-carrying immunoreceptor. *Immunity*, 1999. 11(2):141–51.

27. Day, C.L., et al., PD-1 expression on HIV-specific T cells is associated with T-cell exhaustion and disease progression. *Nature*, 2006. 443(7109):350–54.

28. Trautmann, L., et al., Upregulation of PD-1 expression on HIV-specific CD8+ T cells leads to reversible immune dysfunction. *Nat Med*, 2006. 12(10):1198–202.

29. Urbani, S., et al., PD-1 expression in acute hepatitis C virus (HCV) infection is associated with HCV-specific CD8 exhaustion. *J Virol*, 2006. 80(22):11398–403.

30. Ahmadzadeh, M., et al., Tumor antigen-specific CD8 T cells infiltrating the tumor express high levels of PD-1 and are functionally impaired. *Blood*, 2009. 114(8):1537–44.

31. Sfanos, K.S., et al., Human prostate-infiltrating CD8+ T lymphocytes are oligoclonal and PD-1+. *Prostate*, 2009. 69(15):1694–703.

32. Okazaki, T., et al., A rheostat for immune responses: the unique properties of PD-1 and their advantages for clinical application. *Nat Immunol*, 2013. 14(12):1212–18.

33. Konishi, J., et al., B7-H1 expression on non-small cell lung cancer cells and its relationship with tumor-infiltrating lymphocytes and their PD-1 expression. *Clin Cancer Res*, 2004. 10(15):5094–100.

34. Brown, J.A., et al., Blockade of programmed death-1 ligands on dendritic cells enhances T cell activation and cytokine production. *J Immunol*, 2003. 170(3):1257–66.

35. Flies, D.B. and L. Chen, The new B7s: playing a pivotal role in tumor immunity. *J Immunother*, 2007. 30(3):251–60.

36. Zou, W. and L. Chen, Inhibitory B7-family molecules in the tumour microenvironment. *Nat Rev Immunol*, 2008. 8(6):467–77.

37. Rosenwald, A., et al., Molecular diagnosis of primary mediastinal B cell lymphoma identifies a clinically favorable subgroup of diffuse large B cell lymphoma related to Hodgkin lymphoma. *J Exp Med*, 2003. 198(6):851–62.

38. Iwai, Y., et al., Involvement of PD-L1 on tumor cells in the escape from host immune system and tumor immunotherapy by PD-L1 blockade. *Proc Natl Acad Sci U S A*, 2002. 99(19):12293–97.

39. Iwai, Y., S. Terawaki, and T. Honjo, PD-1 blockade inhibits hematogenous spread of poorly immunogenic tumor cells by enhanced recruitment of effector T cells. *Int Immunol*, 2005. 17(2):133–44.

40. Parsa, A.T., et al., Loss of tumor suppressor PTEN function increases B7-H1 expression and immunoresistance in glioma. *Nat Med*, 2007. 13(1):84–88.

41. Marzec, M., et al., Oncogenic kinase NPM/ALK induces through STAT3 expression of immunosuppressive protein CD274 (PD-L1, B7-H1). *Proc Natl Acad Sci U S A*, 2008. 105(52):20852–57.

42. Green, M.R., et al., Integrative analysis reveals selective 9p24.1 amplification, increased PD-1 ligand expression, and further induction via JAK2 in nodular sclerosing Hodgkin lymphoma and primary mediastinal large B-cell lymphoma. *Blood*, 2010. 116(17):3268–77.

43. Atefi, M., et al., Effects of MAPK and PI3K pathways on PD-L1 expression in melanoma. *Clin Cancer Res*, 2014. 20(13):3446–57.

44. Taube, J.M., et al., Colocalization of inflammatory response with B7-h1 expression in human melanocytic lesions supports an adaptive resistance

mechanism of immune escape. *Sci Transl Med*, 2012. 4(127):127ra37.

45. Wolfle, S.J., et al., PD-L1 expression on tolerogenic APCs is controlled by STAT-3. *Eur J Immunol*, 2011. 41(2):413–24.

46. Kinter, A.L., et al., The common gamma-chain cytokines IL-2, IL-7, IL-15, and IL-21 induce the expression of programmed death-1 and its ligands. *J Immunol*, 2008. 181(10):6738–46.

47. Taube, J.M., et al., Differential expression of immune-regulatory genes associated with PD-L1 display in melanoma: implications for PD-1 pathway blockade. *Clin Cancer Res*, 2015. 21(17):3969–76.

48. Noman, M.Z., et al., PD-L1 is a novel direct target of HIF-1alpha, and its blockade under hypoxia enhanced MDSC-mediated T cell activation. *J Exp Med*, 2014. 211(5):781–90.

49. Mittica, G., et al., Immune checkpoint inhibitors: a new opportunity in the treatment of ovarian cancer? *Int J Mol Sci*, 2016. 17(7).

50. Lipson, E.J., et al., PD-L1 expression in the Merkel cell carcinoma microenvironment: association with inflammation, Merkel cell polyomavirus and overall survival. *Cancer Immunol Res*, 2013. 1(1):54–63.

51. Wimberly, H., et al., PD-L1 expression correlates with tumor-infiltrating lymphocytes and response to neoadjuvant chemotherapy in breast cancer. *Cancer Immunol Res*, 2015. 3(4):326–32.

52. Karim, R., et al., Tumor-expressed B7-H1 and B7-DC in relation to PD-1+ T-cell infiltration and survival of patients with cervical carcinoma. *Clin Cancer Res*, 2009. 15(20):6341–47.

53. Mu, C.Y., et al., High expression of PD-L1 in lung cancer may contribute to poor prognosis and tumor cells immune escape through suppressing tumor infiltrating dendritic cells maturation. *Med Oncol*, 2011. 28(3):682–88.

54. Thompson, R.H., H. Dong, and E.D. Kwon, Implications of B7-H1 expression in clear cell carcinoma of the kidney for prognostication and therapy. *Clin Cancer Res*, 2007. 13(2 Pt 2):709s–15s.

55. Thompson, R.H., et al., PD-1 is expressed by tumor-infiltrating immune cells and is associated with poor outcome for patients with renal cell carcinoma. *Clin Cancer Res*, 2007. 13(6):1757–61.

56. Thompson, R.H., et al., Costimulatory molecule B7-H1 in primary and metastatic clear cell renal cell carcinoma. *Cancer*, 2005. 104(10):2084–91.

57. Thompson, R.H., et al., Tumor B7-H1 is associated with poor prognosis in renal cell carcinoma patients with long-term follow-up. *Cancer Res*, 2006. 66(7):3381–85.

58. Thompson, R.H., et al., B7-H1 glycoprotein blockade: a novel strategy to enhance immunotherapy in patients with renal cell carcinoma. *Urology*, 2005. 66(5 Suppl):10–14.

59. Ohigashi, Y., et al., Clinical significance of programmed death-1 ligand-1 and programmed death-1 ligand-2 expression in human esophageal cancer. *Clin Cancer Res*, 2005. 11(8):2947–53.

60. Wu, C., et al., Immunohistochemical localization of programmed death-1 ligand-1 (PD-L1) in gastric carcinoma and its clinical significance. *Acta Histochem*, 2006. 108(1):19–24.

61. Huang, Y., et al., The prognostic significance of PD-L1 in bladder cancer. *Oncol Rep*, 2015. 33(6):3075–84.

62. Teng, M.W., et al., Classifying cancers based on T-cell infiltration and PD-L1. *Cancer Res*, 2015. 75(11):2139–45.

63. Pages, F., et al., Effector memory T cells, early metastasis, and survival in colorectal cancer. *N Engl J Med*, 2005. 353(25):2654–66.

64. Zhang, L., et al., Intratumoral T cells, recurrence, and survival in epithelial ovarian cancer. *N Engl J Med*, 2003. 348(3):203–13.

65. Fukunaga, A., et al., CD8+ tumor-infiltrating lymphocytes together with CD4+ tumor-infiltrating lymphocytes and dendritic cells improve the prognosis of patients with pancreatic adenocarcinoma. *Pancreas*, 2004. 28(1):e26–31.

66. Schumacher, K., et al., Prognostic significance of activated CD8(+) T cell infiltrations within esophageal carcinomas. *Cancer Res*, 2001. 61(10):3932–36.

67. Eerola, A.K., Y. Soini, and P. Paakko, A high number of tumor-infiltrating lymphocytes are associated with a small tumor size, low tumor stage, and a favorable prognosis in operated small cell lung carcinoma. *Clin Cancer Res*, 2000. 6(5):1875–81.

68. Webster, W.S., et al., Mononuclear cell infiltration in clear-cell renal cell carcinoma independently predicts patient survival. *Cancer*, 2006. 107(1):46–53.

69. Hamanishi, J., et al., Programmed cell death 1 ligand 1 and tumor-infiltrating CD8+ T lymphocytes are prognostic factors of human ovarian cancer. *Proc Natl Acad Sci U S A*, 2007. 104(9):3360–65.

70. Sunshine, J. and J.M. Taube, PD-1/PD-L1 inhibitors. *Curr Opin Pharmacol*, 2015. 23:32–38.

71. Herbst, R.S., et al., Predictive correlates of response to the anti-PD-L1 antibody MPDL3280A in cancer patients. *Nature*, 2014. 515(7528):563–67.

72. Disis, M.L., et al., Avelumab (MSB0010718C; anti-PD-L1) in patients with recurrent/refractory ovarian cancer from the JAVELIN Solid Tumor phase Ib trial: safety and clinical activity. *J Clin Oncol*, 2016. 34(Suppl.):Abstract 5533.

73. Taube, J.M., et al., Association of PD-1, PD-1 ligands, and other features of the tumor immune microenvironment with response to anti-PD-1 therapy. *Clin Cancer Res*, 2014. 20(19):5064–74.

74. Santin, A.D., et al., Phenotypic and functional analysis of tumor-infiltrating lymphocytes compared with tumor-associated lymphocytes from ascitic fluid and peripheral blood lymphocytes in patients with advanced ovarian cancer. *Gynecol Obstet Invest*, 2001. 51(4):254–61.

75. Santin, A.D., et al., Induction of ovarian tumor-specific CD8+ cytotoxic T lymphocytes by acid-eluted peptide-pulsed autologous dendritic cells. *Obstet Gynecol*, 2000. 96(3):422–30.

76. Negus, R.P., et al., Quantitative assessment of the leukocyte infiltrate in ovarian cancer and its relationship to the expression of C-C chemokines. *Am J Pathol*, 1997. 150(5):1723–34.

77. Eisenthal, A., et al., Expression of dendritic cells in ovarian tumors correlates with clinical outcome in patients with ovarian cancer. *Hum Pathol*, 2001. 32(8):803–807.

78. Bachmayr-Heyda, A., et al., Prognostic impact of tumor infiltrating CD8+ T cells in association with cell proliferation in ovarian cancer patients—a study of the OVCAD consortium. *BMC Cancer*, 2013. 13:422.

79. Sato, E., et al., Intraepithelial CD8+ tumor-infiltrating lymphocytes and a high CD8+/regulatory T cell ratio are associated with favorable prognosis in ovarian cancer. *Proc Natl Acad Sci U S A*, 2005. 102(51):18538–43.

80. Curiel, T.J., et al., Specific recruitment of regulatory T cells in ovarian carcinoma fosters immune privilege and predicts reduced survival. *Nat Med*, 2004. 10(9):942–49.

81. Dong, H.P., et al., NK- and B-cell infiltration correlates with worse outcome in metastatic ovarian carcinoma. *Am J Clin Pathol*, 2006. 125(3):451–58.

82. Miyara, M., and S. Sakaguchi, Natural regulatory T cells: mechanisms of suppression. *Trends Mol Med*, 2007. 13(3):108–16.

83. Kryczek, I., et al., Relationship between B7-H4, regulatory T cells, and patient outcome in human ovarian carcinoma. *Cancer Res*, 2007. 67(18):8900–905.

84. Kryczek, I., et al., B7-H4 expression identifies a novel suppressive macrophage population in human ovarian carcinoma. *J Exp Med*, 2006. 203(4):871–81.

85. Mahnke, K., et al., Depletion of CD4+CD25+ human regulatory T cells in vivo: kinetics of Treg depletion and alterations in immune functions in vivo and in vitro. *Int J Cancer*, 2007. 120(12):2723–33.

86. Morse, M.A., et al., Depletion of human regulatory T cells specifically enhances antigen-specific immune responses to cancer vaccines. *Blood*, 2008. 112(3):610–18.

87. Powell, D.J., Jr., et al., Administration of a CD25-directed immunotoxin, LMB-2, to patients with metastatic melanoma induces a selective partial reduction in regulatory T cells in vivo. *J Immunol*, 2007. 179(7):4919–28.

88. Dannull, J., et al., Enhancement of vaccine-mediated antitumor immunity in cancer patients after depletion of regulatory T cells. *J Clin Invest*, 2005. 115(12):3623–33.

89. Rasku, M.A., et al., Transient T cell depletion causes regression of melanoma metastases. *J Transl Med*, 2008. 6:12.

90. Leffers, N., et al., Prognostic significance of tumor-infiltrating T-lymphocytes in primary and metastatic lesions of advanced stage ovarian cancer. *Cancer Immunol Immunother*, 2009. 58(3):449–59.

91. Webb, J.R., et al., PD-L1 expression is associated with tumor-infiltrating T cells and favorable prognosis in high-grade serous ovarian cancer. *Gynecol Oncol*, 2016. 141(2):293–302.

92. Milne, K., et al., Systematic analysis of immune infiltrates in high-grade serous ovarian cancer reveals CD20, FoxP3 and TIA-1 as positive prognostic factors. *PLoS One*, 2009. 4(7):e6412.

93. Wouters, M.C., et al., Treatment regimen, surgical outcome, and t-cell differentiation influence prognostic benefit of tumor-infiltrating lymphocytes in high-grade serous ovarian cancer. *Clin Cancer Res*, 2016. 22(3):714–24.

94. Hwang, W.T., et al., Prognostic significance of tumor-infiltrating T cells in ovarian cancer: a meta-analysis. *Gynecol Oncol*, 2012. 124(2):192–98.

95. Alagkiozidis, I., et al., Increased immunogenicity of surviving tumor cells enables cooperation between liposomal doxorubicin and IL-18. *J Transl Med*, 2009. 7:104.

96. Alagkiozidis, I., et al., Time-dependent cytotoxic drugs selectively cooperate with IL-18 for cancer chemo-immunotherapy. *J Transl Med*, 2011. 9:77.

97. Duluc, D., et al., Tumor-associated leukemia inhibitory factor and IL-6 skew monocyte differentiation into tumor-associated macrophage-like cells. *Blood*, 2007. 110(13):4319–30.

98. Hagemann, T., et al., Ovarian cancer cells polarize macrophages toward a tumor-associated phenotype. *J Immunol*, 2006. 176(8):5023–32.

99. Loercher, A.E., et al., Identification of an IL-10-producing HLA-DR-negative monocyte subset in the malignant ascites of patients with ovarian carcinoma that inhibits cytokine protein expression and proliferation of autologous T cells. *J Immunol*, 1999. 163(11):6251–60.

100. Gottlieb, C.E., et al., Tumor-associated macrophage expression of PD-L1 in implants of high grade serous ovarian carcinoma: a comparison of matched primary and metastatic tumors. *Gynecol Oncol*, 2017. 144(3):607–12.

101. Strickland, K.C., et al., Association and prognostic significance of BRCA1/2-mutation status with neoantigen load, number of tumor-infiltrating lymphocytes and expression of PD-1/PD-L1 in high grade serous ovarian cancer. *Oncotarget*, 2016. 7(12):13587–98.

102. Scarlett, U.K., et al., Ovarian cancer progression is controlled by phenotypic changes in dendritic cells. *J Exp Med*, 2012. 209(3):495–506.

103. Krempski, J., et al., Tumor-infiltrating programmed death receptor-1+ dendritic cells mediate immune suppression in ovarian cancer. *J Immunol*, 2011. 186(12):6905–13.

104. Karyampudi, L., et al., PD-1 blunts the function of ovarian tumor-infiltrating dendritic cells by inactivating NF-□B. *Cancer Res*, 2016. 76(2):239–50.

105. Maine, C.J., et al., Programmed death ligand-1 over-expression correlates with malignancy and

contributes to immune regulation in ovarian cancer. *Cancer Immunol Immunother*, 2014. 63(3):215–24.

106. Darb-Esfahani, S., et al., Prognostic impact of programmed cell death-1 (PD-1) and PD-ligand 1 (PD-L1) expression in cancer cells and tumor-infiltrating lymphocytes in ovarian high grade serous carcinoma. *Oncotarget*, 2016. 7(2):1486–99.

107. Kobel, M., et al., Ovarian carcinoma subtypes are different diseases: implications for biomarker studies. *PLoS Med*, 2008. 5(12):e232.

108. Hamanishi, J., et al., Safety and antitumor activity of anti-PD-1 antibody, nivolumab, in patients with platinum-resistant ovarian cancer. *J Clin Oncol*, 2015. 33(34):4015–22.

109. Topalian, S.L., et al., Mechanism-driven biomarkers to guide immune checkpoint blockade in cancer therapy. *Nat Rev Cancer*, 2016. 16(5):275–87.

110. Hamid, O., et al., Safety and tumor responses with lambrolizumab (anti-PD-1) in melanoma. *N Engl J Med*, 2013. 369(2):134–44.

111. Robert, C., et al., Nivolumab in previously untreated melanoma without BRAF mutation. *N Engl J Med*, 2015. 372(4):320–30.

112. Robert, C., et al., Pembrolizumab versus ipilimumab in advanced melanoma. *N Engl J Med*, 2015. 372(26):2521–32.

113. Larkin, J., et al., Combined nivolumab and ipilimumab or monotherapy in untreated melanoma. *N Engl J Med*, 2015. 373(1):23–34.

114. Garon, E.B., et al., Pembrolizumab for the treatment of non-small-cell lung cancer. *N Engl J Med*, 2015. 372(21):2018–28.

115. Brahmer, J.R., et al., Safety and activity of anti-PD-L1 antibody in patients with advanced cancer. *N Engl J Med*, 2012. 366(26):2455–65.

116. Borghaei, H., et al., Nivolumab versus docetaxel in advanced nonsquamous non-small-cell lung cancer. *N Engl J Med*, 2015. 373(17):1627–39.

117. Motzer, R.J., et al., Nivolumab for metastatic renal cell carcinoma: results of a randomized phase II trial. *J Clin Oncol*, 2015. 33(13):1430–37.

118. Berger, R., et al., Phase I safety and pharmacokinetic study of CT-011, a humanized antibody interacting with PD-1, in patients with advanced hematologic malignancies. *Clin Cancer Res*, 2008. 14(10):3044–51.

119. Topalian, S.L., et al., Safety, activity, and immune correlates of anti-PD-1 antibody in cancer. *N Engl J Med*, 2012. 366(26):2443–54.

120. Mutch, D.G., et al., Randomized phase III trial of gemcitabine compared with pegylated liposomal doxorubicin in patients with platinum-resistant ovarian cancer. *J Clin Oncol*, 2007. 25(19):2811–18.

121. Gordon, A.N., et al., Recurrent epithelial ovarian carcinoma: a randomized phase III study of pegylated liposomal doxorubicin versus topotecan. *J Clin Oncol*, 2001. 19(14):3312–22.

122. Varga, A., et al., Antitumor activity and safety of pembrolizumab in patients with PD-L1 positive advanced ovarian cancer: Interim results from a phase Ib study. *J Clin Oncol*, 2015. 33(Suppl.):Abstract 5510.

123. Sharma, P., and J.P. Allison, The future of immune checkpoint therapy. *Science*, 2015. 348(6230):56–61.

124. Grabosch, S., et al., Abstract 3208: Chemo-induced biology of PD-L1 and in vivo combination immune therapy for ovarian cancer. *Cancer Res*, 2016. 76(14 Suppl.):3208–3208.

125. Grabosch, S., et al., PD-L1 biology in response to chemotherapy in vitro and in vivo in ovarian cancer. *J ImmunoTherap Cancer*, 2015. 3(2):P302.

126. Mesnage, S.J., et al., Neoadjuvant chemotherapy (NACT) increases immune infiltration and programmed death-ligand 1 (PD-L1) expression in epithelial ovarian cancer (EOC). *Ann Oncol*, 2016. 28(3):651–57.

127. Bohm, S., et al., Neoadjuvant chemotherapy modulates the immune microenvironment in metastases of tubo-ovarian high-grade serous carcinoma. *Clin Cancer Res*, 2016. 22(12):3025–36.

128. Mantia-Smaldone, G., et al., The immunomodulatory effects of pegylated liposomal doxorubicin are amplified in BRCA1—deficient ovarian tumors and can be exploited to improve treatment response in a mouse model. *Gynecol Oncol*, 2014. 133(3):584–90.

129. Xu, S., et al., miR-424(322) reverses chemoresistance via T-cell immune response activation by blocking the PD-L1 immune checkpoint. *Nat Commun*, 2016. 7:11406.

130. Mateos-Gomez, P.A., et al., Mammalian polymerase theta promotes alternative NHEJ and suppresses recombination. *Nature*, 2015. 518(7538):254–57.

131. Ceccaldi, R., et al., Homologous-recombination-deficient tumours are dependent on Poltheta-mediated repair. *Nature*, 2015. 518(7538):258–62.

132. Lee, J., et al., Phase I study of the PD-L1 inhibitor, durvalumab (MEDI4736; D) in combination with a PARP inhibitor, olaparib (O) or a VEGFR inhibitor, cediranib (C) in women's cancers (NCT02484404). *J Clin Oncol*, 2016. 34:Abstract 3015.

133. Wrangle, J., et al., Abstract 4619: epigenetic therapy and sensitization of lung cancer to immunotherapy. *Cancer Res*, 2013. 73(8 Suppl.):4619–4619.

134. Li, H., et al., Immune regulation by low doses of the DNA methyltransferase inhibitor 5-azacitidine in common human epithelial cancers. *Oncotarget*, 2014. 5(3):587–98.

135. Chiappinelli, K.B., et al., Inhibiting DNA methylation causes an interferon response in cancer via dsRNA including endogenous retroviruses. *Cell*, 2015. 162(5):974–86.

136. Dear, A.E., Epigenetic modulators and the new immunotherapies. *N Engl J Med*, 2016. 374(7):684–86.

136a. Budczies, J., et al., Pan-cancer analysis of copy number changes in programmed death-ligand 1 (PD-L1, CD274)—associations with gene expression, mutational load, and survival. *Genes, Chromosomes and Cancer*, 2016. 55(8):626–39.

137. Schumacher, T.N. and R.D. Schreiber, Neoantigens in cancer immunotherapy. *Science*, 2015. 348(6230):69–74.

138. Stronen, E., et al., Targeting of cancer neoantigens with donor-derived T cell receptor repertoires. *Science*, 2016. 352(6291):1337–41.

139. Le, D.T., et al., PD-1 Blockade in tumors with mismatch-repair deficiency. *N Engl J Med*, 2015. 372(26):2509–20.

140. Danilova, L., et al., Association of PD-1/PD-L axis expression with cytolytic activity, mutational load, and prognosis in melanoma and other solid tumors. *Proc Natl Acad Sci U S A*, 2016. 113(48):E7769–e7777.

141. Rizvi, N.A., et al., Cancer immunology. Mutational landscape determines sensitivity to PD-1 blockade in non-small cell lung cancer. *Science*, 2015. 348(6230):124–28.

142. Llosa, N.J., et al., The vigorous immune microenvironment of microsatellite instable colon cancer is balanced by multiple counter-inhibitory checkpoints. *Cancer Discov*, 2015. 5(1):43–51.

143. Xiao, Y. and G.J. Freeman, The microsatellite instable subset of colorectal cancer is a particularly good candidate for checkpoint blockade immunotherapy. *Cancer Discov*, 2015. 5(1):16–18.

144. Xiao, X., D.W. Melton, and C. Gourley, Mismatch repair deficiency in ovarian cancer—molecular characteristics and clinical implications. *Gynecol Oncol*, 2014. 132(2):506–12.

145. Bell, D., et al., Integrated genomic analyses of ovarian carcinoma. *Nature*, 2011. 474(7353):609–15.

146. Patch, A.M., et al., Whole-genome characterization of chemoresistant ovarian cancer. *Nature*, 2015. 521(7553):489–94.

147. McAlpine, J.N., et al., BRCA1 and BRCA2 mutations correlate with TP53 abnormalities and presence of immune cell infiltrates in ovarian high-grade serous carcinoma. *Mod Pathol*, 2012. 25(5):740–50.

148. Schumacher, T.N., and N. Hacohen, Neoantigens encoded in the cancer genome. *Curr Opin Immunol*, 2016. 41:98–103.

149. Friedlander, M.L., et al., Molecular profiling of clear cell ovarian cancers: identifying potential treatment targets for clinical trials. *Int J Gynecol Cancer*, 2016. 26(4):648–54.

150. Lastwika, K.J., et al., Control of PD-L1 expression by oncogenic activation of the AKT-mTOR pathway in non-small cell lung cancer. *Cancer Res*, 2016. 76(2):227–38.

151. Qu, Q.X., et al., The increase of circulating PD-L1-expressing CD68(+) macrophage in ovarian cancer. *Tumour Biol*, 2016. 37(4):5031–37.

152. Abiko, K., et al., PD-L1 on tumor cells is induced in ascites and promotes peritoneal dissemination of ovarian cancer through CTL dysfunction. *Clin Cancer Res*, 2013. 19(6):1363–74.

153. Paracchini, L., et al., Regional and temporal heterogeneity of epithelial ovarian cancer tumor biopsies: implications for therapeutic strategies. *Oncotarget*, 2016. http://www.oncotarget.com/index.php?journal=oncotarget&page=article&op=view&path[]=10505&path%5B%5D=33196

11.

GROWTH FACTORS AND THEIR CORRESPONDING RECEPTORS AS TARGETS FOR OVARIAN CANCER THERAPY

Anca Maria Cimpean, Andreea Adriana Jitariu, and Marius Raica

INTRODUCTION

Ovarian cancer remains one of the most common cause of cancer death, not only in less-developed countries but also in those countries with a well-developed health system. Inside malignancy of the ovary, epithelial neoplasms predominate. It is known that epithelial cells with various origins have the ability to secrete growth factors during embryogenesis but also as a response to any damage of the epithelium or during malignancy. Growth factors secretion is followed by regeneration of the epithelial cells from different organs in a controlled manner[1] by inducing the epithelial proliferation, migration, and differentiation. On the other hand, epithelial malignant cells secrete similar growth factors which produce a chaotic, uncontrolled proliferation of neoplastic epithelial cells together with an extensive angiogenesis and lymphangiogenesis-favoring metastasis.[2,3] Most known growth factors, such as fibroblast growth factors (FGFs), platelet-derived growth factors (PDGFs), and vascular endothelial growth factors (VEGFs), were intensely studied in ovarian carcinomas, but their clinical and therapeutic impact are still obscure, and, most probably, therapies targeting these growth factors and/or corresponding receptors does not have the expected efficiency as that observed in pre-clinical models.

THE PDGF BB TYPE IN OVARIAN CANCER

PDGF is a member of the growth factor family that regulates cell growth and division. In a relatively specific way, PDGF plays an important role in the formation of blood vessels during the process of angiogenesis as well as in their growth and maturation. Excessive angiogenesis is a malignant characteristic, but it is also found in the complications of other types of diseases such as diabetes or rheumatoid arthritis. Its chemical structure is that of a dimeric glycoprotein with three isoforms, namely AA, BB, and AB. PDGF is also a potent mitogen factor for mesenchyme-derived cells such as fibroblasts, smooth muscle cells, and glia cells.[4,5] PDGFB is secreted by tumor cells but also by endothelial cells.[6] Its expression in different tumor types determined its study as a potential double-role therapeutic target, namely that of destruction caused to tumor but also the developmental blockage of the adjacent blood vessels. Currently, an anti-PDGF therapy with a large applicability is available especially in oftalmology.

An inhibitor (fovista) with specificity for PDGFB was developed and used on a large scale especially as an inhibitor of angiogenesis in macular degeneration through its stimulating effects on bevacizumab.[7]

The interrelation with VEGF was also observed in ovarian tumors and was reported by Matei and colleagues in 2007.[8] The authors found that PDGF BB induces VEGF secretion in ovarian carcinomas. The authors also noticed that the inhibition of the PDGF cognate receptor using imatinib resulted in a decrease of the serum, immunohistochemical, and molecular levels of VEGF in ovarian carcinomas. Also using an experimental model of ovarian carcinoma that originated from the human tumor cells, Lu and colleagues highlighted the high efficacy of anti-PDGFB therapy through the dual targeting of endothelial cells using bevacizumab and pericytes in an anti-PDGF aptamer.[9]

Recent data continue to support the combined anti-VEGF and anti-PDGF therapy in ovarian cancer.[10] Despite preliminary data that support this combination, the data resulting from in vitro experimental models and, to a lesser extent in vivo, the afferent studies regarding PDGFB expression in ovarian cancers from human tissues are extremely limited; currently the literature cites not more than 14 articles that have PDGFB in these tumor types as their main theme.

OUR RESEARCH EXPERIENCE IN THE EVALUATION OF PDGF BB IN OVARIAN CANCER

Due to the aforementioned aspects, we considered PDGF BB evaluation to be useful on ovarian tumors included in the study as we attempted to confirm our data at a proteic level using molecular methods such as in situ hybridization or RNA quantification on paraffin embedded tissues. This multimodal approach recently published[11] may be useful to complete the microscopic and molecular evaluation of ovarian carcinomas with a possible impact on increasing therapeutic efficacy for such malignant lesions. We found PDGFB expression in the quasinormal ovarian tissue adjacent to the tumor, at the level of the tumor stroma. Stromal cells from normal ovary cortex were positive for PDGFB while for their medullary counterparts PDGFB expression gradually decreased. In the large vessels from the ovarian medulla, PDGFB expression was absent in the endothelial cells lining their lumen and was extremely weak in the ovarian stroma. On the other hand, small size vessels from the ovarian cortex constantly exhibited a positive reaction for PDGF. The intensity of the PDGF B was moderate in the zone located underneath the albuginea of the ovary so that the area that was adjacent to the albicans bodies presented either a low or a negative reaction for PDGFB (Figure 11.1).

PDGF expression in ovarian tumors was detected within the tumor and in the

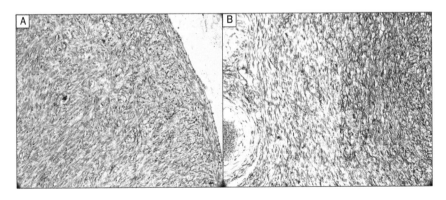

Figure 11.1 PDGF BB in normal human ovary cortex (A) and medulla (B).

peritumoral stroma in 88.1% of cases. Its expression was cytoplasmic and nuclear, dependent on the tumor type and in the tumor cells. At the level of the stroma, an intense reaction was observed in the endothelial cells from the large vessels but also in the stromal cells such as fibroblasts and myofibroblast-like.

In the tumor areas, the nuclear and cytoplasmic expression in the tumor cells was accompanied by PDGFB expression at a nuclear level in the intratumoral blood vessels that were visible, especially in those that were characterized by active angiogenesis. For instance, in a thecoma case we noticed a differential PDGFB expression in the same intratumoral vessel, thus the endothelial cells from the sprouting tip were intensely positive for PDGFB seeming either in direct contact with the positive tumor cells, unlike the endothelial cells lining the rest of the vessels that were negative for PDGFB. In the serous cystadenocarcinoma, PDGFB expression was predominantly cytoplasmic. Very rare zones were characterized by a nuclear expression. PDGF in endometrioid carcinoma is restricted at a cytoplasmic level, but in papillary serous cystadenocarcinomas, the expression is nuclear, cytoplasmic, or combined.

The microscopic evaluation of PDGFB expression evidenced a clear limit between benign and malignant lesions, thus in benign lesions such as thecomas or serous and mucinous cystadenocarcinoma, 22.4% of the total

number of the studied were benign tumors such as serous or mucinous cystadenoma or thecomas, cystic teratoma, dermoid cyst. Out of these, 62.5% did not express PDGFB neither in the stroma nor in the tumor areas. Unlike benign lesions, malignant lesions presented a more intense PDGFB expression with a heterogeneous pattern in both tumor cells and in the tumor stroma. The predominant pattern was a combined nuclear and cytoplasmic one that characterized serous cystadenocarcinomas of the ovary. Regarding PDGFB expression in tumor cells, the majority of cases presented an intense and moderate expression (Figure 11.2). We encountered a low expression, scored +1 or absent in only 7.5%. On the other hand, the stroma exhibited a predominantly low and moderate expression in spite of an intense expression. Moreover, at the level of the tumor stroma, PDGFB expression was found in myofibroblast-like cells and fibroblast-like cells but also in endothelial cells. Out of the total number of studied cases, we observed a strong PDGFB expression (scored +3) in 65.7% of cases; 14.9% presented a +2 PDGFB expression, 7.5% had a low expression (scored +1), and 11.9% out of the total number of analyzed cases did not express PDGFB.

We analyzed PDGFB expression at a nuclear and cytoplasmic level. We found that 35.8% of cases presented a nuclear expression, unlike the 16.4% of the examined blocks that were characterized by a cytoplasmic

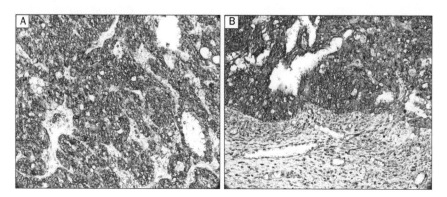

Figure 11.2 Endometrioid type carcinoma, positive with a high intensity for PDGF BB in tumor cells (A) with the pack of expression in tumor stroma, except blood vessels (B).

expression. Despite this, 37.3% exhibited both a nuclear and a cytoplasmic expression, unlike the 10.4% that did not express PDGFB neither at a cytoplasmic level nor at a nuclear level.

We noted that 38.8% presented a strong PDGFB expression in the stroma (scored +3), 14.9% exhibited a stromal PDGFB expression (scored +2), and an equal number (14.9%) of cases that presented a stromal PDGFB expression scored +1; 31.3% of cases did not express PDGFB in the stroma. These analyses were conducted on a study group that included 65.7% malignant tumors, 11.9% of ovarian carcinomas of endometrioid type being separately subject to follow-up, and 22.4% benign tumors. We conducted a comparative analysis of PDGFB expression in the tumor cells compared to pattern distribution of PDGFB expression in the ovarian tumors included in our study. We observed a significant correlation between the intense PDGFB expression in the tumor cells and the nuclear and cellular expression of the PDGFB pattern. We established an extremely significant correlation between PDGFB expression in the tumor cells and the PDGFB pattern of expression (χ^2, $p < 0.001$).

On the other hand, we evaluated the intensity of the PDGFB expression in the tumor cells compared to that of PDGFB expression in the stroma of ovarian tumors. We found a correlation between PDGFB expression in the tumor cells compared to the PDGFB expression in the stroma, indicating a direct proportional increase of the correlation along with the increase of the expression intensity. A statistically significant correlation was established between PDGFB expression in the tumor cells and PDGFB expression in the stroma (χ^2, $p = 0.008$). All of these aspects are summarized in Tables 11.1, 11.2, 11.3 and 11.4.

Due to the intense expression found on immunohistochemically stained specimens, we considered the confirmation of PDGFB expression as useful through hybridization and adjacent molecular techniques.

TABLE 11.1 **THE PROCENTUAL EXPRESSION OF THE PDGF-BB POSITIVE CASES, DEPENDENT BY INTENSITY OF IMMUNOHISTOCHEMICAL EXPRESSION IN TUMOR CELLS**

PDGFB Stromal	No.	%
0	21	31.3
1	10	14.9
2	10	14.9
3	26	38.8
Total	67	100.0

NOTE: PDGF = platelet-derived growth factor.

TABLE 11.2 **DISTRIBUTION OF PDGF-BB EXPRESSION PATTERNS IN OVARIAN TUMORS INCLUDED IN THE STUDY**

PDGF BB Score in Tumor Cells	No. Cases	%
0	8	11.9
1	5	7.5
2	10	14.9
3	44	65.7
Total	67	100.0

NOTE: PDGF = platelet-derived growth factor.

TABLE 11.3 **CASE DISTRIBUTION ACCORDING TO IMMUNOHISTOCHEMICAL SCORE GIVEN FOR STROMAL COMPARTMENT FOR PDGF BB EXPRESSION IN OVARIAN TUMORS**

PDGF BB Immunohistochemical Pattern	No. Cases	%
0	7	10.4
Cytoplasmic	11	16.4
Nuclear	24	35.8
Combined	25	37.3
Total	67	100.0

NOTE: PDGF = platelet-derived growth factor.

TABLE 11.4 INTERRELATION BETWEEN TUMOR STROMAL PDGF BB EXPRESSION

PDGF-BB in Tumor Cells	PDGFB Stromal Cells				
	0	1	2	3	Total
0	7	0	0	1	8
	87.5%	0%	0%	12.5%	100.0%
1	3	1	1	0	5
	60.0%	20.0%	20.0%	0%	100.0%
2	4	2	2	2	10
	40.0%	20.0%	20.0%	20.0%	100.0%
3	7	7	7	23	44
	15.9%	15.9%	15.9%	52.3%	100.0%

NOTE: PDGF = platelet-derived growth factor.

In situ hybridization by applying the RNAscope method for PDGFB revealed a genic amplification of PDGFB in 63.7% of cases. Also, we observed that 28.5% were characterized by a genic amplification that was restricted to the tumor stroma, while the rest presented an amplification that was located in the stromal cells and also in the tumor cells.

The cases in which we obtained a negative immunoreaction were confirmed as negative using in situ hybridization for PDGFB mRNA. The cases that presented a cytoplasmic immunohistochemical reaction in the tumor cells were not confirmed by in situ hybridization. For the cases that were characterized by a combined nuclear and cytoplasmic immunoreaction we obtained the highest hybridization score, with the presence of dotted signals, predominantly at a nuclear level. Also, the majority of cases that were confirmed by means of hybridization exhibited a papillary aspect.

Compared to immunohistochemistry, in situ hybridization detected a heterogeneity of PDGFB overexpression in the tumor cells. We identified tumor cell areas lacking amplification that were mixed with tumor cell areas exhibiting a high PDGFB amplification.

Our results showed the existence of several overexpression patterns. In cases in which the pattern of expression was predominantly nuclear we noted a group-like amplification with amplification dots (dot aggregates), compared to the cases that presented a combined nuclear and cytoplasmic expression, where the dots were scattered with the possibility of their separate count. The stromal amplification in the stromal cells was always weaker compared to the one found in the tumor cells that was present in almost all examined cases. PDGF/mRNA amplification scored 3 was identified in the intratumoral stroma. The same amplification was observed in the peritumoral stroma where myofibroblast-like cells were predominant (Figure 11.3).

PDGF BB EXPRESSION IN OVARIAN CARCINOMA FROM BASIC SCIENCE TO THE CLINIC: WHAT IS MISSING?

Ovarian tumors remain a major problem of women's health, partially due to their insidious evolution and aggressive character and partially due to the absence of an efficient therapy able to improve the prognosis and long-term survival of patients' diagnoses with such malignancies. The current tendencies in ovarian cancer therapy aim toward a multimodal approach and the identification and

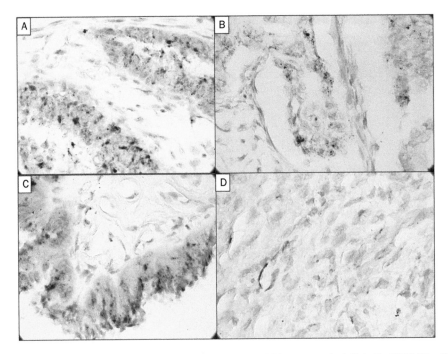

Figure 11.3 PDGF BB mRNA amplification in ovarian cancer certified by RNA scope method. Note the PDGF BB mRNA amplification heterogeneity inside the same tumor (A) and between different ovarian malignant tumors (B, C). Myofibroblast like cells from the stroma had a low amplification for PDGF BB mRNA (D).

usage not only of tumor cells but also of the tumor microenvironment and/or the tumor vasculature as therapeutic targets.[12,13] The addition of inhibitory therapies for growth factors is being assessed; currently the only approved therapy is bevacizumab.[14,15] The partial response of ovarian carcinomas to bevacizumab treatment that is associated with the conventional ovarian cancer therapy determined the reclassification of ovarian cancer through defining molecular groups of prognostic and therapeutic stratification.[16] Recently, lynparza-based therapy, associated with conventional chemotherapy, significantly increased long-term survival prognosis especially for patients with BRCA-type mutations.[17]

Other targeted therapies such as pazopanib, cedirinib, nitedanib, sunitinib, sorafenib, or imatinib[18–22] were also tested for ovarian cancer, but until now none of them received approval to be applied in current medical practice. PDGF/PDGFRbeta axis is less studied in ovarian cancer, paradoxically,

with only 14 research studies reporting their expression in ovarian cancer. The majority of studies made use of PDGFB plasma levels for the stratification of patients with ovarian cancer. Our study revealed PDGFB expression in the tumor cells and in the cells of the tumor stroma. The percentage of PDGFB positive cases is similar to the one described until now in the literature.[23] PDGFB expression in ovarian tumors was reported for the first time by Kacinski and colleagues in 1989.[24] Despite its confirmation through other studies, most of them in vitro,[25] the application of anti-PDGF therapy did not significantly evolve.

Our study attempted a more complex approach of PDGFB evaluation in ovarian cancer. Therefore, we applied immunohistochemical methods, in situ hybridization, and other molecular techniques. Immunohistochemically, in over 80% of the total number of cases, we observed the existence of an immunohistochemical reaction, but, of these, only 63.7% were confirmed as positive using in situ hybridization. This percentage is similar to the one reported in the literature in 2008 on immunohistochemically stained specimens.[26]

The same study presented a series of immunohistochemical images in which PDGF-B expression was both nuclear and cytoplasmic. Our study described three expression patterns for PDGF-B in ovarian carcinomas: nuclear, cytoplasmic and combined, and nuclear and cytoplasmic. This aspect enabled us to validate PDGF BB immunohistochemical expression with subsequent molecular methods. PDGF-B cytoplasmic expression is well known and documented; its nuclear expression is associated with an increase in the tumor progression and aggressiveness, most probably through a hypoxia-induced mechanism. PDGF nuclear expression seems to be regulated by the c-sis system, an aspect that was intensely discussed in metastatic and non-metastatic renal carcinomas.[27,28] It appears that the c-sis/PDGF tandem is implicated in its autocrine effect on tumor cells as it is presented in literature by numerous in vitro and in vivo studies.[29] Moreover, this interrelation is hormonally influenced, an aspect that has not yet been studied in ovarian tumors.[30]

Another incompletely studied and sometimes neglected issue is represented by PDGF-B expression in the tumor stroma. In the tumor stroma, PDGF-B is secreted by fibroblasts and by myofiboblast-type cells.[31] The tumor stroma is regarded as a "malignant" stroma and is implicated in influencing tumor cell behavior as it has already been certified in some molecular forms of breast cancer.[32] In 2006, Lederle and colleagues demonstrated that PDGF BB is intensely expressed in tumor fibroblasts and that its overexpression in tumor fibroblasts increases tumor cell proliferation initially through a transient increase of VEGFA through a paracrine-type mechanism. Moreover, through this mechanism, PDGF BB induces epithelial hyperproliferation thus determining tumor progression.[33]

These aspects were also supported by our results due to the fact that concomitant PDGF-B expression in the stroma and in the tumor cells was certified in over 50% of the cases included in the study. In most cases its expression was nuclear, and this represents another argument for PDGF-B implication in the well-known progression and aggression that are characteristic of ovarian carcinomas. In addition, PDGF-B overexpression was exclusively observed at a nuclear level in the fibroblasts belonging to the tumor stroma.

Our study identified a statistically significant correlation between PDGF-B expression in the stroma and in the tumor cells, thus suggesting a direct interrelation between the two tumoral components and sustains the existence of at least two therapeutic targets that may be neutralized through the application of the same anti-PDGF targeted treatment. The aggressiveness of ovarian carcinomas, which is well documented, is also supported by the nuclear PDGF expression that was identified in our study in over 70% of tumors, associated or not with a cytoplasmic one. Once again, this aspect highlights the implication of PDGF-B in the genesis of ovarian carcinomas but also in therapy resistance.

PDGF-B is expressed in both tumor cells and stromal cells from the tumor stroma of ovarian carcinomas. The overlapping of PDGF-B expression in the stroma and in the tumor cells supports the influence of the stroma on epithelial cell proliferation in ovarian tumors, an aspect that was sustained and significantly correlated from a statistical point of view and reported in our study. It seems that PDGF-B nuclear expression represents an unfavorable prognostic factor in ovarian tumors, but this aspect needs further study. It is mandatory for PDGF-BB immunohistochemical evaluation to be associated with at least one molecular validation method, in situ hybridization, and/or evaluation using other methods such as reverse transcription polymerase chain reaction or PDGF/RNA, respectively. Our results support the application of anti-PDGF-B therapy as an adjuvant therapy, associated with the conventional chemotherapy used in ovarian cancer

FGF/FGFR AXIS IN OVARIAN CANCER: PROGNOSTIC ISSUES AND THERAPEUTIC CHALLENGES

Different experimental studies that used ovarian cancer cell lines[34,35] highlighted the existence of a mutant FGFR and an altered FGF/FGFR axis in ovarian cancer patients.[34] Along with the PDGF family members and their cognate receptors, the FGF/FGFR axis is included among the markers with diagnostic value in ovarian cancer.[36] Using malignant and benign ovarian specimens, borderline ovarian tumors, and healthy control groups, the study conducted by Horala et al.[36] provides multimarker models that include FGF, hepatocyte growth factor, PDGF, follistatin, osteopontin, and leptin in order to ensure a more accurate discrimination between different ovarian lesions. Currently, the molecular mechanisms through which the FGF/FGFR axis promotes ovarian cancer growth, progression, and invasion are incompletely elucidated and controversial, although several clinical and preclinical studies have been focused on this issue over the past years.

Together with other growth factor molecules, FGF is secreted by cancer-associated fibroblasts which are one of the main key players in ovarian cancer progression and invasion.[35] Following FGFR4 phosphorylation, FGF1 determines a cascade of events in which different mitogen-activated protein kinases and epithelial-to-mesenchymal transition associated genes are activated thus promoting ovarian cancer progression.[35] However, FGFR4 is not the only member of the FGF/FGFR family that may be regarded as a potential therapeutic target. FGFR1, FGFR2, and FGFR3 are also important promoters of ovarian cancer progression and may be successfully blocked using selective FGFR inhibitors.[34,37] In order to assess the efficacy of FGFR inhibitors, Tyulyandina et al.[37] used the SKOV3 ovarian cancer cell line that does not express FGF3 but contains tumor cells that are positive for FGFR1 and

FGFR2. Regarding these aspects, alofanib, a novel and selective FGFR2 inhibitor, showed its efficacy in reducing tumor cell growth in several types of cancer such as triple-negative breast cancer, malignant melanoma, and ovarian cancer.[37,38] However, FGFR inhibition alone is not able to ensure ovarian cancer regression. Epithelial ovarian carcinomas are characterized by a synergic Syndecan-1 (SDC-1)–FGF-2 through which malignant cell proliferation and angiogenesis are stimulated.[39] Despite these facts, it appears that the addition of exogenous FGF-2 created the ability to reduce SDC-1 mRNA, thus making the interaction between FGF and other molecules a controversial and somehow paradoxical aspect in ovarian cancer.[39] Moreover, Masoumi-Moghaddam et al.[40] found no statistically significant correlation between FGF expression and the clincopathological features of patients diagnosed with ovarian cancer.

Besides the effects of the FGF/FGFR axis in stimulating the proliferation and migration of ovarian cancer cells, FGF family members are potent promoters of angiogenesis and lymphangiogenesis.[41] FGF-2, along with other growth factor families and different cytokines, is associated with an increased microvessel and microlymphatic vessel density.[41] From this perspective, FGF has been proposed as an anti-angiogenic target, along with PDGF, epidermal growth factor, and VEGF.[38] The use of an anti-VEGF therapeutic strategy in order to inhibit angiogenesis in ovarian cancer specimens leads to different changes in both the tumor and the stromal cells and also in the signaling pathways that ensure tumor growth and progression.[42] Could these changes be represented by increased FGF levels in ovarian tumor cells and tumor-associated fibroblasts? These statements represent another argument that supports the great plasticity of human malignant tumors, including ovarian carcinomas, to a series of stimuli that need further investigation along with the great panel of growth factor families that are implicated in carcinogenesis.

NERVE GROWTH FACTOR AND ENDOCRINE GLAND DERIVED GROWTH FACTOR IN OVARIAN CANCER: POTENTIAL NEW MARKERS FOR PROGNOSIS AND THERAPY

Recently, nerve growth factor (NGF) and its receptors started to be intensely studied in ovarian cancer. It is now certified that NGF promotes proliferation, migration, and differentiation of tumor cells in several malignancies such as esophageal and colon cancer.[43] Discovered first in the nervous system, NGF is involved in the development and normal function of the ovary[44] by allowing the differentiation of precursor cells into primordial follicles and also by allowing the maturation of ovarian follicles.[45] Also, NGF together with VEGF are key players of an intense angiogenic process mandatory for the development of ovarian follicles in normal conditions through tyrosine kinase A receptor.[46–48] Interestingly, the same growth factors induce angiogenesis together with proliferation, migration, and metastasis of malignant cells in ovarian cancer but by uncontrolled and less known mechanisms.[49–51] Various mechanisms have been proposed regarding the involvement of NGF in ovarian tumorigenesis as acting at the epigenetic level or by inducing DNA mutations or chromosomal alterations, and/or by alteration of post-transcriptional or post-translational regulations.[52–55]

But the most neglected growth factor seems to be endocrine gland-derived vascular endothelial growth factor (EG VEGF). EG VEGF, also called prokineticin 1, is known as a regulator of endometrial receptivity and placental development and, together with its receptor, is highly expressed during human folliculogenesis.[56] In the human fetal ovary, EG VEGF is a regulator of germ cell development, and its increased levels induce ERK phosphorylation and elevated COX2 expression in germ cells.[57] Few and scattered data are reported about the involvement of EG VEGF in human ovarian carcinogenesis, but all report a variable overexpression of EG VEGF dependent by tumor type and with a potential impact on prognosis. EG-VEGF is overexpressed mainly in high-grade ovarian carcinomas (type II). Significant differences were registered between the EG-VEGF positive or negative expression and tumor stage and histological subtypes, respectively.[58] Our research group reported that EG-VEGF expression in tumor cells of the epithelial ovarian cancer is a good marker of unfavorable prognosis and could be an attractive therapeutic target in patients with advanced-stage tumors undergoing refractory conventional chemotherapy.[59] Neoplastic cells of the ovarian carcinoma expressed EG-VEGF in 73.33% of the cases, as a cytoplasmic granular product of reaction. We found a strong correlation between the expression of EG-VEGF at the protein level and tumor stage, grade, and microscopic type. The expression of EG-VEGF was found in patients with stage III and IV but not stage II cancer. The majority of serous adenocarcinoma, half of the cases with clear cell carcinoma, and two cases with endometrioid carcinoma showed definite expression in tumor cells. No positive reaction was found in the cases with mucinous carcinoma. Our results showed that EG-VEGF expression is an indicator not only of the advanced stage but also of ovarian cancer progression.[59,60]

CONCLUSIONS AND FUTURE DIRECTIONS

The involvement of growth factors in ovarian carcinogenesis is already proven in pre-clinical studies, but their utility for a better characterization of ovarian cancer is still controversial. A more accurate assessment of growth factors' expression and variability in ovarian cancer may be helpful to define molecular subtypes of ovarian malignant diseases. The definition of molecular subtypes of ovarian cancer, based on growth factors expression together with genetic and epigenetic criteria, may have a strong impact on therapeutic options. To treat each patient in a personalized fashion and not the disease would be the "gold standard" for ovarian cancer in the future.

REFERENCES

1. Kardia E, Mohamed R, and Yahaya BH: Stimulatory secretions of airway epithelial cells accelerate early repair of tracheal epithelium. *Sci Rep 7*: 11732, 2017.
2. Xu CH, He ZH, and Xu H: Association of four genetic polymorphisms in the vascular endothelial growth factor-A gene and development of ovarian cancer: a meta-analysis. *Oncotarget 8*: 73063–78, 2017.
3. Choi HJ, Armaiz Pena GN, Pradeep S, Cho MS, Coleman RL, and Sood AK: Anti-vascular therapies in ovarian cancer: moving beyond anti-VEGF approaches. *Cancer Metastasis Rev 34*: 19–40, 2017.
4. Hannink M, and Donoghue DJ: Structure and function of platelet-derived growth factor (PDGF) and related proteins. *Biochim Biophys Acta 989*: 1–10, 1989.
5. Heldin CH: Structural and functional studies on platelet-derived growth factor. *EMBO J 11*: 4251–59, 1992.
6. Abramsson A, Lindblom P, and Betsholtz C: Endothelial and nonendothelial sources of PDGF-B regulate pericyte recruitment and influence vascular pattern formation in tumors. *J Clin Invest 112*: 1142–51, 2003.
7. Drolet DW, Green LS, Gold L, and Janjic N: Fit for the eye: aptamers in ocular disorders. *Nucleic Acid Ther 26*: 127–46, 2016. doi:10.1089/nat.2015.0573, 2016
8. Matei D, Kelich S, Cao L, Menning N, Emerson RE, Rao J, Jeng MH, and Sledge GW: PDGF BB induces VEGF secretion in ovarian cancer. *Cancer Biol Ther 6*: 1951–59, 2007.
9. Lu C, Shahzad MM, Moreno-Smith M, Lin YG, Jennings NB, Allen JK, Landen CN, Mangala LS, Armaiz-Pena GN, Schmandt R, Nick AM, Stone RL, Jaffe RB, Coleman RL, and Sood AK: Targeting pericytes with a PDGF-B aptamer in human ovarian carcinoma models. *Cancer Biol Ther 9*: 176–82, 2010.
10. Choi HJ, Armaiz Pena GN, Pradeep S, Cho MS, Coleman RL, and Sood AK: Anti-vascular therapies in ovarian cancer: moving beyond anti-VEGF approaches. *Cancer Metastasis Rev 34*: 19–40, 2015.
11. Cimpean AM, Cobec IM, Ceauşu RA, Popescu R, Tudor A, and Raica M: Platelet derived growth factor BB: a "must-have" therapeutic target "redivivus" in ovarian cancer. *Cancer Genomics Proteomics 13*: 511–17, 2016.
12. Hansen JM, Coleman RL, and Sood AK: Targeting the tumour microenvironment in ovarian cancer. *Eur J Cancer 56*: 131–43, 2016.
13. Muggia FM: Intraperitoneal therapy for ovarian cancer. *J Clin Oncol 34*: 882, 2016.
14. Ruscito I, Gasparri ML, Marchetti C, De Medici C, Bracchi C, Palaia I, Imboden S, Mueller MD, Papadia A, Muzii L, and Panici PB: Cediranib in ovarian cancer: state of the art and future perspectives. *Tumour Biol 37*: 2833–39, 2016.
15. Colombo N, Conte PF, Pignata S, Raspagliesi F, and Scambia G. Bevacizumab in ovarian cancer: focus on clinical data and future perspectives. *Crit Rev Oncol Hematol 97*: 335–48, 2016.
16. Symeonides S, and Gourley C: Ovarian cancer molecular stratification and tumor heterogeneity: a necessity and a challenge. *Front Oncol 5*: 229, 2015.
17. Oza AM, Cibula D, Benzaquen AO, Poole C, Mathijssen RH, Sonke GS, Colombo N, Špaček J, Vuylsteke P, Hirte H, Mahner S, Plante M, Schmalfeldt B, Mackay H, Rowbottom J, Lowe ES, Dougherty B, Barrett JC, and Friedlander M: Olaparib combined with chemotherapy for recurrent platinum-sensitive ovarian cancer: a randomised phase 2 trial. *Lancet Oncol 16*: 87–97, 2015.
18. du Bois A, Floquet A, Kim JW, Rau J, del Campo JM, and Friedlander M: Incorporation of pazopanib in maintenance therapy of ovarian cancer. *J Clin Oncol 32*: 3374–82, 2014.
19. Matulonis UA, Berlin S, Ivy P, Tyburski K, Krasner C, Zarwan C, Berkenblit A, Campos S, Horowitz N, Cannistra SA, Lee H, Lee J, Roche M, Hill M, Whalen C, Sullivan L, Tran C, Humphreys BD, and Penson RT: Cediranib, an oral inhibitor of vascular endothelial growth factor receptor kinases, is an active drug in recurrent epithelial ovarian, fallopian tube, and peritoneal cancer. *J Clin Oncol 27*: 5601–606, 2009.
20. Baumann KH, du Bois A, Meier W, Rau J, Wimberger P, Sehouli J, Kurzeder C, Hilpert F, Hasenburg A, Canzler U, Hanker LC, Hillemanns P, Richter B, Wollschlaeger K, Dewitz T, Bauerschlag D, and Wagner U: A phase II trial (AGO 2.11) in platinum-resistant ovarian cancer: a randomized multicenter trial with sunitinib (SU11248) to evaluate dosage, schedule, tolerability, toxicity and effectiveness of a multitargeted receptor tyrosine kinase inhibitor monotherapy. *Ann Oncol 23*: 2265–71, 2012.
21. Hainsworth JD, Thompson DS, Bismayer JA, Gian VG, Merritt WM, Whorf RC, Finney LH, and Dudley BS: Paclitaxel/carboplatin with or without sorafenib in the first-line treatment of patients with stage III/IV epithelial ovarian cancer: a randomized phase II study of the Sarah Cannon Research Institute. *Cancer Med 4*: 673–81, 2015.
22. Safra T, Andreopoulou E, Levinson B, Borgato L, Pothuri B, Blank S, Tiersten A, Boyd L, Curtin J, and Muggia F: Weekly paclitaxel with intermittent imatinib mesylate (Gleevec): tolerance and activity in recurrent epithelial ovarian cancer. *Anticancer Res 30*: 3243–47, 2010.
23. Raica M, and Cimpean AM: Platelet-derived growth factor (PDGF)/PDGF receptors (PDGFR) axis as target for antitumor and antiangiogenic therapy. *Pharmaceuticals 3*: 572–99, 2010.
24. Kacinski BM, Carter D, Kohorn EI, Mittal K, Bloodgood RS, Donahue J, Kramer CA, and

Fischer D: Oncogene expression in vivo by ovarian adenocarcinomas and mixed-mullerian tumors. *Yale J Biol Med 62*: 379–92, 1989.

25. Versnel MA, Haarbrink M, Langerak AW, de Laat PA, Hagemeijer A, van der Kwast TH, van den Berg-Bakker LA, and Schrier PI: Human ovarian tumors of epithelial origin express PDGF in vitro and in vivo. *Cancer Genet Cytogenet 73*: 60–64, 1994.

26. Yamamoto S, Tsuda H, Takano M, Kita T, Kudoh K, Furuya K, Tamai S, and Matsubara O: Expression of platelet-derived growth factors and their receptors in ovarian clear-cell carcinoma and its putative precursors. *Mod Pathol 21*: 115–24, 2008.

27. Song SH, Jeong IG, You D, Hong JH, Hong B, Song C, Jung WY, Cho YM, Ahn H, and Kim CS: VEGF/VEGFR2 and PDGF-B/PDGFR-β expression in non-metastatic renal cell carcinoma: a retrospective study in 1,091 consecutive patients. *Int J Clin Exp Pathol 7*: 7681–89, 2014.

28. Shim M, Song C, Park S, Choi SK, Cho YM, Kim CS, and Ahn H: Prognostic significance of platelet-derived growth factor receptor-β expression in localized clear cell renal cell carcinoma. *J Cancer Res Clin Oncol 141*: 2213–20, 2015.

29. Versnel MA, Hagemeijer A, Bouts MJ, van der Kwast TH, and Hoogsteden HC: Expression of c-sis (PDGF B-chain) and PDGF A-chain genes in ten human malignant mesothelioma cell lines derived from primary and metastatic tumors. *Oncogene 2*: 601–605, 1988.

30. Savolainen-Peltonen H, Loubtchenkov M, Petrov L, Delafontaine P, and Häyry P: Estrogen regulates insulin-like growth factor 1, platelet-derived growth factor A and B, and their receptors in the vascular wall. *Transplantation 77*: 35–42, 2004.

31. Rizvi S, Mertens JC, Bronk SF, Hirsova P, Dai H, Roberts LR, Kaufmann SH, and Gores GJ: Platelet-derived growth factor primes cancer-associated fibroblasts for apoptosis. *J Biol Chem 289*: 22835–49, 2014.

32. Pinto MP, Dye WW, Jacobsen BM, and Horwitz KB: Malignant stroma increases luminal breast cancer cell proliferation and angiogenesis through platelet-derived growth factor signaling. *BMC Cancer 14*: 735, 2014.

33. Lederle W, Stark HJ, Skobe M, Fusenig NE, and Mueller MM: Platelet-derived growth factor-BB controls epithelial tumor phenotype by differential growth factor regulation in stromal cells. *Am J Pathol 169*: 1767–83, 2006.

34. Cha HJ, Choi JH, Park IC, Kim CH, An SK, Kim TJ, and Lee JH: Selective FGFR inhibitor BGJ398 inhibits phophorylation of AKT and STAT3 and induces cytotoxicity in sphere-cultured ovarian cancer cells. *Int J Oncol.* 2017; Epub ahead of print.

35. Sun Y, Fan X, Zhang Q, Shi X, Xu G, and Zou C: Cancer-associated fibroblasts secrete FGF-1 to promote ovarian proliferation, migration and invasion through the activation of FGF-1/FGFR4 signaling. *Tumour Biol 39*(7), 2017. doi:10.1177

36. Horala A, Swiatly A, Matysiak J, Banach P, Nowak-Markwitz E, and Kokot ZJ: Diagnostic value of serum angiogenesis markers in ovarian cancer using multiplex immunoassay. *Int J Mol Sci 18*(1): pii: E123, 2017.

37. Tyulyandina A, Harrison D, Yin W, Stepanova E, Kochenkov D, Solomko E, Peretolchina N, Daeyaert F, Joos JB, Van Aken K, Byakhov M, Gavrilova E, Tjulandin S, and Tsimafeyeu I: Alofanib, an allosteric FGFR2 inhibitor, has potent effects on ovarian cancer growth in preclinical studies. *Invest New Drugs 35*(2): 127–33, 2017.

38. Tsimafeyeu I, Ludes-Meyers J, Stepanova E, Daeyaert F, Kochenkov D, Joose JB, Solomko E, Van Akene K, Peretolchina N, Yin W, Ryabaya O, Byakhov M, and Tjulandin S: Targeting FGFR2 with alofanib (RPT835) shows potent activity in tumor models. *Eur J Cancer 61*: 20–28, 2016.

39. Guo Q, Yang X, Ma Y, and Ma L: Syndecan-1 serves as a marker for the progression of epithelial ovarian carcinoma. *Eur J Gynaecol Oncol 36*(5): 506–13, 2015.

40. Masoumi-Moghaddam S, Amini A, Wei AQ, Robertson G, and Morris DL: Vascular endothelial growth factor expression correlates with serum CA125 and represents a useful tool in prediction of refractoriness to platinum-based chemotherapy and ascites formation in epithelial ovarian cancer. *Oncotarget 6*(29): 28491–501, 2015.

41. Li L, Yu J, Duan Z, and Dang HX: The effect of NFATc1 on vascular generation and the possible underlying mechanism in epithelial ovarian carcinoma. *Int J Oncol 48*(4): 1457–66, 2016.

42. Choi HJ, Armaiz Pena GN, Pradeep S, Cho MS, Coleman RL, and Sood AK: Anti-vascular therapies in ovarian cancer: moving beyond anti-VEGF approaches. *Cancer Metastasis Rev 34*(1): 19–40, 2015.

43. Emoto S, Ishigami H, Yamashita H, Yamaguchi H, Kaisaki S, and Kitayama J: Clinical significance of CA125 and CA72-4 in gastric cancer with peritoneal dissemination. *Gastric Cancer 15*: 154–61, 2012.

44. Streiter S, Fisch B, Sabbah B, Ao A, and Abir R: The importance of neuronal growth factors in the ovary. *Mol Hum Reprod 22*: 3–17, 2016.

45. Chaves RN, Alves AM, Lima LF, Matos HM, Rodrigues AP, and Figueiredo JR: Role of nerve growth factor (NGF) and its receptors in folliculogenesis. *Zygote 21*: 187–97, 2013.

46. Cantarella G, Lempereur L, Presta M, Ribatti D, Lombardo G, Lazarovici P, Zappala G, Pafumi C, and Bernardini R: Nerve growth factor-endothelial cell interaction leads to angiogenesis in vitro and in vivo. *FASEB J 16*: 1307–309, 2002.

47. Calza L, Giardino L, Giuliani A, Aloe L, and Levi-Montalcini R: Nerve growth factor control of neuronal expression of angiogenic and vasoactive factors. *Proc Natl Acad Sci U S A 98*: 4160–65, 2001.

48. Salas C, Julio-Pieper M, Valladares M, Pommer R, Vega M, Mastronardi C, Kerr B, Ojeda SR, Lara HE, and Romero C: Nerve growth factor-dependent

activation of TRKA receptors in the human ovary results in synthesis of follicle-stimulating hormone receptors and estrogen secretion. *J Clin Endocrinol Metab 91*: 2396–403, 2006.

49. Campos X, Muñoz Y, Selman A, Yazigi R, Moyano L, Weinstein-Oppenheimer C, Lara HE, and Romero C: Nerve growth factor and its high-affinity receptor TRKA participate in the control of vascular endothelial growth factor expression in epithelial ovarian cancer. *Gynecol Oncol 104*: 168–75, 2007.

50. Li L, Wang L, Zhang W, Tang B, Zhang J, Song H, Yao D, Tang Y, Chen X, Yang Z, et al: Correlation of serum VEGF levels with clinical stage, therapy efficacy, tumor metastasis and patient survival in ovarian cancer. *Anticancer Res 24*: 1973–79, 2004.

51. Ferrara N, Gerber HP, and LeCouter J: The biology of VEGF and its receptors. *Nat Med 9*: 669–76, 2003.

52. Shen H, Li L, Zhou S, Yu D, Yang S, Chen X, Wang D, Zhong S, Zhao J, and Tang J: The role of ADAM17 in tumorigenesis and progression of breast cancer. *Tumour Biol 37*(12): 15359–70, 2016. doi: 10.1007/s13277-016-5418-y.

53. Girardi S, Tapia V, Kohan K, Contreras H, Gabler F, Selman A, Vega M, and Romero C: ADAM17 and TRKA receptor are involved in epithelial ovarian cancer progression; Proceedings of the 17th World Congress on Advances in Oncology and 15th International Symposium on Molecular Medicine; Hersonissos, Greece. October 11–13, 2012.

54. Romero C, Vallejos C, Gabler F, Selman A, and Vega M: Activation of TRKA receptor by nerve growth factor induces shedding of p75 receptor related with progression of epithelial ovarian cancer; Proceedings of the 23rd Biennial Congress of the European Association for Cancer Research; Munich, Germany. July 5–8, 2014; pp. 5119–20.

55. Vera C, Tapia V, Kohan K, Gabler F, Ferreira A, Selman A, Vega M, and Romero C: Nerve growth factor induces the expression of chaperone protein calreticulin in human epithelial ovarian cells. *Horm Metab Res 44*: 639–43, 2012.

56. Alfaidy N, Hoffmann P, Gillois P, Gueniffey A, Lebayle C, Garçin H, Thomas-Cadi C, Bessonnat J, Coutton C, Villaret L, Quenard N, Bergues U, Feige JJ, Hennebicq S, and Brouillet S: PROK1 level in the follicular microenvironment: a new noninvasive predictive biomarker of embryo implantation. *J Clin Endocrinol Metab 101*: 435–44, 2016.

57. Eddie SL, Childs AJ, Kinnell HL, Brown P, Jabbour HN, and Anderson RA: Prokineticin ligands and receptors are expressed in the human fetal ovary and regulate germ cell expression of COX2. *J Clin Endocrinol Metab 100*: E1197–205, 2015.

58. Lozneanu L, Avădănei R, Cîmpean AM, Giuşcă SE, Amălinei C, and Căruntu ID: Relationship between the proangiogenic role of EG-VEGF, clinicopathological characteristics and survival in tumoral ovary. *Rev Med Chir Soc Med Nat Iasi 119*: 461–65, 2015.

59. Bălu S, Pirtea L, Gaje P, Cîmpean AM, and Raica M. The immunohistochemical expression of endocrine gland-derived-VEGF (EG-VEGF) as a prognostic marker in ovarian cancer. *Rom J Morphol Embryol 53*: 479–83, 2012.

60. Corlan AS, Cîmpean AM, Jitariu A-A, Melnic E, and Raica M: Endocrine gland-derived vascular endothelial growth factor/prokineticin-1 in cancer development and tumor angiogenesis. *Int J Endocrinol 2017*: 3232905, 2017.

12.

UNIQUE CHALLENGES FACING IMMUNOTHERAPY OF METASTATIC OVARIAN CANCER

Michelle N. Messmer, Colleen S. Netherby, and Scott I. Abrams

INTRODUCTION

The course of ovarian tumorigenesis is highly complex and ultimately reflects dynamic and complex interactions between the transformed cell and its microenvironment. Interestingly, a major component of the host microenvironment is the immune system, a network of specialized cells adapted to respond to "dangerous" or "foreign" substances that are endowed with the capacity to eliminate such threats. The immune system can indeed be a powerful weapon to halt and, perhaps, eradicate neoplastic growth or progression. However, in the case of neoplasia, including ovarian cancer, such cells have developed a number of "escape" mechanisms that can limit the effectiveness of anti-tumor immune attack. This chapter addresses the nature and consequences of the immune system-ovarian tumor interaction: on the one hand, how ovarian cancer cells antagonize anti-tumor immunity and, on the other hand, the design of therapeutic interventions to engage and bolster anti-tumor immune responses.

IMMUNOLOGY BASICS

Immune cells play critically important roles in neoplasia. Chronic inflammation caused by inappropriately triggered immune responses can drive genetic or epigenetic changes contributing to tumorigenesis and has been implicated as a potential causative factor in ovarian cancer. However, evidence has shown that the immune system is also able to protect against neoplastic disease; the presence of certain immune cells can be a positive prognostic indicator while patients with suppressed immune responses have a higher tumor incidence. These observations support the theory of "immune surveillance," which states that the immune system is continuously surveying the host not only for invading pathogens but also for cells that become transformed or cancerous. Within this theory, scientists have now elaborated three phases of the interactions between host immune cells and developing neoplastic cells. In the first phase, known as "elimination," as soon as a potential cancer cell arises, the immune system is able to recognize the cell as atypical and destroy it. In cases where the immune system fails to completely eradicate all atypical cells, the immune system can still restrain their growth through a phase known as "equilibrium." Essentially, this represents a stage when pro-tumor and anti-tumor factors are balanced against each other. The final phase of the immune cell-cancer cell interaction is called "escape." In this phase, cancer cells surviving the initial two stages of immune surveillance have adopted one or more mechanisms to suppress or evade immune responses, allowing these cells to "escape" the control of the immune system and grow as malignant tumors. In essence, this theory states that a successful malignant lesion has undergone immune-mediated selective pressure, collectively termed "cancer immunoediting." Thus, the tumor that ultimately emerges has been sculpted from the start to resist the immune system, which explains why designing effective cancer immunotherapies remain a daunting task (discussed later).

Immunity can be divided into two primary types of responses: innate and adaptive. Innate immune responses are considered rapid, often occurring on the scale of minutes to hours, and are considered relatively nonspecific. Receptors on innate immune cells bind to ligands common across a variety of pathogens or disease states and then immediately signal these cells to kill the target through intracellular (engulfing) or extracellular mechanisms. Adaptive immune responses require a longer time frame to develop. This is because cells of the adaptive immune response require special instruction, or "licensing," in order to recognize their targets, called "antigens," and respond accordingly. Adaptive immune cells are thus highly specific and effective killers. An additional benefit to adaptive immune responses is the development of immune memory. Once adaptive immune cells have found their targets and successfully eliminated the threat, the immune cells remain vigilant. If the same target returns, it takes much less time for the adaptive immune cells to respond.

Before exploring the specific ways the immune system can protect against ovarian cancer, it is important to understand the various types of cells involved in host immunity. Cells of the immune system are broadly called leukocytes, or white blood cells. These cells can be classified into various subsets based on their development during hematopoiesis, as well as their function acquired during later stages of differentiation. Figure 12.1 shows the major cellular subsets and their roles

relevant to tumor immunity. Flow cytometry, a major technique used in studying these cells, is highlighted in Box 12.1.

Adaptive immune responses are associated with the greatest protection from tumor development or progression. The major cells of the adaptive immune system are B cells and T cells. Monocytes, which give rise to macrophages and populations of dendritic cells (DCs), play important roles in bridging the innate and adaptive immune systems. These phagocytic cells internalize antigen and then process it to instruct B cells or T cells to recognize their targets. "Recognition" refers to the complementary binding of a receptor protein on the immune cell with its corresponding ligand on the target cell, leading to immune activation. Cells that present antigen for recognition are thus termed "antigen presenting cells" (APCs).

B cells accomplish recognition via cell surface immunoglobulins, which are able to bind to a large range of targets including proteins, fats, and sugars. Immature B cells express such structures on their cell surface to sample their environment. Once this B cell receptor interacts with its complementary antigen, the B cell receives a signal to mature into a plasma cell and begins secreting immunoglobulins, termed antibodies, into the blood. Antibodies strongly and specifically bind to the same antigens that triggered this process in the first place. Once in circulation, these antibodies then bind either to cells bearing the corresponding antigens, including tumor cells, or their secreted soluble products, such as toxins, which also harbor the corresponding antigens. Antibody-antigen binding promotes at least three major immune functions important in cancer immunology: (a) enhanced phagocytosis of the antigen by macrophages, (b) activation of the complement system leading to the destruction of the antigen-bearing targets, and (c) inducing a type of cell killing known as antibody dependent cellular cytotoxicity (ADCC) by macrophages and natural killer (NK) cells. These functions are discussed in more detail throughout the chapter.

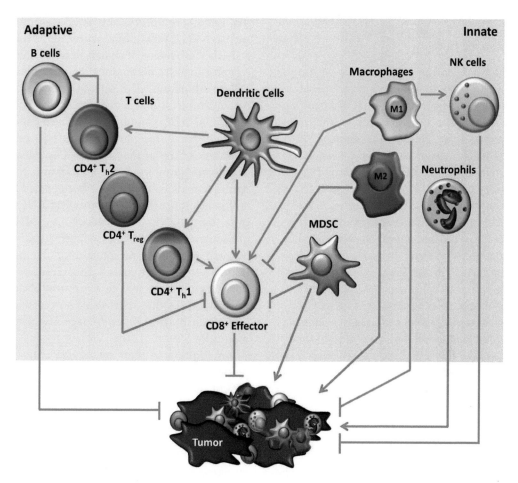

Figure 12.1 Major cell types of the adaptive and innate immune systems that are involved in the host-tumor interaction. Dendritic cells form the bridge between the adaptive and innate immune response. Dendritic cells initiate T-cell activation through antigen processing and presentation and provide the requisite costimulatory signals to drive the differentiation and expansion of various CD4+ T helper subsets as well as CD8+ cytotoxic T cells. CD8+ T cells are a major effector of tumor cell killing, but their activities can be suppressed by Treg cells, MDSCs, or M2 macrophages. B cells also rely on CD4+ T helper cells for their anti-tumor function. M1 macrophages, through the production of IFN-γ, contribute to or enhance CD8+ cytotoxic T-cell activity as well as NK-cell-mediated killing. Subsets of neutrophils are also associated with tumor-promoting activities via mechanisms that remain less understood. Green lines depict anti-tumor responses, whereas red lines depict pro-tumor responses. Arrow heads indicate positive actions, while cross hatches indicate negative actions.

T cells recognize antigen via the T-cell receptor in a more restricted manner. All humans express major histocompatibility complex (MHC) proteins called human leukocyte antigens (HLA). HLA can be divided into two types: class I is expressed on all nucleated cells of the body, while class II expression is restricted to APCs. Proteins are continuously being recycled inside of cells; small fragments of these proteins, termed peptides, are reserved for presentation by class I molecules. Once these peptides in association with class I are presented on the surface of a cell, such as a cancer cell, they can act as antigens for T cells. MHC class II molecules also bind peptides, but their peptides are typically derived from proteins that were internalized by APCs, such as when an antibody-coated bacteria is engulfed by a macrophage or when a DC takes up cellular debris from a dead/dying cancer cell. T-cell receptors specifically recognize

BOX 12.1 IDENTIFYING CELLS OF THE IMMUNE SYSTEM

The most common current technique used to rapidly identify cells of the immune system is called "flow cytometry." This technique allows investigators to identify cell populations based on their surface molecules, or markers, which are often given a "cluster of differentiation" (CD) designation followed by a number. For example, CD3 is a marker expressed by all T cells in the host, while expression of the markers CD4 and CD8 divide T cells into two different populations with different effector functions. CD8$^+$ T cells recognize peptides presented by MHC class I molecules and are the primary effector cells most strongly associated with cell-mediated killing. CD4$^+$ T cells recognize peptides presented by MHC class II and can be further divided based on the types of effector molecules they produce and the unique transcription factors they express which govern their differentiation into distinct subsets which regulate the immune response. B cells are broadly defined by expression of CD19 or CD20, while macrophages are predominately CD11b$^+$ and DCs are CD11c$^+$. There is some overlap of certain markers between classes of cells, and these markers can also have functional significance in addition to their use for phenotypic identification.

the combination of MHC molecules with peptides but will not respond to peptide alone or to "empty" MHC molecules without peptides bound. Small inheritable variations in the MHC molecules can be used to distinguish one individual from another and are the determining factor used for tissue-typing patients prior to organ transplantation. These differences in MHC molecules impact the variety of antigens individuals are able to recognize, which can have important consequences in disease.

Granulocytes, or cells containing granules, and NK cells are major cells of the innate immune system. NK cells express two families of receptors, activating receptors such as NKG2D and inhibitory receptors such as KIR. The balance of signals between these receptor families determines the outcome of NK cell function. The activating receptors recognize stress-associated molecules such as MICA, MICB, and ULBP1-3. Signaling through these receptors causes NK cell-mediated killing of the target cell by release of cytolytic granules. NK cells can also recognize and kill cells that have been coated by antibodies through Fc receptors, via ADCC. Importantly, NK cells recognize MHC molecules and MHC-associated ligands through inhibitory receptors that dampen these activating signals. This inhibitory signaling prevents NK cells from attacking normal tissues that may also be expressing low levels of stress- or damage-associated molecules.

In addition to their specialized antigen-presenting roles, macrophages play other important roles in determining immune responses. These cells are capable of recognizing antibody-antigen complexes using Fc receptors that interact with a specific part of the antibody molecule and ingesting such immune complexes through a process termed opsonization. Once the complexes have been internalized, they are degraded for presentation on MHC molecules. Macrophages can also internalize dying, or apoptotic, cells and can clear away other cellular debris. Macrophages, as well as DCs, express a number of receptors to detect molecules associated with damage (DAMPs) or with pathogens (PAMPs). Receptor activation causes these cells to produce a range of effector molecules as well as express different phenotypic or functional markers. Based on these characteristics, macrophages have been dichotomized into M1 or M2 phenotypes. M1 responses are necessary for host defense against infection and cancer and are characterized by the production of activating signals for NK cells, recruitment and activation of CD8$^+$ T cells, and direct killing of intracellular pathogens. M2 responses, instead, are important for wound healing such as promoting tissue regeneration and suppression of further destruction by immune cells. The global macrophage response in a particular disease setting usually falls along the continuum of these two extremes.

As part of the wound healing program, M2 macrophages express enzymes called matrix metalloproteinases that are able to remodel the extracellular environment by degrading connective tissue proteins. Macrophages also produce growth factors such as vascular endothelial growth factor (VEGF) to promote a process known as angiogenesis, or the formation of new blood vessels, to restore blood flow to the injured tissues. As discussed later, these aspects of wound healing are exploited in cancer, including ovarian cancer. Altogether, given this profile, M2 responses are thought to be counterproductive to host defense against cancer.

As discussed, receptor-based recognition of ligands by cells of the immune system often results in the production of effector molecules. The most predominant of these molecules are cytokines and chemokines. Cytokines and chemokines are small proteins critically important in cell signaling/activation and cell migration, respectively, and support communication between cells. Such proteins are released by cells either in a local or paracrine manner and then influence the behavior or recruitment of other cells. Often, signaling by one cytokine on a target cell will induce the production of a secondary cytokine, which can then have additional effects on yet another cell. In this way, cytokines form signaling networks of two or more cytokines that work in conjunction to exert their overall influence. An example of such a network formed by tumor necrosis factor alpha (TNF-α), interleukin (IL)-6, and CXCL12 are described later in this text.

IMMUNE RESPONSES IN OVARIAN CANCER PATIENTS

Immunogenicity describes the ability of a cell or other molecule to stimulate an immune response against itself. For a long time, ovarian cancer was not considered to be an immunogenic tumor type. However, previous definitions of immunogenicity, or the ability to stimulate adaptive immune responses, relied on experiments in mouse models that did not fully appreciate the extent that tumor-host interactions can shape the immune response. Indeed, many human tumors are now widely accepted to be immunogenic.[1] Specifically in ovarian cancer, several important studies have highlighted how important the immune system can be in prolonging patient survival, especially regarding the association of T cells with the malignancy (Box 12.2).

It is well known that CD8+ T cells are required for antitumor immunity in most solid tumor types, while CD4+ T cells can either play a supportive function or, alternatively, a suppressive function depending on the type of CD4+ T cell present. However, T-cell function is greatly dependent on the ability to interact with the target. Thus, researchers have identified tumor-infiltrating lymphocytes (TILs) as a better prognostic marker than simply measuring lymphocytes in the blood. Specifically, T cells present within intraepithelial regions of ovarian tumors, as defined by either CD3 or CD8 expression, are associated with significantly increased overall survival. Patients without TILs present have a hazard ratio of approximately 2, representing twice the risk of dying from their disease.[4] Evidence has shown that TILs are not just silent cells invading the tumor tissue; these T cells show several markers of effector function. Tumors with high numbers of TILs have higher levels of interferon-gamma (IFN-γ)-induced cytokines to support anti-tumor immune responses. Profiling tumors from patients with low or high rates of T-cell infiltration have identified two genes associated with more TIL accumulation: (a) higher expression of the transcription factor IRF1 to drive MHC class I expression and (b) chemokine receptor CXCR6 to enable enhanced T-cell proliferation.[5]

BOX 12.2 IMPORTANCE OF T-CELL INFILTRATION IN OVARIAN CARCINOMA

Zhang et al.[2] published one of the first studies showing the prognostic importance of T cells infiltrating ovarian tumors in *The New England Journal of Medicine* in 2003. Sections of patients' tumors were stained with antibodies specific for CD3 and scored based on the localization and frequency of TILs. TIL[+] patients had an abundance of CD3[+] T cells within tumor islets, as well as within tumor stroma compared to TIL[−] patients where T cells were either absent or restricted to the peritumoral stroma. Stratifying ovarian cancer patients by their TIL status revealed a significant survival advantage for those with detectable TILs.

Further studies by Sato et al.[3] delved deeper into the association between TILs and ovarian cancer prognosis, focusing on specific T-cell subsets. In Figure 12.2 (left), Panel A shows staining for CD3, the pan T-cell marker, in brown. Panel B shows staining for CD8, the marker associated with cytotoxic T cells. Panel C shows the staining for CD4, which identifies subsets of cells that are associated with helper functions but also Treg subsets. Further analysis for markers of the Treg cell subset are shown in Panel D. CD25 is a surface marker (brown) while FoxP3 (deep pink) is a master transcription factor controlling Treg cell development and function. In this study, the ratio of CD8[+] effector T cells to Treg cells was investigated as a prognostic marker, and again showed a significant survival advantage for patients with a higher ratio of CD8:Tregs cells (Figure 12.2, right).

Importantly, these T cells show evidence of effector function. IFN-γ and IL-2 are several-fold higher in tumor tissue with TILs present compared to non-TIL-associated tumors. IL-2 is an important cytokine that supports T cell survival and proliferation. IFN-γ is secreted by activated T cells and NK cells and has a number of effects on target cells to enhance their susceptibility to T cell killing including increasing expression of MHC molecules. IFN-γ is also associated with direct anti-proliferative and anti-angiogenic effects on ovarian tumors.

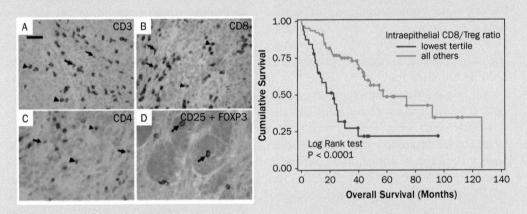

Figure 12.2 Association between TILs and ovarian cancer patient survival. Adapted with permission from Sato E, Olson SH, Ahn J, et al. Intraepithelial CD8+ tumor-infiltrating lymphocytes and a high CD8+/regulatory T cell ratio are associated with favorable prognosis in ovarian cancer. *Proc Natl Acad Sci U S A.* 2005; 102(51): 18538–43. Top: From Figure 1C-F. Bottom: From Figure 2H. Copyright (2005) National Academy of Sciences, USA.

A role for the second major lymphoid cell type, B cells, in modulating ovarian cancer immunity remains is less understood but remains an emerging area of investigation. B cells, as producers of antibody, are not required to directly infiltrate tumors to produce effector function. Thus, studies associating tumor-infiltrating B cells with improved survival have yielded mixed results. A certain subset of B cells expressing CD20 has been identified to correlate with CD8[+] T-cell infiltration of the tumor, where they are often co-localized, and are implicated in either recruiting T cells or modulating their activity.[5] Several studies have shown that antibodies in the peripheral blood of ovarian cancer patients recognize tumor antigens, such as MAGE.[6] Recognition of such antigens on tumor cells can lead to tumor cell destruction. Importantly, the presence of such antibodies, or "humoral" responses, correlates with improved prognosis.

Studies have identified several antigens from ovarian cancer samples that are capable of stimulating immune responses. These antigens fall into two broad categories, either tumor-specific antigens (TSAs) or tumor-associated antigens (TAAs). TSAs include antigens that are exclusive to the malignancy, often due to specific genetic or epigenetic alterations that occurred during the process of oncogenesis. TAAs are derived from proteins that are differentially expressed in tumor tissue when compared to normal tissue. This includes proteins that are expressed when they would not normally be present, proteins that are expressed at much higher levels compared to normal, or proteins that are posttranslationally modified differently in tumor compared to normal tissues. Antigens associated with ovarian cancer are summarized in Table 12.1. Unfortunately, not all patients develop detectable "spontaneous," or pre-existing, immune responses against their tumors. Several mechanisms have been exploited by tumors to prevent generation of such immune responses. In addition, some TAAs may actually contribute directly to suppressing anti-tumor immune responses.

Effector cells of the innate arm of the immune response are also not well correlated with improvements in overall survival. Almost all ovarian cancers express high levels of the stress ligands MICA, MICB, and ULBP2, yet the presence of NK cells has been associated with poor prognosis for metastatic ovarian cancer.[5] However, this may be due to expression of immune suppressive molecules by the tumor that inhibit NK cell killing, rather than a pro-tumor role for the NK cells.

Such immune-suppressive molecules are discussed in more detail later.

It is important to understand that while many underlying biologic processes unite ovarian tumors into particular classes that express shared antigens, an individual tumor also carries a library of unique antigens. Conventional therapies for ovarian cancer such as first-line platinum-based chemotherapies or second-line irradiation cause massive tumor cell death through disruptive mechanisms. This type of cell death triggers warning signals to the immune system and recruits cells such as macrophages and DCs to the tumor site that can internalize and process the antigens to then activate T-cell responses. Such responses are important in fighting residual disease to prevent recurrence and disease appearing at metastatic sites. Immune status prior to therapeutic intervention has thus been investigated as a prognostic marker for response to chemotherapy. However, for many patients, several factors stand in the way of generating productive host immunity following these conventional therapies.

ROADBLOCKS TO IMMUNITY IN OVARIAN CANCER

The host employs several mechanisms to reduce collateral damage of an activated immune response. The ability to suppress responses once a pathogen is cleared is necessary to avoid generalized tissue destruction. These checkpoints to immune activation also exist to prevent potentially life-threatening autoimmunity. However, since cancer cells arise from self-tissues and therefore are closely related to normal cells, they are able to benefit from these same "protective" mechanisms. The roadblocks to antitumor immune responses can be grouped into four broad mechanisms: (a) loss or downregulation of tumor antigen, (b) production of immunosuppressive cytokines, (c) expression of immune suppressive molecules, and (d) recruitment of suppressive

TABLE 12.1 OVARIAN CANCER ASSOCIATED ANTIGENS

Type	Example Antigens	Freq.	Refs
Cancer-Testis Antigens	**Melanoma antigen gene (MAGE):** High expression correlates with tumor differentiation and stage.	50%	5,11
	NY-ESO-1: Normally expressed by germ cells, normal function unknown; originally identified as a tumor antigen in esophageal cancer.	43% EOC	5,7
	Sperm protein 17 (SP17): High expression results in enhanced migration and chemoresistance.	70%	5,10
Growth, Activating Receptors	**Her2/neu:** Transmembrane glycoprotein, tyrosine kinase activity.	5%–66%	5,7
	Epithelial cell adhesion molecule (EpCAM): Type I membrane glycoprotein expressed in almost all epithelial cell membranes, overexpressed across all ovarian cancer types.	70%–90%	5,8
	IGFBP-2: Binds and regulates insulin-like growth factor -1 and 2 to regulate cell proliferation, differentiation, and apoptosis; expressed by normal tissue but increased in cancer.	~80%	5
Tumor Suppressors	**P53:** Most common single mutation in ovarian cancer; loss of wild-type p53 or mutations resulting in gain-of-oncogenic function. Presence of antibodies against p53 predicts survival.	50% overexpress	5,7
	BRCA1 and 2: Required for maintenance of chromosomal stability.	10%–15%	9
Tumor Micro-Environment	**Vascular endothelial growth factor (VEGF):** Modulator of angiogenesis and vascular permeability. Also plays an important role in normal ovarian function; intrafollicular VEGF increases early in ovulation, followed by vascular regression at the end of the ovulation cycle. High expression contributes to increased tumor angiogenesis and poor survival in ovarian cancer.	Elevated in most	14
	B7-H4: Serves as a negative regulator of T-cell function during immune regulation, and its expression by myeloid cells and plasmacytoid dendritic cells is elevated during the first trimester of pregnancy and in the luteal phase of ovulation.	85%	12
	Colony-stimulating factor 1 (CSF1), CSF1 receptor (CSF1R): Critical for monocyte development during hematopoiesis and involved in immune regulation during placental development.	75% primary, 69% metastatic, receptor: 92% primary, 83% metastatic	13
Mucins	**MUC1:** Present in healthy and cancer tissue but differentially glycosylated; levels of anti-muc1 antibodies inversely correlate with ovarian cancer risk factors.		5,7
	MUC4: Less known about its biology; mediates epithelial-to-mesenchymal transition, but no known association between expression and outcome.	>90% malignant ovarian cancer	5
	CA-125 (MUC16): Overexpressed on surface of tumors and shed into the blood and peritoneal cavity; presence is used as a tumor marker for monitoring growth and recurrence of disease.	50%–80%	5
Other Abnormal Expressed Molecules	**Folate receptor alpha (FRα):** Normally restricted to apical surface of kidney tubule epithelium where it recovers folate from the urine; overexpressed by many epithelial cancers and 90-fold higher in non-mucinous ovarian cancer cells compared to normal epithelia.	70%–80%	5
	Mammaglobin B: Typically associated with mammary gland; independently correlates with better outcomes.	~50%	5
	Human epididymis protein 4 (HE4): Normally restricted to epididymis, endometrial glands, and respiratory tract.	Early and late stage, 90% of serous	15
	Mesothelin: Normally restricted to mesothelial cells; overexpressed by many cancers but ovarian cancer expression is highest, particularly by non-mucinous subtypes. Potentially biologically important for pathogenesis—associated with increased chemoresistance and poor survival.		5

NOTE: EOC = epithelial ovarian cancer.

immune cells. Additionally, physical barriers within the tumor microenvironment can contribute to immune suppression. Each of these mechanisms is discussed later, with examples of each as identified in ovarian cancer.

LOSS OR DOWNREGULATION OF TUMOR ANTIGEN

As discussed earlier, a number of antigens have been identified in association with ovarian cancer. The presence of these antigens can serve as prognostic indicators of patients who may benefit from certain immunotherapies such as specific antigen-based vaccines. However, the selection of a TAA for targeted therapy must be done rationally. Once an immune response against a particular antigen is initiated, the cancer cells come under selective pressure to lose, or reduce expression of, that antigen. Thus, if the antigen does not provide a survival advantage, cells expressing that antigen will be eliminated, leaving behind cells no longer expressing that antigen. However, in cases where the antigens arise from proteins required for cancer cell survival, certain mechanisms can be employed to "hide" the antigen from the immune response. As discussed earlier, antigens must undergo processing, or the specific cleavage of a larger protein into smaller peptide sequences, inside a cell before they can be presented by the MHC system. This stepwise process is regulated by the expression of several proteins, as well as expression of the MHC proteins themselves. Ovarian cancer cells have been shown to decrease the expression of these proteins such as the transporter associated with antigen processing as well as MHC. Indeed, loss of these proteins is associated with increasing disease stage for ovarian cancer patients.[16] In this way, cancer cells can still benefit from their mutated proteins while effector T cells will no longer be able to recognize that the antigen is present. However, this solution is imperfect since T cells are not the only effector cells of the immune system; loss of MHC expression may render tumor cells susceptible to NK-cell mediated killing. This mix of selective pressures results in a tenuous balance between reducing antigen or MHC expression and evading NK cell-mediated destruction.

PRODUCTION OF IMMUNE SUPPRESSIVE CYTOKINES

Interactions between ovarian cancer cells and host-derived immune cells result in the production of a number of significant cytokines within the tumor microenvironment that can both drive tumor progression while simultaneously suppressing immune responses. As described earlier, cytokines fit into larger signaling networks. In ovarian cancer, a number of cytokine networks have been identified that effectively suppress anti-tumor immune responses. One such network is formed by TNF-α, IL-6, and CXCL12.[5] The effects of TNF-α strongly depend on the dose and duration of exposure; high, acute doses may promote tumor regression while low, chronic exposure may promote tumor progression. Although immune cells are a major source of TNF-α, this cytokine can also be synthesized by ovarian tumors. Using RNA silencing to reduce TNF-α production, such cells grow normally in culture, but, when they are introduced to mice, this results in decreased tumor burden. This suggests the ovarian cancer cells do not benefit directly from TNF-α expression but through an indirect mechanism.

Intratumoral TNF-α expression is highly correlated with increased expression of IL-6 and CXCL12. High expression of IL-6 has been detected within ovarian tumors, and high serum concentrations of IL-6 are associated with reduced survival of ovarian cancer patients. IL-6 is also often detected in the malignant ascites of ovarian cancer patients. IL-6 regulates several pathways associated with inducing proliferation of tumor cells, promoting angiogenesis and decreasing the sensitivity of tumor cells to apoptotic signals.

IL-6 is also implicated in elevating the level of platelets often observed in ovarian cancer.

Chemokines describe a subset of cytokines characterized by their ability to induce chemotaxis, or directed movement or migration along a chemical gradient, by responder cells. They act as signals to draw cells to a particular site. Ovarian cancer cells can constitutively express the chemokine receptor CXCR4. Expression of CXCR4 is correlated with lymph node metastasis in ovarian cancer patients.[17] The ligand for CXCR4 is CXCL12, which can be produced by other cells in the tumor microenvironment as well as by some ovarian cancer cells. In addition to migration associated with this receptor-ligand interaction, signaling through CXCR4 can have important intracellular consequences. Blocking CXCL12 and CXCR4 interactions in mouse models increases survival, induces tumor cell apoptosis, and reduces recruitment of immune suppressive T cells, (i.e., regulatory T cells [Treg] cells).

Ligation of CXCR4 by CXCL12 also results in increased production of VEGF.[18] VEGF is a product of both ovarian cancer cells as well as immune suppressive cells recruited to tumor tissue. VEGF is well recognized as a key player in the wound-healing process. It acts to stimulate angiogenesis, or the growth of new blood vessels, following injury. Due to the rapid proliferation of tumor cells, there is a large demand for nutrients supplied by these new blood vessels. However, these blood vessels are often disordered due to the excessive production of VEGF by tumor-associated cells. The resulting intratumoral blood flow is often sporadic and does not allow larger materials or substances, such as immune cells or even some antibodies and drugs, to pass through. Indeed, despite a high level of vascularity, most solid tumors show areas of hypoxia, or low oxygen, and high internal pressures which favor tumor cell survival.

Another important cytokine produced by ovarian cancer cells is granulocyte-colony stimulating factor (G-CSF). As the name indicates, G-CSF stimulates the production and mobilization of granulocytic cells from the bone marrow, particularly during acute, systemic infections. However, in cancer, the overexpression of G-CSF can result in the production of myeloid-derived suppressor cells (MDSCs), which are discussed in later. Importantly, some ovarian cancers also express the receptor for G-CSF and can thus respond to this cytokine as an autocrine growth factor.

The cytokine milieu is thus responsible for modulating immune responses within ovarian cancer patients as well as the growth of the tumor cells themselves. It should be noted that there is a great amount of variability in this milieu among cancer patients. The propensity to produce certain cytokines can depend on a patient's particular genetic background, as well as the unique set of mutations that underlie her ovarian tumor. Screening ovarian cancer patients for differences in their germline, or normal genetic sequence, has revealed several polymorphisms or variations in additional cytokine-associated genes that could be predictive of ovarian cancer survival.[5] Understanding the effects of these polymorphisms on cytokine expression and their novel signaling networks for immune regulation can identify new targets for therapy.

EXPRESSION OF IMMUNE SUPPRESSIVE MOLECULES

Cytokines are not the only molecules able to modulate immune responses. In the late 1980s to mid-1990s, scientists first identified molecules expressed on the surface of immune cells that can actually suppress T-cell activation and/or function.[19] These molecules are described as immune "checkpoints" and are turned on when normal cells are exposed to certain inflammatory stimuli. Expression of these molecules prevents excessive tissue damage once immune responses are initiated. Since the tumor microenvironment is in a nearly constant state of inflammation, cancer cells are able to utilize the system to avoid immune destruction. Major examples of these immune suppressive molecules are discussed later. Just as in other solid cancers, these molecules have been identified in the context of ovarian cancer and are currently under investigation as therapeutic targets in preclinical or clinical studies.

The first molecule identified as an immune checkpoint was cytotoxic T-lymphocyte associated protein-4 (CTLA-4). CTLA-4 is an immune suppressive molecule expressed on the surface of Treg cells and at a low level on effector T cells. The expression of this molecule is important at the initiation phase of an immune response. After a naïve T cell is stimulated, CTLA-4 is expressed on the cell surface and competes with CD28 (an activating receptor) to bind co-stimulatory ligands, CD80 or CD86 on APCs. This competition reduces the activating signals received by the T cell to dampen its proliferative or effector functions. Once the T cells migrate to the tumor microenvironment, a large presence of Treg cells provide continuous signaling through CTLA-4 to suppress T-cell activation after antigen recognition.[20] Other molecules that are involved at comparable points in immune activation have since been identified with similar suppressive functions.

A second major set of checkpoint molecules include the "death receptors," programmed death-1 (PD-1) and first apoptosis signal (Fas). These receptors play important roles in development and normal cellular turnover but also have specific functions in constraining immune responses. PD-1 is expressed by activated T cells, particularly during development in the thymus. The ligands for PD-1, PD-L1, and PD-L2 are increased on inflamed tissues, including some cancer cells. PD-L1 expression specifically is increased on ovarian cancer tissues compared to normal ovarian tissue. Signaling through PD-1 inhibits cytokine production, cytolytic activity, and T-cell proliferation.

Fas receptor binding to its cognate ligand, Fas ligand (FasL), induces apoptosis. T cells express FasL after they are activated.

Expression of FasL by T cells constitutes an important mechanism for killing target cells expressing Fas receptor. However, Fas also forms a feedback loop to control T-cell responses. Upon activation, T cells begin to express Fas receptor but are initially resistant to apoptosis. The longer they remain activated, though, the more sensitive T cells become to Fas-induced apoptosis. Overexpression of FasL on cancer cells can stimulate apoptosis of tumor-infiltrating lymphocytes. Interestingly, ovarian cancer cells appear to be resistant to Fas-mediated killing. Indeed, ovarian cancer cells have been shown to secrete soluble FasL, and binding of the ligand to the receptor on ovarian cancer cells paradoxically promotes tumor growth through activation of a distinct set of proliferative, rather than death-inducing, signals.

The molecules described here are primarily membrane-bound receptor-ligand pairs. However, ovarian cancer cells also produce soluble factors that can suppress immune responses. Exposure to the inflammatory cytokine, IFN-γ, can lead to the production of the enzyme idoleamine 2,3-dioxygenase (IDO) by tumor cells. IDO catalyzes the conversion of tryptophan into kynurenine. Activated T cells and NK cells are extremely dependent on tryptophan to undergo cellular proliferation and to maintain their effector function and are thus inhibited when tryptophan is depleted due to high IDO levels. In addition, the byproduct kynurenine can be toxic to these cells. IDO also promotes development of Treg cells, which are discussed later, due to a reduced requirement for tryptophan by these cells. IDO expression occurs in over 50% of serous, clear-cell, and endometrioid ovarian cancers and is associated with reduced overall and progression-free survival. This correlates with a reduced ratio of CD8+ T to Treg cells and is also associated with resistance to paclitaxel therapy.

Certain TAAs can be directly involved in promoting tumor growth through suppression of immune responses. For example, the ovarian cancer antigen CA-125, also known as MUC16, has been shown to have immune suppressive properties. CA-125 is a highly glycosylated membrane-bound protein that can be overexpressed by ovarian cancer cells. This overexpression results in steric hindrance to NK cell binding to tumor cells, which is required for recognition and NK cell–mediated killing. CA-125 can also be shed into the blood, with the concentration reflecting tumor burden, and can serve as a biomarker for disease recurrence and resistance to therapy. It is not yet clear, however, whether soluble CA-125 also has immune suppressive functions.

RECRUITMENT OF SUPPRESSIVE IMMUNE CELLS

The combination of cytokines and immune suppressive molecules described in the last two sections create an inhospitable environment for effector T cells and instead promote the recruitment and survival of cells whose primary function is immune suppression. Just as for the molecules discussed previously, these cells are ordinarily required in healthy individuals to prevent autoimmunity, but, in the case of cancer, they can sustain the neoplastic process by suppressing host immunity. Suppressive cell subsets from both the myeloid and lymphoid lineages have been associated with poorer ovarian cancer patient outcomes.

Myeloid cells make up the major proportion of tumor-infiltrating suppressive cells. These include macrophages, tolerogenic DCs, and MDSCs. As discussed in the section on immunology basics, macrophages normally occupy healthy tissues where they sample the surrounding environment surveying for pathogens or damaged cells. They can elicit a range of responses, with pure M1 or M2 phenotypes representing the most extreme and diametrically opposing polarization states. The M2-like responses are most strongly associated with a poor prognosis in ovarian cancer. Staining for the pan macrophage marker, CD68, alone did not show an association between macrophage infiltration

and ovarian cancer survival; however, stratification using more specific markers for M2 responses such as CD206 and CD163 revealed an increased risk in cancer progression for patients with high M2-like macrophages in their tumors.[5]

DCs are a common component of normal tissues. However, in the cancer setting, DCs take on aberrant properties due to the presence of tumor-derived factors. Ovarian cancers produce high levels of the cytokine IL-10, which can alter the differentiation of DCs to suppress their ability to activate T cells.[5] Additionally, DCs within the tumor express high levels of suppressive molecules such as PD-L1, which can be used to further suppress T-cell activation within the tumor. Murine models of ovarian cancer have shown improved antitumor immunity after depletion of certain subsets of DCs. Despite what is broadly known about impaired DC numbers/function in cancer, the DC-ovarian cancer axis still remains understudied.

As in many other types of solid tumors, ovarian cancer causes patients to have increased numbers of immature or otherwise abnormal myeloid cells in their blood. These cells, MDSCs, inhibit T-cell activation and proliferation. This is accomplished by a number of mechanisms such as reduced antigen processing and presentation, reduced expression of co-stimulatory molecules, and reduced cytokine expression necessary to drive T-cell expansion. MDSCs also express suppressive cytokines, such as TGF-β, IL-10, and other molecules that promote tumor growth such as matrix metalloproteinases necessary for stromal remodeling as tumors progress to metastatic disease. MDSCs are also a potential source of VEGF. MDSCs are thought to arise in response to various types of tumor-derived factors, such as G-CSF, GM-CSF, or M-CSF, resulting in morphologically and phenotypically heterogeneous populations comprised of subsets reflecting granulocytic, monocytic, or even more immature myeloid cell types.

A final myeloid subset associated with immune suppression is the neutrophil. These cells are largely expanded in cancer and sometimes can be confused with granulocytic MDSCs. Recently, the ratio of neutrophils to lymphocytes has been proposed as a novel prognostic marker in cancer patients. Patients with advanced ovarian cancer and high preoperative neutrophil-to-lymphocyte ratio had decreased overall survival.[8] However, the direct suppressor function of these neutrophils is difficult to determine due to the overlap with certain MDSC subsets.

The major suppressive lymphoid cell type is the Treg cell. Treg cells are a specific type of T cell (identified as CD4+CD25+FoxP3+) that patrol normal and inflamed tissues and work to "turn off" activated T cells that might damage healthy tissue. Cytokines produced by macrophages and MDSCs can recruit Treg cells into the tumor, and, once there, Treg cells produce TGF-β and IL-10 to directly suppress the cytotoxicity of effector T cells. In contrast to prolonged survival seen with CD8+ TILs, tumor-infiltrating Treg cells correlate with reduced survival and increased tumor metastasis in ovarian cancer patients.[8] In fact, the ratio between CD8+ T cells and Treg cells in the tumor microenvironment can be an effective prognostic marker. Treg cells inversely correlate with effector cytokines IL-2, IFN-γ, and TNF-β within ovarian cancers.

PHYSICAL BARRIERS TO IMMUNE RESPONSES

In most ovarian cancer patients, spontaneous tumor-specific T cells can be detected in the peripheral blood, and yet this does not always correlate with TILs. Indeed, T cells are often observed on the outside edges of ovarian tumors, apparently unable to gain access to the tumor cells they are seeking to destroy.

The process by which T cells cross endothelial barriers to enter inflamed tissue is termed "extravasation" and is controlled by a specific sequence of molecular events. Lymphocytes travel through the blood until receiving signals from cytokines or chemokines that draw them to sites of inflammation. Endothelial cells can be activated by inflammatory signals, such as damage- or pathogen-associated molecules or inflammatory cytokines (i.e., TNF-α). Activation of endothelial cells causes them to express molecules called selectins that tether lymphocytes to the surface of the endothelia. This initiates a process of rolling by the lymphocyte along the surface of the vasculature until the lymphocytes interact with integrins which bind with higher affinity to arrest lymphocytes on the surface of the endothelia. Following arrest, the lymphocyte begins to spread and then transmigrate across the endothelial cell barrier, exiting the blood and entering the tissue.

Expression of MHC and other co-stimulatory markers on the surface of endothelial cells assist T cells in their migration toward their specific antigen-bearing targets. However, endothelial cells in cancer tend to have reduced expression of these molecules. Additionally, endothelial cells within tumors have been shown to express programmed death ligands (of the PD-L family) and FasL to inhibit T-cell activity. These endothelial cells also produce soluble inhibitors of T-cell activation, such as prostaglandin-E2, TGF-β, IL-10, and IDO.

Importantly, by the time most ovarian cancer patients are diagnosed, their disease is likely to have already metastasized. The primary sites for metastasis of ovarian cancers are the liver, lungs, and peritoneal cavity. These tissues are sites where MDSCs and other suppressive myeloid cells accumulate and potentially contribute to immune suppression, enabling metastatic deposits to further colonize and proliferate.

IMMUNOTHERAPY AS A THERAPEUTIC APPROACH IN METASTATIC OVARIAN CANCER

Several immunotherapeutic approaches are currently under investigation in ovarian cancer. These immunotherapies include both active and passive approaches.[21] Active immunotherapy describes methods designed to trigger endogenous (or de novo) immune responses within an ovarian cancer patient, using the patients' own immune system to combat disease. Passive immunotherapy is the delivery of immune effector cells or molecules to the patient without needing to rely on the patient's own immune system to generate an anti-cancer response. Generally, active immunotherapy is considered to be a more long-term modality since it does not require the repeated administration of exogenous immune-activating products. However, passive immunotherapy is considered to be a more effective option for patients that would be considered immune-compromised either due to concomitant chemotherapies or to the underlying nature of neoplastic disease progression.

Immunotherapies can also be categorized as antigen specific or antigen non-specific. Antigen-specific therapies focus on identified TSAs or TAAs as targets of the intervention while non-specific interventions, such as the delivery of inflammatory cytokines or the use of antibodies for checkpoint blockade, do not rely on defined antigens and instead stimulate a global immune response which likely includes an antigen-specific component. This section discusses the full range of current immunotherapies being investigated for use in ovarian cancer patients (Table 12.2).

ANTIBODIES

A major advance in passive immuno-therapeutic approaches has been the development of synthetically generated antibodies directed against tumor-associated molecules. The technology for generating therapeutically effective antibodies began with the development of hybridomas. This process utilizes immortal cells fused to antibody-producing plasma cells to generate a steady supply of antibodies in the cell culture supernatant. These antibodies are then purified and processed into therapeutic biologics. Genetic modifications to these antibody-producing cells have allowed for customization of these antibodies to include mouse-human chimeras and fully humanized antibodies, as well as human antibodies fused with other proteins and/or chemotherapeutics.

While the use of these antibodies has shown to be effective in preventing metastasis or reducing the size and scope of metastatic lesions in the setting of residual disease, antibodies are not as effective when the disease burden is more advanced. This may be due to reduced permeation of the tissue by the antibodies or other physical barriers to trafficking of immune cells necessary for ADCC. Antibodies developed for cancer therapy are enumerated in Table 12.2 and include both antibodies directed against cell surface antigens, as well as antibodies directed against cytokines and other immune suppressive molecules. Antibodies targeting cell surface receptors elicit responses in two ways, both by blocking receptor-ligand interactions and by targeting bound cells for immune destruction. Antibodies directed against soluble factors result in their clearance from the blood and the tumor microenvironment to inhibit their activity.

Rather than just relying on exogenous administration of antibodies as passive immunotherapies, vaccines targeting antigens to stimulate B cells for antibody production have also been developed. One vaccine showing potential clinical benefit was generated using a chimeric peptide to induce anti-Her2/neu antibodies. This peptide includes the Her2/neu epitope as well as a promiscuous T-cell epitope from the measles virus to stimulate CD4$^+$ T helper cells to promote antibody production.

IMMUNE CHECKPOINT INHIBITORS

An important class of bioactive antibodies merits their own discussion due to their unique mode of action. Rather than being targeted against tumor-specific molecules, these antibodies specifically interact with cells of the immune system to impede inhibitory feedback signaling discussed earlier. These antibodies are called "checkpoint inhibitors" for their ability to promote

TABLE 12.2 OVARIAN CANCER IMMUNOTHERAPIES IN CLINICAL TRIALS

Type	Examples	Function	Type of Immunity[21]				Refs
			Active	Passive	Specific	Nonspecific	
Antibodies	Bevacizumab	Anti-VEGF; blocks VEGF signaling to inhibit angiogenesis		X	X		22
	Catumaxomab	Bispecific to EpCAM and T cell CD3; recruits T cells to EpCAM overexpressing tumors and enhances T cell and NK cell-mediated cytolysis	X	X	X	X	5, 8, 22
	Cetuximab, panitumumab	Anti-EGFR; blocks EGFR signaling and speeds receptor internalization		X	X		22
	RG7155	Anti-CSF1R; to deplete tumor associated macrophages, CSF1R expressing tumor cells	X	X	X		22
	Farletuzumab	Binds FRα to reduce tumor growth		X	X		5
	Trastuzumab, pertuzumab	Antibodies against Her2/neu to inhibit Her2/neu-mediated cell proliferation		X	X		5
	Abagovomab	Mirrors the structure of CA-125; used to induce antigen specific immunity	X		X		5, 8
	Oregovomab	Binds to CA-125 to induce antibody dependent cytotoxicity		X	X		5, 8
	Siltuximab	Binds to IL-6 to reduce the IL-6 in circulation	X			X	5
Checkpoint Inhibitors	Ipilumumab, termelimumab	Anti-CTLA-4 antibodies; deplete Treg cells, inhibit CTLA-4 signaling		X		X	5, 7, 20
	Nivolumab, pidilizumab, pembrolizumab	PD-1 blocking antibodies to inhibit PD-1 signaling	X	X		X	20, 22
	BMS-936559, MPDL3280A, MEDI4736	PD-L1 blocking antibodies	X	X		X	20

(continued)

TABLE 12.2 CONTINUED

Type	Examples	Function	Type of Immunity[21]				Refs
			Active	Passive	Specific	Nonspecific	
Adoptive Cell Transfer	Ex vivo expanded T cells	Harvested from the tumor or collected from peripheral blood and then expanded or stimulated using specific tumor antigens		X	X		5, 8
	CAR T cells	Transgenically made to express receptors for tumor antigens that bypass the requirement for HLA presentation to the TCR		X	X		5, 8
	NK cells	Efforts to both expand the cells ex vivo as well as pharmacologic boost their effects in vivo		X		X	8
	DC vaccines	DC are either pulsed with antigenic proteins or made to express these proteins using viral vectors in combination with cytokines and other approaches.	X		X		5, 8, 22
Other	Recombinant cytokines	Various cytokines in development to stimulate immune responses.	X			X	7, 8
	Immune stimulating drugs	Various targets. Ex. 1-methyl-tryptophan (1MT)—chemical inhibitor of IDO; ATRA—chemical inducer of DC maturation	X			X	5, 22

NOTE: VGEF = vascular endothelial growth factor ; EpCAM = epithelial cell adhesion molecule; NK = natural killer; EGFR = epidermal growth factor receptor; FRα = folate receptor alpha; CSF1R = colony-stimulating factor 1 receptor; IL = interleukin; Treg = regulatory T cells; CAR = chimeric antigen receptor; HLA = human leukocyte antigens; TCR = T cell receptor; IDO = idoleamine 2,3-dioxygenase; ATRA = all-trans retinoic acid; DC = dendritic cells.

CD8+ T cell effector function despite an immune-suppressive tumor microenvironment. For their ability to allow endogenous immune responses to flourish, these antibodies could also be considered a form of active immunotherapy against non-specific immune targets. The effectiveness of these antibodies has been shown in a number of cancer models but is only recently being studied in the context of ovarian cancer.

Since these antibodies nondiscriminatorily block both normal and neoplastic inhibitory feedback mechanisms, the most common immune-related side effects are associated with loss of tolerance to the host tissues leading to the development of autoimmune reactions. These can have serious clinical consequences with symptoms including fatigue, colitis, diarrhea, pneumonitis, arthralgia, rash, nausea, vomiting, anorexia, pruritis, and headache. Generally, though, the extent and instance of adverse events related to these approaches are much less than those associated with conventional chemotherapy. However, these antibodies may still be prone to the same drawbacks discussed earlier; in the setting of extensive primary disease, they have limited effectiveness. This may be due to the inability of these antibodies to effectively permeate the tumor, which is necessary to relieve cell-contact mediated immune suppressive mechanisms.

ADOPTIVE CELL THERAPY

Suppression of immune cell proliferation is considered to be a major limiting factor to effective immune responses in cancer patients. One of the approaches to circumvent this problem is the activation of cells, such as the important effector CD8+ T cells, outside of the host and then returning them to the patient. Several clinical trials have adopted different mechanisms to expand these T cells ex vivo. Usually this process includes repeated exposure of these T cells to a tumor antigen in the presence of IL-2, a cytokine that promotes T-cell survival and proliferation. By this technique, the number of antigen-specific T cells can be greatly expanded prior to transfer. In some patients, this boost in antigen-specific T-cell numbers has shown some benefit. Unfortunately, repeated antigen exposure is also associated with increasing markers of T-cell exhaustion, when T cells become less responsive to their antigens. Additionally, these T cells would likely remain vulnerable to the same inhibiting feedback mechanisms within the tumor microenvironment. Finally,

this ex vivo culture of antigen-specific T cells is not successful in all patients, particularly if the antigen used for expanding these T cells is not expressed on the patient's tumor.

To combat the problems of T-cell exhaustion and susceptibility to immune suppression, a new technology was developed whereby a portion of an antibody molecule was fused to T-cell receptor signaling motifs, referred to as a chimeric antigen receptor (CAR), and then expressed in T cells derived from the patient. The first generation of CAR T cells tested in ovarian cancer included a FR-alpha receptor antibody coupled to the signaling motif of the Fc receptor gamma chain. Transfer of these cells into patients proved to be safe, but they appeared to have no clinical activity. It was found that this first generation of CAR T cells did not persist for long following transfer, a common limitation to adoptive cell transfer therapies. A second generation of CAR T cells has been developed for ovarian cancer, which now includes an anti-FR-alpha antibody fused with the CD3zeta chain and 4-1BB costimulatory domain.[8] These cells have been shown to have longer persistence following transfer and may have clinical efficacy.

T cells are not the only immune effector cells that have been adoptively transferred into ovarian cancer patients. An additional approach has incorporated NK cells for therapy. These NK cells were treated ex vivo with IL-2 for activation. However, these cells were only found to have transient persistence. Methods to prolong their persistence or to better induce endogenous NK responses are under investigation.

DC-BASED VACCINES

DCs, the primary bridge between innate and adaptive immune responses, can be an effective target for therapeutic intervention. Many approaches have been developed to utilize the DC antigen processing and presentation abilities including methods to expand DCs ex vivo before adoptive transfer to the patient, often in combination with specially targeted antigens as a vaccine.

Multiple formulations of antigen delivery have been tested.[22] The most straightforward approach includes the resection of the patient's primary tumor followed by lysis of the cells to produce a "whole tumor cell lysate" vaccine containing all of the potential antigens expressed by the tumor. However, this mixture of proteins and other cellular components may include immune-suppressive molecules. Once specific immunogenic proteins are identified, these proteins can be synthetically produced. Unfortunately, purified whole proteins do not induce strong immune responses on their own once they are separated from other inflammatory molecules. Thus, adjuvants are required to activate DCs to drive efficient antigen processing and presentation. DCs, after internalizing these proteins, degrade them in order to present the immunogenic peptide epitopes on their surface. One drawback to this approach is that once the protein inside the cell has been fully degraded, the source of immunogenic peptides is gone. Several groups have developed either bacterial or viral vectors for delivery of tumor antigens to DCs. Using these vector-based approaches, there is a more persistent source of protein for antigen processing and presentation.

A particular drawback to these approaches is their reliance on DCs to effectively process the internalized or exogenously expressed antigens. In the cancer setting, DCs can be impaired in their ability to process antigens. To circumvent this issue, researchers have also developed vaccines using shortened peptide sequences that retain the antigenic epitopes but require minimal to no processing by the DCs. Indeed, in the most basic format, these peptides can bind to unoccupied MHC class I molecules on the cell surface and be presented immediately without requiring any internalization. This approach, however, still requires the use of adjuvants to drive the expression of co-stimulatory molecules.

Targeting DCs for their ability to present antigens to effector cells has been shown to be particularly effective in cases of residual disease, once the immune suppressive tumor microenvironment has been dampened following surgery or chemotherapy. To expand the utility of these approaches, several groups have begun to combine DC vaccines with other therapies such as bevacizumab to block angiogenesis, with ex vivo-expanded T cells, or in combination with lymphodepletion to reduce Treg cells.

OTHER IMMUNOLOGICALLY IMPORTANT APPROACHES

Additional pharmacologic approaches exist to modulate the immune response in cancer patients. These approaches generally are characterized as non-specific, as their use can stimulate an endogenous response within the host directed against their own tumor antigens. These new drugs can be both biologically (protein based) and chemically (e.g., small molecules) derived.

Cytokines, as discussed earlier, are signaling molecules that can dramatically impact immune responses. Just as tumors produce immune suppressive cytokines, researchers are investigating the use of stimulatory cytokines to promote immune activation. Using recombinant technologies, several companies have developed cytokine-based therapies that are either in clinical trials or already in clinical use. Each recombinant cytokine has a differential effect on immune cell function and can be influenced by the presence of other cytokines within a cancer patient. Thus, the effectiveness of a particular cytokine-based therapy can be largely disease-specific. Only two cytokines have been approved by the Food and Drug Administration (FDA) as monotherapies in cancer: IL-2 and IFN-α. However, IL-2 as a monotherapy in ovarian cancer has historically only had modest effects.[23] IFN-α has been investigated as part of maintenance therapy as well as in combination with other immunotherapeutic approaches but is not considered effective as a primary therapy.[24] Additional cytokines have been investigated in early-stage clinical trials, including IFN-γ, GM-CSF, IL-7, IL-12, IL-15, IL-18, and IL-21.[7] IFN-γ has been tested in the first-line therapy of ovarian cancer patients and shown to improve progression-free and overall survival but has not been approved by the FDA for use in cancer therapy.[25] As we have discussed, cytokines can be potent modulators of immune responses and are often associated in signaling networks such that administration of a single cytokine can elicit myriad effects. Thus, therapeutic administration of these cytokines has the potential to induce a variety of adverse side effects associated with unrestrained inflammation. Patients undergoing these therapies must therefore be closely monitored.

Novel therapies are being investigated to chemically target the immune suppressive mechanisms described earlier. An example of this approach includes 1-methyl-tryptophan, a chemical inhibitor of the immune suppressive IDO. Another approach includes the use of all-trans retinoic acid to stimulate differentiation of immature myeloid cells, such as MDSCs into DCs and improving the antigen-presenting capabilities of the myeloid compartment.

Finally, our understanding of conventional chemotherapy has advanced in recent years to include an immune-mediated component to explain susceptibility to these therapies. The extensive amount of tumor cell death induced following treatments such as platinum-based agents releases a wave of antigens and other DAMPs that can stimulate endogenous immune responses. Studies are underway to investigate combinatorial treatments that take advantage of these fundamental immune mechanisms.

SUMMARY AND FUTURE PERSPECTIVES

Immune responses can be powerful tools in controlling tumor growth and preventing tumor progression as well as metastasis. These responses are shaped both by the underlying genetic background of the patient as well as by the patient's own unique tumor biology. Understanding the immune roadblocks that exist in ovarian cancer patients will allow researchers to develop better immune interventions to improve treatment outcomes. Because many of these approaches, especially those that rely on specific tumor antigens, require knowledge of this biology, a great push has been made to incorporate more patient screening for tailor-made vaccines. Additionally, screening for underlying immune responses to tumors could assist in determining the course of treatment that might be most effective. The presence of spontaneous effector T-cell responses could suggest that conventional therapies may be beneficial on their own, while a lack of these T cells may require a more synthetic or artificial intervention such as adoptive transfer of CAR T cells. It is likely that most patients will be best served by an optimized combination of conventional therapies with innovative therapies to boost immune responses.

ACKNOWLEDGMENTS

SIA was supported by National Institute of Health/National Cancer Institute grants R01CA140622 and R01CA172105; Department of Defense, W81XWH-11-1-0394. CSN was supported by National Institutes of Health grant T32CA085183.

REFERENCES

1. Blankenstein T, Coulie PG, Gilboa E, Jaffee EM. The determinants of tumour immunogenicity. *Nat Rev Cancer.* 2012;12(4):307–13.
2. Zhang L, Conejo-Garcia JR, Katsaros D, et al. Intratumoral T cells, recurrence, and survival in epithelial ovarian cancer. *N Engl J Med.* 2003;348(3):203–13.
3. Sato E, Olson SH, Ahn J, et al. Intraepithelial CD8+ tumor-infiltrating lymphocytes and a high CD8+/regulatory T cell ratio are associated with favorable prognosis in ovarian cancer. *Proc Natl Acad Sci U S A.* 2005;102(51):18538–43.

4. Hwang WT, Adams SF, Tahirovic E, Hagemann IS, Coukos G. Prognostic significance of tumor-infiltrating T cells in ovarian cancer: a meta-analysis. *Gynecol Oncol.* 2012;124(2):192–98.

5. Knutson KL, Karyampudi L, Lamichhane P, Preston C. Targeted immune therapy of ovarian cancer. *Cancer Metastasis Rev.* 2015;34(1):53–74.

6. Daudi S, Eng KH, Mhawech-Fauceglia P, et al. Expression and immune responses to MAGE antigens predict survival in epithelial ovarian cancer. *PLoS One.* 2014;9(8):e104099.

7. Zakharia Y, Rahma O, Khleif SN. Ovarian cancer from an immune perspective. *Radiat Res.* 2014;182(2):239–51.

8. Bronte G, Cicero G, Sortino G, et al. Immunotherapy for recurrent ovarian cancer: a further piece of the puzzle or a striking strategy? *Expert Opin Biol Ther.* 2014;14(1):103–14.

9. Nelson BH. New insights into tumor immunity revealed by the unique genetic and genomic aspects of ovarian cancer. *Curr Opin Immunol.* 2015;33:93–100.

10. Chiriva-Internati M, Wang Z, Salati E, Timmins P, Lim SH. Tumor vaccine for ovarian carcinoma targeting sperm protein 17. *Cancer.* 2002;94(9):2447–53.

11. Zhang S, Zhou X, Yu H, Yu Y. Expression of tumor-specific antigen MAGE, GAGE and BAGE in ovarian cancer tissues and cell lines. *BMC Cancer.* 2010;10:163.

12. Smith JB, Stashwick C, Powell DJ Jr. B7-H4 as a potential target for immunotherapy for gynecologic cancers: a closer look. *Gynecol Oncol.* 2014;134(1):181–89.

13. Chambers SK. Role of CSF-1 in progression of epithelial ovarian cancer. *Future Oncol.* 2009;5(9):1429–40.

14. Hata K, Watanabe Y, Nakai H, Hata T, Hoshiai H. Expression of the vascular endothelial growth factor (VEGF) gene in epithelial ovarian cancer: an approach to anti-VEGF therapy. *Anticancer Res.* 2011;31(2):731–37.

15. Chang X, Ye X, Dong L, et al. Human epididymis protein 4 (HE4) as a serum tumor biomarker in patients with ovarian carcinoma. *Int J Gynecol Cancer.* 2011;21(5):852–58.

16. Vitale M, Pelusi G, Taroni B, et al. HLA class I antigen down-regulation in primary ovary carcinoma lesions: association with disease stage. *Clin Cancer Res.* 2005;11(1):67–72.

17. Wang J, Cai J, Han F, et al. Silencing of CXCR4 blocks progression of ovarian cancer and depresses canonical Wnt signaling pathway. *Int J Gynecol Cancer.* 2011;21(6):981–87.

18. Liang Z, Brooks J, Willard M, et al. CXCR4/CXCL12 axis promotes VEGF-mediated tumor angiogenesis through Akt signaling pathway. *Biochem Biophys Res Commun.* 2007;359(3):716–22.

19. Monteiro J. Timeline: checkpoint blockade. *Cell.* 2015;162(6):1434.

20. Wang DH, Guo L, Wu XH. Checkpoint inhibitors in immunotherapy of ovarian cancer. *Tumour Biol.* 2015;36(1):33–39.

21. Galluzzi L, Vacchelli E, Bravo-San Pedro JM, et al. Classification of current anticancer immunotherapies. *Oncotarget.* 2014;5(24):12472–508.

22. Chester C, Dorigo O, Berek JS, Kohrt H. Immunotherapeutic approaches to ovarian cancer treatment. *J Immunother Cancer.* 2015;3:7.

23. Santoiemma PP, Powell DJ Jr. Tumor infiltrating lymphocytes in ovarian cancer. *Cancer Biol Ther.* 2015;16(6):807–20.

24. Lawal AO, Musekiwa A, Grobler L. Interferon after surgery for women with advanced (stage II-IV) epithelial ovarian cancer. *Cochrane Database Syst Rev.* 2013;6:Cd009620.

25. Windbichler GH, Hausmaninger H, Stummvoll W, et al. Interferon-gamma in the first-line therapy of ovarian cancer: a randomized phase III trial. *Br J Cancer.* 2000;82(6):1138–44.

13.

CLINICAL TRIALS OF OVARIAN CANCER IMMUNOTHERAPY AND FUTURE DIRECTIONS

Justin M. Drerup, Curtis A. Clark, and Tyler J. Curiel

INTRODUCTION

Ovarian cancer (OC) is thought to result from uncontrolled growth of epithelial cells surrounding the ovaries, stromal cells, or ova, although specific cells of origin for various histologic types are incompletely understood.[1] Epithelial OC is by far the most common OC subtype, and all discussion in this chapter refers to epithelial OC. Nearly 80% of OC patients present with regional or distant OC metastasis, and, although OC responds well to initial chemotherapy and surgical debulking, more than half of patients succumb to chemoresistant relapse within five years of diagnosis. Immunotherapy could be a viable treatment modality[2-9] as there are a number of immunogenic OC-associated antigens that provoke detectable and specific T-cell responses.[10-19] Intratumoral CD8+ T-cell density positively correlates with OC patient survival, a seminal finding that supports the role of anti-tumor immunity in slowing OC progression.[20] However, in spite of abundant evidence that immune therapy could be effective for OC, clinical trials have been, at best, humbling with only modest successes. The earliest attempts at immunotherapy for OC unsuccessfully employed intraperitoneal instillations of anti-human milk fat globulin-1 antibodies in 1987,[21] which was among the very first uses of antibodies as cancer immunotherapy. A number of similar attempts followed, most notably with failure of the anti-CA-125 antibody oregovomab.

Although many anecdotal reports of newer immunotherapy approaches indicate positive patient outcomes and high-profile successes in other solid tumors (e.g., melanoma and lung cancer), there is currently no Food and Drug Administration (FDA)–approved immune therapy for OC. Nonetheless, new data suggests that effective, tolerable OC immunotherapy could be developed. A more complete understanding of OC immunopathogenesis, OC rejection antigens, the role of immune-suppressive regulatory T cells and immature myeloid cells, and dysfunctional immune co-signaling help identify new and possibly more effective approaches to activate anti-OC immunity. As with chemotherapy, combination immunotherapies appear more promising than single agents. An important area for future trials is to determine optimal combinations of immunotherapy, cytotoxics, targeted inhibitors, radiation therapy, or surgery with the ultimate goal of developing comprehensive, multimodal, and potentially curative OC treatment regimens. Here we describe the current state of OC immunotherapy clinical trials and comment on future directions.

CHEMOTHERAPY AS IMMUNOTHERAPY

Several cytotoxic agents act as immune modulators and can reduce immunosuppressive cells or increase tumor immunogenicity.

Fludarabine[22] or cyclophosphamide[23] can deplete immunopathogenic regulatory T cells. 5-fluorouracil can deplete cancer-promoting myeloid-derived suppressor cells in preclinical models.[24] Anthracyclines can promote immune surveillance by causing release of tumor antigens by tumor cell lysis or release of danger signals, such as high-mobility group box 1.[25] Thus, chemotherapy is a rational adjunct to immune therapy to increase tumor immunogenicity or impair immune suppressive cells.

MONOCLONAL ANTIBODIES

Anti-Milk Fat Globulin-1

Nearly three decades ago, intraperitoneal radiolabeled anti-milk fat globulin antibodies were tested as OC immunotherapy,[21] where dose of irradiation correlated with occasional treatment responses. Further trials continued to establish the safety of intraperitoneal antibody instillation, demonstrating that this could be a viable route to concentrate drug at the site of OC tumors.[26] A Phase II trial of [90]yttrium-labeled anti-human milk fat globulin-1 in 25 patients failed to produce meaningful objective responses, and dose escalation produced myelosuppression that limited this approach.[27]

However, [90]yttrium-labeled anti-human milk fat globulin-1 was later tested in 52 patients in combination with surgical debulking and chemotherapy.[28] Twenty-one of 52 patients had no evidence of disease at therapy cessation, with a median survival of 35 months that compared favorably to historical controls. A seven-year follow-up corroborated potential efficacy.[29] Further trials indicate that a major limitation was the inability of anti-milk fat globulin 1 to control distant relapses that reduced any advantages conferred by reduction of intraperitoneal tumor burden.[30]

Farletuzumab

Farletuzumab is a humanized anti-folate receptor-α antibody (folate receptor is elevated in many OCs) that does not inhibit folate transport but stimulates antibody-mediated cytotoxicity against folate receptor-expressing cells. Phase I and II trials demonstrated safety and activity in chemoresistant OC patients.[31,32] Fifty-four OC patients received weekly farletuzumab alone or combined with carboplatin with paclitaxel or docetaxel.[31] Farletuzumab monotherapy was well tolerated and did not potentiate side effects typically seen with chemotherapeutics. Of 47 patients on farletuzumab plus chemotherapy, 38 (80.9%) normalized CA-125. Complete or partial response rates were 75% with farletuzumab plus cytotoxics. Thus, farletuzumab alone might be poorly effective, but combination with carboplatin plus a taxane was thought to merit additional consideration in the context of chemoresistant relapsed patients. Very disappointingly, chemotherapy followed by farletuzumab failed to improve progression-free or overall survival at two doses in a recently published Phase III trial of 1,100 platinum-resistant OC patients,[33] although survival trended to be improved in patients with the lowest tumor burden (as indicated by pre-farletuzumab CA-125 levels).

Catumaxomab

Catumaxomab targets epithelial cell adhesion molecule (EpCAM)–expressing tumor cells thought to mediate ascites accumulation. It is approved in Europe but not the United States to treat malignant ascites. Adverse effects include fever, nausea, vomiting, and abdominal pain. A Phase IIIb study demonstrated that 25 mg prednisolone mitigated adverse events.[34] Because catumaxomab is a rat-mouse hybrid antibody, xenoantibodies could modulate its efficacy. OC patients treated with catumaxomab exhibited increased latency to subsequent paracentesis as expected but surprisingly also experienced significantly increased median overall survival.[35]

IMMUNE CHECKPOINT INHIBITORS

Compared to any other immunotherapy, immune checkpoint blockade antibodies have accumulated the most evidence of increased patient overall survival and long-term responses in solid tumors. Highly anticipated clinical trial successes culminated in the FDA approval of ipilimumab (anti-CTLA-4), pembrolizumab (anti-PD-1), and nivolumab (anti-PD-1) for melanoma and non-small cell lung cancer (and, very recently, avelumab [anti-PD-L1] for advanced bladder cancer). These checkpoint inhibitors block negative regulatory signals from PD-L1[+] cancer cells or antigen-presenting cells that cause T-cell exhaustion,[36] although very recent preclinical studies demonstrate that cancer-cell intrinsic PD-1/PD-L1 signaling is directly advantageous for tumor growth, independent of immunity.[37,38] Thus, direct effects on tumor are potential additional mechanisms of action for PD-1 or PD-L1 blocking antibodies. Due to these unprecedented trial successes, antibodies targeting several other checkpoint proteins are now in various stages of preclinical and clinical development, including against Tim3, LAG-3, or TIGIT. Tremelimumab, like ipilimumab, is a fully human anti-CTLA-4 checkpoint antibody. Ipilimumab became the first approved checkpoint inhibitor following Phase III trials demonstrating efficacy against metastatic or unresectable melanoma.[39] Anecdotal ipilimumab efficacy against OC prompted an ongoing Phase II trial of ipilimumab in treatment-resistant OC (NCT01611558). Ipilimumab has significant immune-related side effects that include off-target inflammation that is occasionally life-threatening but generally resolves after administration of corticosteroids or immune-suppressive monoclonal antibodies (e.g., infliximab). Tremelimumab (in Phase III trials for melanoma) could have similar efficacy with reduced toxicities. Avelumab, an anti-PD-L1 antibody, was recently FDA approved for bladder cancer and multiple studies continue to provide a rationale for PD-L1 as a therapeutic target in many cancer types.[40] BMS-936559 is a fully human monoclonal antibody that prevents PD-L1 from ligating its known cognate receptors, PD-1 and CD80. It demonstrated safety in a Phase I trial that included 17 OC patients.[40] Adverse events occurred in 91% of 207 total patients. However, just 6% halted therapy due to side effects. Common adverse events included fatigue, infusion reactions, diarrhea, arthralgia, pruritis, rash, nausea, and headache. Immune-related adverse events (rash, hypothyroidism, hepatitis, sarcoidosis, diabetes mellitus, endophthalmitis, myasthenia gravis) were observed in 81 patients (39%). Objective responses among OC patients were generally modest and only observed at the highest dose of 10 mg/kg: one patient (6%) with a partial response and three (18%) with stable disease (>24 weeks). Anti-PD-L1 is currently being tested in multiple clinical trials as monotherapy or in combination with other immune-modulating antibodies. A Phase I/II clinical trial will test anti-PD-L1 alone in patients with advanced, treatment-refractory solid tumors, including OC (NCT01693562). Several other trials examine the combination of anti-PD-L1 with anti-CTLA-4, anti-PD-1, or anti-OX-40 (an agonistic antibody that stimulates T cell activation) (NCT02205333, NCT02118337, NCT02261220). Pembrolizumab (anti-PD-1 antibody) is currently under investigation in a Phase 1b trial for patients with biomarker-positive solid tumors, including OC (NCT02054806).

In OC, there is some evidence that clear cell histology is more immunotherapy sensitive versus the more common high-grade serous histology. For example, one of two patients with clear cell OC experienced a complete clinical response in a trial of nivolumab for platinum-refractory disease.[41] In a Phase 1b trial of the anti-PD-L1 antibody avelumab in OC, two of two patients with clear cell histology had partial clinical responses.[42]

CD137 (4-1BB) is a stimulatory immune checkpoint protein that promotes T-cell responsiveness. In preclinical OC models, anti-CD137 plus anti-Tim3[43] or anti-PD-1[44] improved immune and clinical responses. Anti-CD137 has moved into Phase I human clinical trials that include patients with OC.[45] Urelumab targets CD137 through agonistic stimulation and has also entered early clinical trials against solid tumors, including OC as a single agent (NCT01471210) or combined with anti-PD-1 (NCT02253992). Antibodies blocking LAG-3, another T-cell checkpoint protein, recently entered Phase I/II clinical trials for patients with solid tumors, including OC (NCT01968109).

Oregovomab

The OC tumor-associated antigen CA-125 is used as a biomarker for treatment responses. Oregovomab, a murine IgG1 monoclonal antibody that complexes with CA-125 in vivo, can prime dendritic cells (DCs),[46] activating anti-tumor T cells.[47] In a Phase III study of 373 OC patients[48], oregovomab used as maintenance after first-line therapy was well tolerated, although without significant clinical efficacy, causing initial abandonment. However, as previous reports indicated immune-boosting effects,[46–48] renewed interest in oregovomab prompted current use in combination with first-line chemotherapy (carboplatin plus paclitaxel) in a Phase II randomized trial of advanced OC (NCT01616303). In addition to clinical end points, this study will also assess immune-modulating effects of anti-CA-125.

Abagovomab

The anti-idiotypic CA-125 murine monoclonal antibody, abagovomab,[49] is proposed to function by inducing anti-CA-125 antibodies. The most common adverse events were minor injection site pain, myalgia, and fever in a Phase I trial of 42 OC patients randomized to intramuscular versus subcutaneous abagovomab vaccination (2.0 or 0.2 mg four times every two weeks, plus two additional monthly vaccinations). In addition to anti-CA-125 antibodies, human anti-mouse antibodies (irrespective of dose or administration route) were detected in all patients.[50] Abagovomab as maintenance therapy (2 mg or placebo initially administered every two weeks for six weeks, followed by maintenance vaccinations every four weeks until recurrence), induced a robust anti-CA-125 response without increase in recurrence-free or overall survival in a recent Phase III trial (the MIMOSA study) of 888 patients with stage III or IV OC[51] in complete clinical remission after front-line surgery plus platinum/taxane chemotherapy. Patients were treated for 450 days on average, and minor adverse events were similar to those in the Phase I trial. Subsequent studies confirmed the inability to extend overall survival in OC[52] or to expand CA-125-specific CD8+ T cells. Nonetheless, as elevated CA-125-specific CD8+ T cells can predict increased survival,[52] stimulation of CA-125-specific cytotoxic lymphocyte responses remains a viable OC treatment strategy.

Volociximab

Targeting the integrin subunit AAB1, volociximab is a chimeric IgG4 monoclonal antibody with anti-neoangiogenic properties by blocking interaction of α5β1integrin with fibronectin.[53] In a Phase II trial of 16 patients with platinum-resistant OC or primary peritoneal cancer,[54] intravenous volociximab (15 mg/kg weekly until disease progression or treatment intolerance) elicited stable disease in one patient at eight weeks, but all others progressed. Headache and fatigue were common adverse events in 75% of patients, while posterior leukoencephalopathy syndrome, pulmonary embolism, and hyponatremia were possible study-related, serious but reversible adverse events in three patients. Results from this trial have incited additional investigations.

Amatuximab

Mesothelin is a tumor differentiation antigen overexpressed in certain cancers including OC[55] and is a thus a candidate OC treatment target. In a Phase I trial of 24 patients with mesothelin-expressing tumors including OC, the chimeric anti-mesothelin monoclonal antibody MORAb-009 (amatuximab) effected stable disease in 11 patients,[56] prompting an ongoing Phase II trial in mesothelioma patients.

Tocilizumab/Siltuximab

Interleukin (IL)-6 in immunopathologic in diverse cancers[57] and plays varied immunopathogenic roles in OC.[58,59] Tocilizumab is a humanized anti-IL-6 receptor antibody tested for tumor cachexia[60] and mitigation of cytokine release symptoms in adoptive T-cell therapy.[61] A Phase I trial tested tocilizumab plus chemotherapy in 23 OC patients,[62] finding it to be safe and tolerable. Objective responses were observed in 11 of 21 evaluable patients (6 stable disease, 3 progressive disease). Likewise, the anti-IL-6 antibody siltuximab is being explored as therapy for numerous carcinomas, hematologic malignancies, and cachexia.[63] Siltuximab was evaluated in a Phase I/II trial of patients with solid tumors (including 29 OC patients)[64] and was well tolerated but without clinical efficacy. Various trials are currently underway, including use in cancer, evaluating anti-IL-6 and anti-IL-6 receptor antibodies.

OTHER MONOCLONAL ANTIBODY CLINICAL TRIALS IN PROGRESS

Immunotherapy is being tested in a wide-range and number of clinical trials involving solid tumors. In one study involving platinum-resistant OC patients, the cytotoxic agent MMAE is being tested as a drug/antibody conjugate that targets the type II sodium-phosphate cotransporter, which is overexpressed on many ovarian and lung cancers (NCT01991210). In Phase I/II trials in patients with platinum-resistant OC, demcizumab and OM-P52M51 antibodies are being investigated in their ability to inhibit Notch-dependent cancer cell-intrinsic growth pathways by targeting delta-like ligand-4 or Notch1, respectively (NCT01952249 and NCT01778439). In a multicenter Phase I/II trial, monoclonal antibodies specific for Trop-2, which is overexpressed in many epithelial carcinomas and preclinical studies implicate its role in cancer cell invasion, survival, and stemness,[65] are being tested in patients with epithelial cancers, including OC (NCT01631552). Antibody-based therapy for cancer has been previously reviewed in detail.[66]

ADDITIONAL APPROACHES

Targeting detrimental regulatory T cells in human malignancies, including OC, remains a practical therapeutic strategy. Our recent report of a Phase I clinical trial using denileukin diftitox fusion toxin demonstrated the potential benefit of reducing regulatory T cells and eliciting enhanced anti-tumor immunity in human cancer, in which a significant partial clinical response in one patient with metastatic OC was observed. In a subsequent Phase II trial of 28 OC patients, administration of denileukin diftitox (12 µg/kg every three to four weeks) was well tolerated with no more than grade 2 toxicities (most commonly fatigue, fever, myalgias) but failed clinically, despite reducing blood regulatory T (Treg) cells.[67] We recently reported preclinical findings that immune checkpoint blockade greatly enhances denileukin diftitox clinical efficacy, including in OC,[68] which has encouraged ongoing studies of combination strategies. Our preclinical studies have also suggested that anti-CD73 could improve clinical efficacy of adoptive T-cell transfer in

OC[69] and demonstrated that age[70] and sex[71] alter immunotherapy outcomes, significant factors generally not taken into account in immunotherapy trial design.

CYTOKINES

INTERFERON-α

Type I interferons (primarily interferons α, β, and ω) were originally identified as anti-viral proteins[72] but have subsequently been found to block malignant cell proliferation. Studies of type I interferons in human cancer have primary focused on interferon-α and using relatively high doses that directly inhibit tumor cell replication, despite significant toxicities that limit clinical applications.[73] Initially evaluated in the early 1980s as one of the first OC immunotherapy approaches, intraperitoneal interferon-α exhibited only modest clinical efficacy.[74,75] A Phase II study of 14 OC patients demonstrated that interferon-α could be administered intraperitoneally in combination with cis-platinum as salvage therapy when optimal surgical debulking was not obtainable. This approach was tolerable with indications of clinical efficacy,[76] but intraperitoneal interferon-α also failed to manage malignant OC ascites.[77]

Interferon-α improved paclitaxel clinical efficacy in a preclinical OC mouse model.[78] In vitro, interferon-α upregulated OC cell human leukocyte antigen class I,[79] indicating the potential for enhanced anti-tumor immune recognition, whereas potential OC antigen targets such as HMFG1 and HMFG2 were downregulated, altogether emphasizing that multiple factors must be considered when designing combination therapies.

In our subsequent and ongoing studies, interferon-α at low, immune-modulating doses improved the immune and clinical efficacy of denileukin diftitox used to deplete regulatory T cells in a mouse OC model and in two of two OC patients, with manageable toxicities.[80] As an additional possible mechanism of action, interferon-α reduces proliferation of human OC stem cells[81] that play major roles in initiation, perpetuation, and development of cancer treatment resistance. Expression of interferon-β by engineered adenoviruses was used as gene therapy in an early-phase clinical trial that included two OC patients,[82] in which one patient demonstrated stable disease two months after treatment ended. However, both patients died within five months of treatment initiation. Despite generation of anti-tumor antibodies, development of neutralizing anti-adenovirus antibodies, a well-known limitation of repeated adenovirus administrations, reduced interferon-β levels after the second adenovirus infusion.

INTERFERON-γ

By 1992, interferon-γ was established to treat OC,[83] and by 1996, intraperitoneal administration of interferon-γ elicited some promising preliminary results.[84] Interferon-γ in combination with front-line chemotherapy was confirmed to improve OC survival.[85] In combination with interleukin-2, interferon-γ was studied with infusion of tumor-infiltrating lymphocytes in OC. Either alone or combined with interleukin-2, interferon-γ upregulated tumor cell human leukocyte antigen class I and class II expression,[86] potentially improving tumor immunogenicity. Two of 22 OC patients receiving cytokine treatments also received tumor-infiltrating lymphocyte adoptive transfer after ex vivo expansion, and one of these two had disease stabilization lasting >6 months. In combination with IL-2 therapy, interferon-γ activated CD8[+] T cells but also stimulated expression of possibly immunosuppressive IL-10 and TGF-β.

Interferon-γ to boost antibody-dependent cellular cytotoxicity was investigated in a Phase I clinical trial of 25 possibly chemotherapy-sensitive OC patients with recurrent measurable disease. Administration of GM-CSF (starting at 400 µg/day subcutaneously) for seven days plus interferon-γ (100 μg subcutaneously, on days 5 and 7), before and after intravenous carboplatin (AUC 5) increased activation of blood monocytes but without definitive alteration of antibody-dependent cellular cytotoxicity.[87]

Interferon-γ significantly improved survival in mouse OC xenograft models, while administration of the matrix metalloprotease inhibitor batimastat but not carboplatin enhanced survival with interferon-γ.[88] In vitro, interferon-γ downregulated Her2 and inhibited cell proliferation in multiple human OC lines[89] and augmented OC cell susceptibility to CA-125 (tumor)-specific CD8+ T cell-mediated cytotoxicity.[90] Thus, interferons deserve additional consideration in immunotherapy trials in OC.

INTERLEUKIN-2

IL-2, first identified as an in vitro T-cell growth factor, is among the first effective cancer immunotherapies.[91] It exerts modest anti-cancer activity in melanoma and renal cell carcinoma, among other cancers.[92] During its initial human trials, a small fraction of patients (with aggressive cancers that failed all prior therapies) exhibited long-term cancer-free survival (putative cures), an immunotherapy first. A major limitation of IL-2 therapy is toxicity due to vascular leak syndrome caused by stimulation of IL-2 receptor on endothelial cells, as well as IL-2-mediated expansion of immune suppressive regulatory T cells in OC.[93] Because IL-2 was later found to be a Treg growth and differentiation factor, combining IL-2 with specific Treg depletion could be useful clinically. Low-dose IL-2 plus retinoic acid was tested in an OC cohort.[94] Five-year progression-free survival and overall survival rates were 29% and 38%, respectively, in 65 patients. Notable observations included a lowering of vascular endothelial growth factor and augmentation of lymphocyte and natural killer

(NK) cell numbers. In a Phase II trial of 31 chemoresistant OC patients,[95] intraperitoneal IL-2 elicited minor clinical efficacy but with few major adverse events, indicating this route of administration could be superior to intravenous IL-2. In 24 patients so assessed, there were four complete and two partial clinical responses with overall survival positively correlating with cytokine-expressing cytotoxic T-cell numbers. A combination of IL-2 plus erythropoietin was tested in peripheral blood stem cell transplants for breast cancer and OC. Myeloid cell recovery was improved, but there were no significant immune benefits.[96]

IL-2/anti-IL-2 cytokine-antibody complexes can harness the ability of IL-2 to stimulate effector T and NK cells but avoid Treg expansion and vascular leak syndrome. In preclinical studies, when IL-2 is complexed with anti-IL-2 antibodies that occlude the CD25-binding moiety of IL-2, IL-2 will stimulate only low-affinity IL-2 receptor, and thus there is predominantly expansion of effector, but not regulatory, immune cells, which has reduced tumor burden in several mouse cancer models.[97] Development of clinical-grade CD122-specific anti-IL-2/IL-2 complexes will be an important area of future development for cancer immunotherapy with IL-2. We recently reported that a CD122-directed IL-2 complex (targeting the intermediate-affinity IL-2 receptor) improved anti-cancer immunity, reduced tumor growth, and improved survival in an aggressive model of mouse OC,[98] providing rationale for translation of IL-2 complexes into OC trials.

TUMOR NECROSIS FACTOR α

Tumor necrosis factor alpha (TNF-α) induces cancer cell apoptosis and boosts anticancer immunity. A fusion protein of TNF-α and the tripeptide asparagine-glycine-arginine (NGR-hTNF) selectively binds CD13, a molecule overexpressed on tumor blood vessels. NGR-hTNF has higher potency versus native

TNF-α and reduces toxicities. Thirty-seven patients with platinum-resistant OC received a median four cycles of NGR-hTNF.[99] Partial clinical responses were achieved in 8 (23%), and stable disease was achieved in 15 (43%). Common side effects included weakness, leukopenia, anemia, nausea, neutropenia (including one instance of febrile neutropenia), chills, constipation, and vomiting. Nonetheless, <10% of these adverse events were attributed to NGR-hTNF. In contrast, preclinical data now suggest that TNF-α promotes OC cell-intrinsic growth in humans and mouse OC cell lines.[100,101] Thus, TNF-α inhibitors (of which some are already FDA approved) warrant testing as OC therapy.

IL-18

In mouse models, recombinant IL-18 (SB-485232) improves antitumor immunity when combined with PEGylated liposomal doxorubicin. SB-485232 was used with PEGylated liposomal doxorubicin in a Phase I study of patients with recurrent OC. Sixteen patients were treated with four PEGylated liposomal doxorubicin cycles (40 mg/m^2) every 28 days, in combination with dose-escalated SB-485232 on cycle days 2 and 9. Eighty-two percent of patients were platinum-resistant/refractory and heavily pretreated. SB-485232 was well tolerated. PEGylated liposomal doxorubicin did not affect SB-485232 biologic activity, and SB-485232 did not alter toxicities of doxorubicin. Thirty-eight percent of patients had stable disease, but improved clinical responses were modest.[102]

A summary of recent selected clinical trials using antibodies, immunotoxins, or cytokines is presented in Table 13.1.

OTHER TREATMENTS

PEPTIDE VACCINES

Although the mutational load in OC is low compared to many epithelial carcinomas,

a number of tumor-associated antigens have been identified. Thus, there is potential to elicit beneficial anti-tumor immunity. Identified OC tumor-associated antigens to date include HER2/neu, MUC1,[10] membrane folate receptor,[12] NY-ESO-1,[11] folate binding protein (gp38),[13] mesothelin,[15,16] TAG-72,[14] milk fat globulin-1,[21] sialyl-Tn,[17,18] and OA3.[19]

A significant limitation of peptide vaccines is that they are recognized in the context of specific major histocompatibility complex molecules and thus will generally not be widely applicable. Using peptide library vaccines or rapid synthesis of patient-specific peptides are currently being investigated for cancers generally and could help overcome this limitation.[103]

NY-ESO-1

NY-ESO-1 is a cancer/testis antigen found in some OCs. It was delivered in vaccinia or fowlpox vectors and given to 22 patients with advanced OC in clinical remission.[104] One intradermal dose of NY-ESO-1-vaccinia vector followed by monthly subcutaneous NY-ESO-1-fowlpox vector increased NY-ESO-1 specific antibodies. Median duration of progression-free survival and median overall survival were 21 months and 4 years, respectively, with no major adverse events.

In a Phase I trial with 12 patients with relapsed OC, the epigenetic modifier decitabine and liposomal doxorubicin were combined with an NY-ESO-1 vaccine. Treatment was safe and with manageable adverse events. Vaccination augmented NY-ESO-1-specific antibodies as well as antibodies to additional distinct OC tumor antigens. Stable disease or partial clinical response was observed in 6 of 10 patients,[105] prompting further studies.

p53

p53 overexpression is common in selected OC types. p53 peptide vaccination in

TABLE 13.1 **SELECTED RECENT CLINICAL TRIALS IN OC THAT USE ANTIBODIES/IMMUNOTOXINS OR CYTOKINES**

Clinical Trial Approach	Clinical Trial	No. OC Patients	Objective Responses	Reference or Trial ID
Antibodies and Immunotoxins	Phase II trial of farletuzumab (anti-folate receptor) ± carboplatin or a taxane, 2013	54	44–CR/PR, 10–PD or N/A	31
	Phase I trial of farletuzumab, 2010	25	9–SD, 15–PD, 1–N/A	32
	Phase II trial of ipilimumab (anti-CTLA-4) ongoing	N/A	N/A	NCT01611558
	Phase I trial of BMS-936559 (anti-PD-L1), 2012	17	1–PR, 3–SD, 13–PD	42
	Phase II trial of oregovomab ± paclitaxel or paclitaxel/carboplatin, ongoing	N/A	N/A	NCT01616303
	Phase III trial of abagovomab (anti-CA-125 idiotype), 2013	888	No change in recurrence free or overall survival	51
	Phase II trial of volociximab (anti-α5β1 integrin), 2011	16	1–SD, 15–PD	54
	Phase I trial of amatuximab (MORAb-009, anti-mesothelin), 2010	4	0–CR/PR	56
	Phase 0/I trial of denileukin diftitox (IL-2/diphtheria fusion toxin)	4	1–PR	67
	Phase II trial of denileukin diftitox, 2014	28	26–PD 2–SD	67
	Phase III trial of farletuzumab in platinum-resistant OC patients	1100	Failed to improve overall and PFS	33
	Phase I trial of siltuximab (anti-IL-6 receptor) in solid tumors, including OC	29	No objective responses occurred	64
	Phase I/II trial of anti-PD-L1 in solid tumors including OC, ongoing	N/A	N/A	NCT01693562
	Combination immunotherapy with anti-PD-L1, anti-CTLA-4, anti-PD-1, and anti-OX40 for solid tumors including OC, ongoing	N/A	N/A	NCT02205333, NCT02118337, NCT02261220
	Phase 1b trial of anti-PD-1 (pembrolizumab) for solid tumors including OC, ongoing	N/A	N/A	NCT02054806
	Phase I of urelumab alone or in combination with anti-PD-1 for solid tumors including OC, ongoing	N/A	N/A	NCT01471210 NCT02253992
	Phase I of anti-LAG-3 in solid tumors including OC, ongoing	N/A	N/A	NCT01968109

(continued)

TABLE 13.1 CONTINUED

Clinical Trial Approach	Clinical Trial	No. OC Patients	Objective Responses	Reference or Trial ID
Cytokines	Phase II trial of NGR-hTNF+ doxorubicin, 2012	35	8–PR, 15–SD, 7–PD	99
	Phase I trial of IL-18 + pegylated liposomal doxorubicin, 2013	15	1–PR, 6–SD, 8–PD	102
	Phase II trial of denileukin diftitox plus subcutaneous pegylated interferon-α	3	2–SD 1–PD	80
	Phase II trial of intraperitoneal IL-2 instillation in platinum resistant OC patients	24	4–CR 2–PR	95

NOTE: OC = ovarian cancer; PD = progressive disease; IR = initial response; CR = complete response; CCR = continued clinical response; PR = partial response; SD = stable disease; NED = no evidence of disease; NR = no response; N/A = not available; PFS = progression-free survival; OS = overall survival.

addition to IL-2, GM-CSF and montanide adjuvant was tested in patients with stage II or IV or recurrent OC with p53 overexpression. Vaccination augmented anti-p53 immunity (p53-specific T cells and interferon-γ) in 9 of 13 patients.[106] Vaccination using subcutaneous versus intravenous p53-pulsed DC infusion with IL-2 to boost T-cell function was assessed. Comparable immunity was demonstrated by either vaccine route.[106] Thus, subcutaneous vaccination could be a logistically easier route for further trials. Clinical data were not reported in this trial. It was also noted that IL-2 augmented blood Treg numbers. As Tregs can defeat OC-specific immunity[9], more work on this adjuvant approach is needed. In a separate Phase II trial, a long synthetic p53 peptide was assessed in recurrent OC. This peptide induced antigen-specific T cells but without clear clinical benefit, even when combined with chemotherapy.[107]

NATURALLY OCCURRING CANCER PEPTIDES

DPX-0907 (DepoVax) is a peptide adjuvant that is oil based. In a Phase I trial of patients with advanced-stage breast cancer, prostate cancer, or OC, naturally occurring HLA A2-expressed cancer peptides (from cell lines) in this vaccine were well tolerated and immunogenic when DPX-0907 as adjuvant was used.[108] The most common adverse effect was injection-site reactions. Polyfunctional T cells, including in OC patients, were generated, leading to more studies in progress (NCT01416038).

Carcinoembryonic Antigen Glypican-3

A GPC3-derived peptide vaccine in incomplete Freund's adjuvant was tested in a Phase II OC trial. Patients were vaccinated biweekly six times and then every six weeks until they progressed clinically. Two partial clinical responses were observed in chemorefractory OC patients.[109]

Carcinoembryonic Antigen and MUC1

In a Phase I clinical trial, 25 patients were primed using vaccinia virus expressing the costimulatory molecules CD80, intercellular adhesion molecule 1, and lymphocyte function-associated antigen 3, and the cancer antigens CEA and MUC-1 (PANVAC-V). Immunity was boosted with fowlpox expressing the same molecules (PANVAC-F). Treatments were well tolerated except for some significant local vaccine reactions. CEA-specific and/or MUC-1-specific immunity was elicited in 9 of 16 patients. One patient with clear cell OC had a clinical response lasting 18 months.[110]

In a follow-up trial, 26 patients received monthly PANVAC vaccinations. The major toxicity again was injection-site reactions. The trial included 14 OC patients. Their median time to progression was two months (range 1–6), and their median overall survival was 15 months, with one complete clinical response. An OC patient who was also treated in the original Phase I trial had a durable response lasting 38 months. The best clinical responses generally occurred in patients with limited tumor burden and fewer lines of prior chemotherapy.[111]

5T4 Antigen

Preclinical mouse models showed that viral delivery of tumor antigen caused regression of 5T4-expressing tumors in a CD4+ T-cell dependent manner.[112] TroVax is the tumor-associated antigen 5T4 delivered in a modified vaccinia virus Ankara vector[113] previously tested in prostate cancer,[114] renal cell cancer,[115] and melanoma[116] with only modest results. It is now in a Phase II trial for asymptomatic relapsed OC patients, with disease progression as the primary outcome (NCT01556841). A similar trial is underway in the United Kingdom.

PEPTIDE VACCINE TRIALS IN PROGRESS

There are several antigens that elicit measurable, specific T-cell responses that could mediate immune rejection of OC. FANG is a patient-autologous tumor cell vaccine that is modified to secrete GM-CSF (promoting DC uptake and migration) and shRNA-knockdown of furin (which prevents furin activation of immune-suppressive TGF-β). Early Phase I studies demonstrated safety and increases in surrogates of tumor-specific T-cell activation with FANG vaccine. A Phase II trial still underway is testing FANG in combination with bevacizumab (anti-VEGF antibody) in patients with stage III or IV OC (NCT01551745). CDX-1401 is an antibody/vaccine conjugate that targets NY-ESO-1 to DCs by covalent attachment to an anti-DEC-205 (DC marker) antibody. Indolamine-2,3-dioxygenase 1 (IDO1) promotes the formation of tryptophan metabolites that inhibit anticancer immunity. A small molecule IDO1 inhibitor is currently in a Phase II trial for patients with advanced OC (NCT02042430) after a successful Phase I pilot that demonstrated safety and tolerability. A Phase I/II trial is testing CDX-1401 plus a toll-like receptor 3 agonist and an IDO1 inhibitor in patients with OC in remission (NCT02166905). Vaccines against E39 and J65, both folate binding proteins overexpressed in OC, are being tested in a Phase Ib trial in OC patients in remission (NCT02019524). A vaccine developed against Her2 is being tested in a Phase I trial with solid tumors, including OC (NCT01376505).

ADOPTIVE CELL TRANSFERS

DCs

DC effects in cancer therapy have been extensively reviewed.[117] Tumor antigen-pulsed DC adoptive transfer improves anti-tumor immunity through anti-tumor T-cell activation. Eleven advanced-stage OC patients in a Phase I/II trial were treated with DC pulsed with Her2/neu, telomerase, and pan T helper cell stimulating (PADRE) peptides either with or without low-dose cyclophosphamide to deplete Tregs.[118] Infusions were generally well tolerated. The most common adverse events were low-grade hypersensitivity reactions. Elicited anti-tumor immunity was only modest. However, only 1 of 11 patients died within three years of vaccination. In the other 10 patients, 3 developed chemotherapy-responsive recurrences and the other 7 remained disease-free. Another trial tested autologous whole tumor lysate-pulsed DC plus bevacizumab, cyclophosphamide, and autologous tumor lysate-primed T cells in recurrent OC patients.[119] Transfusions were well tolerated. Two of six patients had partial clinical responses, and two others had stable disease. Blood Tregs were reduced and tumor-specific T cells were increased in the four patients with experienced clinical benefit. Long-term follow-up results from this trial are expected shortly.

A Phase II trial of 10 patients with minimal residual OC were given subcutaneous autologous tumor lysate-pulsed DC plus the adjuvant, keyhole limpet hemocyanin and low-dose IL-2.[120] Three of 10 patients had complete clinical remissions for 38 to 83 months. A third patient had a complete remission but then relapsed after 50 months. Distinct measures of anti-tumor immunity increased. In patients experiencing clinical benefit, immune outcomes were improved including NK cell activity, $T_H 1$-stimulating interferon-γ^+ T cells, and IL-12, and immunosuppressive TGF-β was reduced. A Phase I trial of an autologous NY-ESO-1-pulsed DC vaccine in combination with the immune-modulator sirolimus (rapamycin) (NCT01522820) is underway for epithelial cancers including OC.

DC/Tumor Cell Fusions

Reinfusion of DC fused to OC cells could present a wider array of tumor antigens versus tumor alone. The concept of DC/tumor cell fusion has been tested in various preclinical models[121,122] but not in human OC trials to date to our knowledge.

T Cells

Adoptive transfer of tumor-reactive T cells is a promising approach for future clinical trials, as advances in gene editing technology now allow for reprogramming

T-cell specificity toward tumor-associated antigens. Recent technologies have been reviewed.[123,124] Seven patients with recurrent local OC in a Phase I trial received repeated cycles of intraperitoneal infusions of autologous MUC1 peptide-stimulated cytotoxic T cells.[125] Infusions were well tolerated, multiple versus single infusions were equally effective, and clinical benefit was observed only in one patient, but she remained disease-free >12 years. Another trial from the same group gave intraperitoneal MUC-1 peptide-stimulated PBMCs to seven OC patients with recurrent local disease. Adoptively transferred cells were largely CD4$^+$CD25$^+$ and expressed interferon-γ and IL-10.[126] Patients with longer survival had durable levels of IL-10 and interferon-γ producing T cells in peripheral blood, suggesting that cytokines produced by adoptively transferred T cells contributed to long-term survival, although larger numbers and more studies are required to draw conclusions.

TILs

TILs are likely to be enriched in tumor-specific T cells and lend themselves well to ex vivo expansion for autologous reinfusion in patients with pre-existing tumor inflammation. However, there are few published trials testing TIL as therapy in OC. One group tested autologous TILs in combination with chemotherapy. OC patients receiving TIL plus chemotherapy had superior three-year survival rates compared to chemotherapy alone. Therapies utilizing transduced T cells conferring greater tumor specificity have gained in popularity after the underwhelming clinical responses observed with unmodified TIL in numerous cancer types.

Recombinant T Cell Receptors or Chimeric Antigen Receptor Transduced T Cells

Recombinant T cell receptors (TCRs) give T cells MHC-dependent specificity.

Chimeric antigen receptor (CAR) T cells are engineered to express surface tumor-antigen specific antibody components. These surface fragments are fused to intracellular activation proteins (e.g., CD3ζ, OX40, 4-1BB) and recognize antigens independent of their cognate MHC-peptide complex through the antibody recognition site. A preclinical study found that NKG2D-specific CAR T cells protected against different OC tumors even though only 7% expressed NKG2D.[127] CAR T cell efficacy in solid tumors is limited compared to impressive efficacy in leukemia/lymphoma patients due to inefficient tumor homing. Advances in understanding which T cell-attracting chemokines are enriched in OC could improve the efficacy of adoptive T-cell therapy in OC.[128] Ex vivo stimulation of CD3/CD28 could upregulate chemokine receptors that promote migration of tumor-specific T cells to the OC tumor mass.[128]

CAR T cells with folate receptor-α specificity and downstream CD3ζ plus CD137 co-stimulating domains protected from established OC in a mouse model. A Phase I trial of OC patients with recurrent disease using folate receptor-α–specific CAR (CD3ζ-CD137) T cells is planned.[129] We recently reported that follicle stimulating hormone receptor is a useful target for CAR T cell treatment of OC in a preclinical model.[130]

An ongoing Phase II trial uses lentivirus to transduce autologous T cells with an NY-ESO-1 specific TCR. NY-ESO-1 specific T cells will be reinfused into patients with solid tumors, including OC, after cyclophosphamide preconditioning and adjunct therapy with NY-ESO-1-pulsed DCs and IL-2 (NCT01697527). CAR T cells specific for the VEGF receptor 1 are being tested in a Phase I/II trial for patients with metastatic cancer, including OC (NCT01218867). A Phase I/II trial is now testing autologous NY-ESO-1-specific TCR-transgenic T cells in patients with treatment-refractory OC. (NCT01567891). CAR T cells specific for mesothelin, which is overexpressed in pancreatic and OC, are being used in a Phase I study of metastatic mesothelin-positive cancers (NCT02159716).

ONCOLYTIC VIRUSES

Modified viruses that preferentially kill cancer cells or confer susceptibility to other drugs are another promising mode of immune therapy for OC. Myxoma virus infects human cancer cells while sparing normal tissue and is oncolytic in rodent models, reviewed elsewhere,[131] and has demonstrated oncolytic activity against ascites-derived human OC cells ex vivo.[132] However, there are no published OC trials utilizing myxoma virus. In vitro, reovirus is oncolytic against human OC cells.[133] Neutralizing antibodies in malignant ascites can inactivate reovirus oncolytic activity, prompting approaches to overcome this limitation by loading reovirus onto immature DCs or lymphokine-activated killer cells.[134] A Phase I trial of reovirus in platinum-resistant OC patients is ongoing (NCT00602277). A Phase I trial demonstrated the safety of an oncolytic measles virus that expresses the sodium/iodide symporter after intraperitoneal injection where a 26-month overall survival in this small cohort was observed, with no dose-limiting toxicities.[135] An ongoing Phase I/II study is using intraperitoneal injected mesenchymal stem cells infected with oncolytic measles virus encoding thyroidal sodium/iodide symporter in patients with recurrent OC (NCT02068794). An ongoing study with oncolytic herpes simplex virus in patients with advanced OC uses a herpes virus vector to force tumor expression of thymidine kinase followed by treatment with valacyclovir (a thymidine kinase inhibitor) to kill transduced tumor cells (NCT01997190).

A summary of recent selected clinical trials using vaccines, adoptive cell transfers, and oncolytic viruses is presented in Table 13.2.

Clinical Trial Approach	Clinical Trial	No. OC Patients	Objective Responses	Reference or Trial ID
Vaccines	Phase II trial of recombinant vaccinia and fowlpox vaccines expressing NY-ESO-1, 2012	22	21 mos PFS, 4 year OS	104
	Phase II trial of subcutaneous or intravenous p53 peptide vaccination, 2012	13	4.2 mos PFS, 40.8 mos OS	106
	Phase II trial of p53-synthetic long peptide vaccine, 2012	20	No increase in OS	107
	Phase II trial of Trovax (5T4 antigen in vacinnia virus vector) for asymptomatic relapsed OC, ongoing	N/A	N/A	NCT01556841
	Phase II FANG vaccine for stage III or IV OC patients, ongoing	N/A	N/A	NCT01551745
	Phase I/II trial of CDX-1401 (DC-targeted NY-ESO-1) with TLR3 agonist and IDO-1 inhibitor for OC patients in remission, ongoing	N/A	N/A	NCT02166905
	Phase Ib trial of E39/J65 (folate binding proteins) vaccine for OC patients in remission, ongoing	N/A	N/A	NCT02019524
	Phase I trial of Her2 vaccine for solid tumors including OC, ongoing	N/A	N/A	NCT01376505
Adoptive Cell Transfers	Phase II trial of p53-pulsed dendritic cells vaccine, 2012	6	8.7 mos PFS, 29.6 mos OS	106
	Phase I/II vaccination trial of Her2/neu, telomerase, and PADRE peptide-pulsed DCs ± cyclophosphamide, 2012	11	90% 3 year OS, NED in 6 pts at 3 yrs	118
	Phase I trial of autologous tumor lysate-pulsed dendritic cells + bevacizumab, cyclophosphamide, and autologous tumor lysate-primed T cells, 2013	6	2–PR, 2–SD, 2–PD	119
	Pilot study of MUC1-primed cytotoxic T lymphocyte transfer, 2012	7	1–CR, 6–PD	125,126
	Phase I trial of anti-mesothelin CAR T cells, ongoing	N/A	N/A	NCT02159716
	Phase I trial of anti-mesothelin CAR T cells + chemotherapy, ongoing	N/A	N/A	NCT01583686
	Phase I trial of anti-VEGFR2 CD8$^+$ CAR T cells + chemotherapy, ongoing	N/A	N/A	NCT01218867

TABLE 13.2 **CONTINUED**

Clinical Trial Approach	Clinical Trial	No. OC Patients	Objective Responses	Reference or Trial ID
Oncolytic Viruses	Phase I trial of CA-125- or Na/I symporter-expressing measles virus, ongoing	N/A	N/A	NCT00408590
	Phase I/II trial of Na/I symporter-expressing measles virus infected mesenchymal stem cells, ongoing	N/A	N/A	NCT02068794
	Phase II trial of thymidine kinase-inactivated vaccinia virus, ongoing	N/A	N/A	NCT02017678
	Phase I/II trial of oncolytic adenovirus, ongoing	N/A	N/A	NCT02028117
	Phase II trial of oncolytic reovirus, ongoing	N/A	N/A	NCT02028117
	Phase I trial of oncolytic reovirus, ongoing	N/A	N/A	NCT00602277
	Phase I trial of thymidine kinase transducing herpesvirus vector plus valacyclovir	N/A	N/A	NCT01997190

NOTE: OC = ovarian cancer; PD = progressive disease; IR = initial response; CR = complete response; CCR = continued clinical response; PR = partial response; SD = stable disease; NED = no evidence of disease; NR = no response; N/A = not available; PFS = progression-free survival; OS = overall survival; pts = patients.

CONCLUSION

Advances in the identification of numerous cancer immunotherapeutic targets and in the translation of novel agents has produced great excitement in the potential of immunotherapy to become the next pillar of treatment in the oncologist's arsenal. In the case of OC, there are currently no FDA-approved immunotherapies, but ongoing preclinical studies and clinical trials continue to generate promising leads. Within the next decade, it is reasonable to expect that important advances in OC immunotherapy will be made, leading to important Phase II and III trials and possible FDA approval of immunotherapy for OC. Promising leads from CAR T cell trials and combinations of immune checkpoint inhibitors could lead to important advances. With the recognition that tumor mutational burden is generally directly proportional to immunogenicity, and that OC has a low mutational burden relative to other carcinomas, strategies to boost OC immunogenicity (e.g., epigenetic modifiers, targeting viruses, interferons) could become

important adjuncts and deserve additional study. Because OC also has relatively few conserved tumor antigens, strategies to personalize immunotherapy (e.g., whole tumor vaccines, peptides from individual tumor proteomic analyses) deserve more attention. In this regard, the concept that certain OC subtypes are more immunogenic (such as clear cell histologies) deserves additional attention. Checkpoint inhibitors successful in other carcinomas are showing only modest effects thus far in OC. Perhaps other checkpoint inhibitors will be more effective, or OC-specific adjuncts will be useful and needed. For example, we have shown how Treg depletion improves anti-PD-L1 effects in an OC preclinical model. Other OC-specific immune dysfunctional attributes deserve additional attention to determine if there are clinically exploitable leads, as we expect. For example, myeloid cells appear particularly dysfunctional in OC.[8,136,137] We recently showed that tumor-intrinsic PD-L1 induces novel immunopathogenesis in OC[138] and in collaboration with the Conejo-Garcia group that estrogens have off-tumor detrimental effects on OC myeloid cells,[139] both concepts of which are clinically actionable. Because of a lack of curative salvage treatment options for chemorefractory OC, every clinician should counsel patients about referral to clinical trials, including OC immunotherapy trials, and patients should ask their treating physicians about clinical trial options.

REFERENCES

1. Matulonis UA, Sood AK, Fallowfield L, Howitt BE, Sehouli J, Karlan BY. Ovarian cancer. *Nat Rev Dis Primers.* 2016;2:16061.
2. Ioannides CG, Fisk B, Pollack MS, Frazier ML, Taylor Wharton J, Freedman RS. Cytotoxic T-cell clones isolated from ovarian tumour infiltrating lymphocytes recognize common determinants on non-ovarian tumour clones. *Scand J Immunol.* 1993;37(4):413–24.
3. Peoples GE, Goedegebuure PS, Smith R, Linehan DC, Yoshino I, Eberlein TJ. Breast and ovarian cancer-specific cytotoxic T lymphocytes recognize the same HER2/neu-derived peptide. *Proc Natl Acad Sci U S A.* 1995;92(2):432–36.
4. Wagner U, Schlebusch H, Kohler S, Schmolling J, Grunn U, Krebs D. Immunological responses to the tumor-associated antigen CA125 in patients with advanced ovarian cancer induced by the murine monoclonal anti-idiotype vaccine ACA125. *Hybridoma.* 1997;16(1):33–40.
5. Disis ML, Gooley TA, Rinn K, et al. Generation of T-cell immunity to the HER-2/neu protein after active immunization with HER-2/neu peptide-based vaccines. *J Clin Oncol.* 2002;20(11):2624–32.
6. Knutson KL, Schiffman K, Cheever MA, Disis ML. Immunization of cancer patients with a HER-2/neu, HLA-A2 peptide, p369-377, results in short-lived peptide-specific immunity. *Clin Cancer Res.* 2002;8(5):1014–18.
7. Qian HN, Liu GZ, Cao SJ, Feng J, Ye X. The experimental study of ovarian carcinoma vaccine modified by human B7-1 and IFN-gamma genes. *Int J Gynecol Cancer.* 2002;12(1):80–85.
8. Curiel TJ, Wei S, Dong H, et al. Blockade of B7-H1 improves myeloid dendritic cell-mediated antitumor immunity. *Nature Med.* 2003;9(5):562–67.
9. Curiel TJ, Coukos G, Zou L, et al. Specific recruitment of regulatory T cells in ovarian carcinoma fosters immune privilege and predicts reduced survival. *Nature Med.* 2004;10(9):942–49.
10. Vlad AM, Kettel JC, Alajez NM, Carlos CA, Finn OJ. MUC1 immunobiology: from discovery to clinical applications. *Adv Immunol.* 2004;82:249–93.
11. Diefenbach CS, Gnjatic S, Sabbatini P, et al. Safety and immunogenicity study of NY-ESO-1b peptide and montanide ISA-51 vaccination of patients with epithelial ovarian cancer in high-risk first remission. *Clin Cancer Res.* 2008;14(9):2740–48.
12. Coliva A, Zacchetti A, Luison E, et al. 90Y Labeling of monoclonal antibody MOv18 and preclinical validation for radioimmunotherapy of human ovarian carcinomas. *Cancer Immunol Immunother.* 2005;54(12):1200–13.
13. Mantovani LT, Miotti S, Menard S, et al. Folate binding protein distribution in normal tissues and biological fluids from ovarian carcinoma patients as detected by the monoclonal antibodies MOv18 and MOv19. *Eur J Cancer.* 1994;30A(3):363–69.
14. Thor A, Gorstein F, Ohuchi N, Szpak CA, Johnston WW, Schlom J. Tumor-associated glycoprotein (TAG-72) in ovarian carcinomas defined by monoclonal antibody B72.3. *J Natl Cancer Inst.* 1986;76(6):995–1006.
15. Chang K, Pastan I. Molecular cloning of mesothelin, a differentiation antigen present on mesothelium, mesotheliomas, and ovarian cancers. *Proc Natl Acad Sci U S A.* 1996;93(1):136–40.
16. Cheng WF, Huang CY, Chang MC, et al. High mesothelin correlates with chemoresistance and poor survival in epithelial ovarian carcinoma. *Br J Cancer.* 2009;100(7):1144–53.
17. Inoue M, Ogawa H, Nakanishi K, Tanizawa O, Karino K, Endo J. Clinical value of sialyl Tn antigen in patients with gynecologic tumors. *Obstet Gynecol.* 1990;75(6):1032–36.
18. Sandmaier BM, Oparin DV, Holmberg LA, Reddish MA, MacLean GD, Longenecker BM. Evidence of a cellular immune response against sialyl-Tn in breast and ovarian cancer patients after high-dose chemotherapy, stem cell rescue, and immunization with Theratope STn-KLH cancer vaccine. *J Immunother.* 1999;22(1):54–66.
19. Campbell IG, Freemont PS, Foulkes W, Trowsdale J. An ovarian tumor marker with homology to vaccinia virus contains an IgV-like region and multiple transmembrane domains. *Cancer Res.* 1992;52(19):5416–20.
20. Zhang L, Conejo-Garcia JR, Katsaros D, et al. Intratumoral T cells, recurrence, and survival in epithelial ovarian cancer. *N Engl J Med.* 2003;348(3):203–13.
21. Epenetos AA, Munro AJ, Stewart S, et al. Antibody-guided irradiation of advanced ovarian cancer with intraperitoneally administered radiolabeled monoclonal antibodies. *J Clin Oncol.* 1987;5(12):1890–99.
22. Beyer M, Kochanek M, Darabi K, et al. Reduced frequencies and suppressive function of CD4+CD25hi regulatory T cells in patients with chronic lymphocytic leukemia after therapy with fludarabine. *Blood.* 2005;106(6):2018–25.
23. Motoyoshi Y, Kaminoda K, Saitoh O, et al. Different mechanisms for anti-tumor effects of low- and high-dose cyclophosphamide. *Oncol Rep.* 2006;16(1):141–46.
24. Vincent J, Mignot G, Chalmin F, et al. 5-Fluorouracil selectively kills tumor-associated myeloid-derived suppressor cells resulting in enhanced T

cell-dependent antitumor immunity. *Cancer Res.* 2010;70(8):3052–61.

25. Apetoh L, Mignot G, Panaretakis T, Kroemer G, Zitvogel L. Immunogenicity of anthracyclines: moving towards more personalized medicine. *Trends Mol Med.* 2008;14(4):141–51.

26. Riva P, Marangolo M, Lazzari S, et al. Locoregional immunotherapy of human ovarian cancer: preliminary results. *Int J Rad Appl Instrum B.* 1989;16(6):659–66.

27. Stewart JS, Hird V, Snook D, et al. Intraperitoneal yttrium-90-labeled monoclonal antibody in ovarian cancer. *J Clin Oncol.* 1990;8(12):1941–50.

28. Hird V, Maraveyas A, Snook D, et al. Adjuvant therapy of ovarian cancer with radioactive monoclonal antibody. *Br J Cancer.* 1993;68(2):403–406.

29. Epenetos AA, Hird V, Lambert H, Mason P, Coulter C. Long term survival of patients with advanced ovarian cancer treated with intraperitoneal radioimmunotherapy. *Int J Gynecol Cancer.* 2000;10(S1):44–46.

30. Oei AL, Verheijen RH, Seiden MV, et al. Decreased intraperitoneal disease recurrence in epithelial ovarian cancer patients receiving intraperitoneal consolidation treatment with yttrium-90-labeled murine HMFG1 without improvement in overall survival. *Int J Cancer.* 2007;120(12):2710–14.

31. Armstrong DK, White AJ, Weil SC, Phillips M, Coleman RL. Farletuzumab (a monoclonal antibody against folate receptor alpha) in relapsed platinum-sensitive ovarian cancer. *Gynecol Oncol.* 2013;129(3):452–58.

32. Konner JA, Bell-McGuinn KM, Sabbatini P, et al. Farletuzumab, a humanized monoclonal antibody against folate receptor alpha, in epithelial ovarian cancer: a phase I study. *Clin Cancer Res.* 2010;16(21):5288–95.

33. Vergote I, Armstrong D, Scambia G, et al. A randomized, double-blind, placebo-controlled, phase III study to assess efficacy and safety of weekly farletuzumab in combination with carboplatin and taxane in patients with ovarian cancer in first platinum-sensitive relapse. *J Clin Oncol.* 2016;34(19):2271–78.

34. Sehouli J, Pietzner K, Wimberger P, et al. Catumaxomab with and without prednisolone premedication for the treatment of malignant ascites due to epithelial cancer: results of the randomised phase IIIb CASIMAS study. *Med Oncol.* 2014;31(8):76.

35. Ott MG, Marme F, Moldenhauer G, et al. Humoral response to catumaxomab correlates with clinical outcome: results of the pivotal phase II/III study in patients with malignant ascites. *Int J Cancer.* 2012;130(9):2195–203.

36. Pardoll DM. The blockade of immune checkpoints in cancer immunotherapy. *Nat Rev Cancer.* 2012;12(4):252–64.

37. Kleffel S, Posch C, Barthel SR, et al. Melanoma Cell-Intrinsic PD-1 Receptor functions promote tumor growth. *Cell.* 2015;162(6):1242–56.

38. Clark CA GH, Pandeswara S, Sareddy GR, Yuan B, Hurez V, Li R, Vadlamudi R, Curiel TJ. Tumor-intrinsic B7-H1 in melanoma and ovarian cancer regulates mTOR, autophagy and tumor growth. *J Immunol.* 2016;196 (1 Suppl.): Abstract 144.9.

39. Hodi FS, O'Day SJ, McDermott DF, et al. Improved survival with ipilimumab in patients with metastatic melanoma. *N Engl J Med.* 2010;363(8):711–23.

40. Brahmer JR, Tykodi SS, Chow LQ, et al. Safety and activity of anti-PD-L1 antibody in patients with advanced cancer. *N Engl J Med.* 2012;366(26):2455–65.

41. Hamanishi J, Mandai M, Ikeda T, et al. Safety and antitumor activity of anti-PD-1 antibody, nivolumab, in patients with platinum-resistant ovarian cancer. *J Clin Oncol.* 2015;33(34):4015–22.

42. ML D, MR P, Pant S ea. Avelumab (MSB0010718C), an anti-PD-L1 antibody, in patients with previously treated, recurrent or refractory ovarian cancer: a phase Ib, open-label expansion trial. Paper presented at the American Society of Clinical Oncology meeting, Chicago, 2015.

43. Guo Z, Cheng D, Xia Z, et al. Combined TIM-3 blockade and CD137 activation affords the long-term protection in a murine model of ovarian cancer. *J Transl Med.* 2013;11:215.

44. Wei H, Zhao L, Li W, et al. Combinatorial PD-1 blockade and CD137 activation has therapeutic efficacy in murine cancer models and synergizes with cisplatin. *PLoS One.* 2013;8(12):e84927.

45. Vinay DS, Kwon BS. Immunotherapy of cancer with 4-1BB. *Mol Cancer Ther.* 2012;11(5):1062–70.

46. Berek JS. Immunotherapy of ovarian cancer with antibodies: a focus on oregovomab. *Expert Opin Biol Ther.* 2004;4(7):1159–65.

47. Ehlen TG, Hoskins PJ, Miller D, et al. A pilot phase 2 study of oregovomab murine monoclonal antibody to CA125 as an immunotherapeutic agent for recurrent ovarian cancer. *Int J Gynecol Cancer.* 2005;15(6):1023–34.

48. Berek J, Taylor P, McGuire W, Smith LM, Schultes B, Nicodemus CF. Oregovomab maintenance monoimmunotherapy does not improve outcomes in advanced ovarian cancer. *J Clin Oncol.* 2009;27(3):418–25.

49. Pfisterer J, Harter P, Simonelli C, et al. Abagovomab for ovarian cancer. *Expert Opin Biol Ther.* 2011;11(3):395–403.

50. Sabbatini P, Dupont J, Aghajanian C, et al. Phase I study of abagovomab in patients with epithelial ovarian, fallopian tube, or primary peritoneal cancer. *Clin Cancer Res.* 2006;12(18):5503–10.

51. Sabbatini P, Harter P, Scambia G, et al. Abagovomab as maintenance therapy in patients with epithelial ovarian cancer: a phase III trial of the AGO OVAR, COGI, GINECO, and GEICO—the MIMOSA study. *J Clin Oncol.* 2013;31(12):1554–61.

52. Buzzonetti A, Fossati M, Catzola V, Scambia G, Fattorossi A, Battaglia A. Immunological response induced by abagovomab as a maintenance therapy in patients with epithelial ovarian

cancer: relationship with survival-a substudy of the MIMOSA trial. *Cancer Immunol Immunother.* 2014;63(10):1037–45.

53. Almokadem S, Belani CP. Volociximab in cancer. *Expert Opin Biol Ther.* 2012;12(2):251–57.

54. Bell-McGuinn KM, Matthews CM, Ho SN, et al. A phase II, single-arm study of the anti-alpha5beta1 integrin antibody volociximab as monotherapy in patients with platinum-resistant advanced epithelial ovarian or primary peritoneal cancer. *Gynecol Oncol.* 2011;121(2):273–79.

55. Hassan R, Bera T, Pastan I. Mesothelin: a new target for immunotherapy. *Clin Cancer Res.* 2004;10(12 Pt 1):3937–42.

56. Hassan R, Cohen SJ, Phillips M, et al. Phase I clinical trial of the chimeric anti-mesothelin monoclonal antibody MORAb-009 in patients with mesothelin-expressing cancers. *Clin Cancer Res.* 2010;16(24):6132–38.

57. Taniguchi K, Karin M. IL-6 and related cytokines as the critical lynchpins between inflammation and cancer. *Semin Immunol.* 2014;26(1):54–74.

58. Coward J, Kulbe H, Chakravarty P, et al. Interleukin-6 as a therapeutic target in human ovarian cancer. *Clin Cancer Res.* 2011;17(18):6083–96.

59. Kryczek I, Zou L, Rodriguez P, et al. B7-H4 expression identifies a novel suppressive macrophage population in human ovarian carcinoma. *J Exp Med.* 2006;203(4):871–81.

60. Berti A, Boccalatte F, Sabbadini MG, Dagna L. Assessment of tocilizumab in the treatment of cancer cachexia. *J Clin Oncol.* 2013;31(23):2970.

61. Maude SL, Barrett D, Teachey DT, Grupp SA. Managing cytokine release syndrome associated with novel T cell-engaging therapies. *Cancer J.* 2014;20(2):119–22.

62. Dijkgraaf EM, Santegoets SJ, Reyners AK, et al. A phase I trial combining carboplatin/doxorubicin with tocilizumab, an anti-IL-6R monoclonal antibody, and interferon-alpha2b in patients with recurrent epithelial ovarian cancer. *Ann Oncol.* 2015;26(10):2141–49.

63. Middleton K, Jones J, Lwin Z, Coward JI. Interleukin-6: an angiogenic target in solid tumours. *Crit Rev Oncol Hematol.* 2014;89(1):129–39.

64. Angevin E, Tabernero J, Elez E, et al. A phase I/II, multiple-dose, dose-escalation study of siltuximab, an anti-interleukin-6 monoclonal antibody, in patients with advanced solid tumors. *Clin Cancer Res.* 2014;20(8):2192–204.

65. Shvartsur A, Bonavida B. Trop2 and its overexpression in cancers: regulation and clinical/therapeutic implications. *Genes Cancer.* 2015;6(3-4):84–105.

66. Scott AM, Wolchok JD, Old LJ. Antibody therapy of cancer. *Nat Rev Cancer.* 2012;12(4):278–87.

67. Thibodeaux SR, Barnett B, Wall S, et al. Denileukin diftitox depletes regulatory T cells without clinical benefit in advanced stage epithelial ovarian carcinoma. Paper presented at the American Association of Immunologists meeting, 2014; abstract 1944021.

68. Murthy K, Sareddy G, Hurez V, et al. B7-H1 blockade improves efficacy of regulatory T cell depletion as cancer immunotherapy by reducing Treg regeneration, possibly through tumor B7-H1 effects. Paper presented at the American Association of Immunologists meeting, 2014; abstract number 1944036.

69. Jin D, Fan J, Wang L, et al. CD73 on tumor cells impairs antitumor T-cell responses: a novel mechanism of tumor-induced immune suppression. *Cancer Res.* 2010;70(6):2245–55.

70. Hurez V, Daniel BJ, Sun L, et al. Mitigating age-related immune dysfunction heightens the efficacy of tumor immunotherapy in aged mice. *Cancer Res.* 2012;72(8):2089–99.

71. Lin PY, Sun L, Thibodeaux SR, et al. B7-H1-dependent sex-related differences in tumor immunity and immunotherapy responses. *J Immunol.* 2010;185(5):2747–53.

72. Pestka S, Krause CD, Walter MR. Interferons, interferon-like cytokines, and their receptors. *Immunol Rev.* 2004;202:8–32.

73. Kirkwood J. Cancer immunotherapy: the interferon-alpha experience. *Semin Oncol.* 2002;29(3 Suppl 7):18–26.

74. Berek JS, Hacker NF, Lichtenstein A, et al. Intraperitoneal recombinant alpha-interferon for "salvage" immunotherapy in stage III epithelial ovarian cancer: a Gynecologic Oncology Group Study. *Cancer Res.* 1985;45(9):4447–53.

75. Bezwoda WR, Seymour L, Dansey R. Intraperitoneal recombinant interferon-alpha 2b for recurrent malignant ascites due to ovarian cancer. *Cancer.* 1989;64(5):1029–33.

76. Nardi M, Cognetti F, Pollera CF, et al. Intraperitoneal recombinant alpha-2-interferon alternating with cisplatin as salvage therapy for minimal residual-disease ovarian cancer: a phase II study. *J Clin Oncol.* 1990;8(6):1036–41.

77. Stuart GC, Nation JG, Snider DD, Thunberg P. Intraperitoneal interferon in the management of malignant ascites. *Cancer.* 1993;71(6):2027–30.

78. Tedjarati S, Baker CH, Apte S, et al. Synergistic therapy of human ovarian carcinoma implanted orthotopically in nude mice by optimal biological dose of pegylated interferon alpha combined with paclitaxel. *Clin Cancer Res.* 2002;8(7):2413–22.

79. Metcalf KS, Selby PJ, Trejdosiewicz LK, Southgate J. Culture of ascitic ovarian cancer cells as a clinically relevant ex vivo model for the assessment of biological therapies. *Eur J Gynaecol Oncol.* 1998;19(2):113–19.

80. Thibodeaux SR, Hurez V, Wall S, et al. Interferon-α augments the clinical efficacy of regulatory T cell depletion in ovarian cancer through direct and indirect T cell effects. Paper presented at the American Association of Immunologists annual meeting, Pittsburgh, PA, 2014; abstract number 1943855.

81. Moserle L, Indraccolo S, Ghisi M, et al. The side population of ovarian cancer cells is a primary

target of IFN-alpha antitumor effects. *Cancer Res.* 2008;68(14):5658–68.

82. Sterman DH, Recio A, Haas AR, et al. A phase I trial of repeated intrapleural adenoviral-mediated interferon-beta gene transfer for mesothelioma and metastatic pleural effusions. *Mol Ther.* 2010;18(4):852–60.

83. Chen JT, Hasumi K, Masubuchi K. Interferon-alpha, interferon-gamma and sizofiran in the adjuvant therapy in ovarian cancer—a preliminary trial. *Biotherapy.* 1992;5(4):275–80.

84. Pujade-Lauraine E, Guastalla JP, Colombo N, et al. Intraperitoneal recombinant interferon gamma in ovarian cancer patients with residual disease at second-look laparotomy. *J Clin Oncol.* 1996;14(2):343–50.

85. Windbichler GH, Hausmaninger H, Stummvoll W, et al. Interferon-gamma in the first-line therapy of ovarian cancer: a randomized phase III trial. *Br J Cancer.* 2000;82(6):1138–44.

86. Freedman RS, Kudelka AP, Kavanagh JJ, et al. Clinical and biological effects of intraperitoneal injections of recombinant interferon-gamma and recombinant interleukin 2 with or without tumor-infiltrating lymphocytes in patients with ovarian or peritoneal carcinoma. *Clin Cancer Res.* 2000;6(6):2268–78.

87. Apte SM, Vadhan-Raj S, Cohen L, et al. Cytokines, GM-CSF and IFNgamma administered by priming and post-chemotherapy cycling in recurrent ovarian cancer patients receiving carboplatin. *J Transl Med.* 2006;4:16.

88. Burke F, East N, Upton C, Patel K, Balkwill FR. Interferon gamma induces cell cycle arrest and apoptosis in a model of ovarian cancer: enhancement of effect by batimastat. *Eur J Cancer.* 1997;33(7):1114–21.

89. Marth C, Muller-Holzner E, Greiter E, et al. Gamma-interferon reduces expression of the protooncogene c-erbB-2 in human ovarian carcinoma cells. *Cancer Res.* 1990;50(21):7037–41.

90. Madiyalakan R, Yang R, Schultes BC, Baum RP, Noujaim AA. OVAREX MAb-B43.13:IFN-gamma could improve the ovarian tumor cell sensitivity to CA125-specific allogenic cytotoxic T cells. *Hybridoma.* 1997;16(1):41–45.

91. Rosenberg SA. IL-2: the first effective immunotherapy for human cancer. *J Immunol.* 2014;192(12):5451–58.

92. Antony GK, Dudek AZ. Interleukin 2 in cancer therapy. *Curr Med Chem.* 17(29):3297–302.

93. Wei S, Kryczek I, Edwards RP, et al. Interleukin-2 administration alters the CD4+FOXP3+ T-cell pool and tumor trafficking in patients with ovarian carcinoma. *Cancer Res.* 2007;67(15):7487–94.

94. Recchia F, Di Orio F, Candeloro G, Guerriero G, Piazze J, Rea S. Maintenance immunotherapy in recurrent ovarian cancer: long term follow-up of a phase II study. *Gynecol Oncol.* 116(2):202–207.

95. Vlad AM, Budiu RA, Lenzner DE, et al. A phase II trial of intraperitoneal interleukin-2 in patients with platinum-resistant or platinum-refractory ovarian cancer. *Cancer Immunol Immunother.* 2010;59(2):293–301.

96. Perillo A, Pierelli L, Battaglia A, et al. Administration of low-dose interleukin-2 plus G-CSF/EPO early after autologous PBSC transplantation: effects on immune recovery and NK activity in a prospective study in women with breast and ovarian cancer. *Bone Marrow Transplant.* 2002;30(9):571–78.

97. Boyman O, Surh CD, Sprent J. Potential use of IL-2/anti-IL-2 antibody immune complexes for the treatment of cancer and autoimmune disease. *Exp Opinion Biol Therapy.* 2006;6(12):1323–31.

98. Drerup JM PA, Chen W, Clark CA, Curiel TJ. Manipulation of IL-2 signals by IL-2/antibody complex and CD25 blockade improves tumor immunity, reprograms regulatory T cells, and augments CD8+ central memory in an ovarian cancer model. *J Immunol.* 2016;196(1 Suppl.):Abstract 212.22.

99. Lorusso D, Scambia G, Amadio G, et al. Phase II study of NGR-hTNF in combination with doxorubicin in relapsed ovarian cancer patients. *Br J Cancer.* 2012;107(1):37–42.

100. Charles KA, Kulbe H, Soper R, et al. The tumor-promoting actions of TNF-alpha involve TNFR1 and IL-17 in ovarian cancer in mice and humans. *J Clin Invest.* 2009;119(10):3011–23.

101. Rei M, Goncalves-Sousa N, Lanca T, et al. Murine CD27(-) Vgamma6(+) gammadelta T cells producing IL-17A promote ovarian cancer growth via mobilization of protumor small peritoneal macrophages. *Proc Natl Acad Sci U S A.* 2014;111(34):E3562–70.

102. Simpkins F, Flores A, Chu C, et al. Chemoimmunotherapy using pegylated liposomal Doxorubicin and interleukin-18 in recurrent ovarian cancer: a phase I dose-escalation study. *Cancer Immunol Res.* 2013;1(3):168–78.

103. Mirshahidi S, Kramer VG, Whitney JB, et al. Overlapping synthetic peptides encoding TPD52 as breast cancer vaccine in mice: prolonged survival. *Vaccine.* 2009;27(12):1825–33.

104. Odunsi K, Matsuzaki J, Karbach J, et al. Efficacy of vaccination with recombinant vaccinia and fowlpox vectors expressing NY-ESO-1 antigen in ovarian cancer and melanoma patients. *Proc Natl Acad Sci U S A.* 2012;109(15):5797–802.

105. Odunsi K, Matsuzaki J, James SR, et al. Epigenetic potentiation of NY-ESO-1 vaccine therapy in human ovarian cancer. *Cancer Immunol Res.* 2014;2(1):37–49.

106. Rahma OE, Ashtar E, Czystowska M, et al. A gynecologic oncology group phase II trial of two p53 peptide vaccine approaches: subcutaneous injection and intravenous pulsed dendritic cells in high recurrence risk ovarian cancer patients. *Cancer Immunol Immunother.* 2012;61(3):373–84.

107. Leffers N, Vermeij R, Hoogeboom BN, et al. Long-term clinical and immunological effects of p53-SLP(R) vaccine in patients with ovarian cancer. *Int J Cancer.* 2012;130(1):105–12.

108. Karkada M, Berinstein NL, Mansour M. Therapeutic vaccines and cancer: focus on DPX-0907. *Biologics*. 2014;8:27–38.

109. Suzuki S, Shibata K, Kikkawa F, Nakatsura T. Significant clinical response of progressive recurrent ovarian clear cell carcinoma to glypican-3-derived peptide vaccine therapy: two case reports. *Hum Vaccin Immunother*. 2014;10(2):338–43.

110. Gulley JL, Arlen PM, Tsang KY, et al. Pilot study of vaccination with recombinant CEA-MUC-1-TRICOM poxviral-based vaccines in patients with metastatic carcinoma. *Clin Cancer Res*. 2008;14(10):3060–69.

111. Mohebtash M, Tsang KY, Madan RA, et al. A pilot study of MUC-1/CEA/TRICOM poxviral-based vaccine in patients with metastatic breast and ovarian cancer. *Clin Cancer Res*. 2011;17(22):7164–73.

112. Harrop R, Ryan MG, Myers KA, Redchenko I, Kingsman SM, Carroll MW. Active treatment of murine tumors with a highly attenuated vaccinia virus expressing the tumor associated antigen 5T4 (TroVax) is CD4+ T cell dependent and antibody mediated. *Cancer Immunol, Immunother*. 2006;55(9):1081–90.

113. Rowe J, Cen P. TroVax in colorectal cancer. *Hum Vaccin Immunother*. 2014;10(11):3196–200.

114. Harrop R, Chu F, Gabrail N, Srinivas S, Blount D, Ferrari A. Vaccination of castration-resistant prostate cancer patients with TroVax (MVA-5T4) in combination with docetaxel: a randomized phase II trial. *Cancer Immunol Immunother*. 2013;62(9):1511–20.

115. Hawkins RE, Macdermott C, Shablak A, et al. Vaccination of patients with metastatic renal cancer with modified vaccinia Ankara encoding the tumor antigen 5T4 (TroVax) given alongside interferon-alpha. *J Immunother*. 2009;32(4):424–29.

116. Kaufman HL, Taback B, Sherman W, et al. Phase II trial of Modified Vaccinia Ankara (MVA) virus expressing 5T4 and high dose Interleukin-2 (IL-2) in patients with metastatic renal cell carcinoma. *J Transl Med*. 2009;7:2.

117. Palucka K, Banchereau J. Dendritic-cell-based therapeutic cancer vaccines. *Immunity*. 2013;39(1):38–48.

118. Chu CS, Boyer J, Schullery DS, et al. Phase I/II randomized trial of dendritic cell vaccination with or without cyclophosphamide for consolidation therapy of advanced ovarian cancer in first or second remission. *Cancer Immunol Immunother*. 2012;61(5):629–41.

119. Kandalaft LE, Powell DJ, Jr., Chiang CL, et al. Autologous lysate-pulsed dendritic cell vaccination followed by adoptive transfer of vaccine-primed ex vivo co-stimulated T cells in recurrent ovarian cancer. *Oncoimmunology*. 2013;2(1):e22664.

120. Baek S, Kim YM, Kim SB, et al. Therapeutic DC vaccination with IL-2 as a consolidation therapy for ovarian cancer patients: a phase I/II trial. *Cell Mol Immunol*. 2015;12(1):87–95.

121. Gong J, Nikrui N, Chen D, et al. Fusions of human ovarian carcinoma cells with autologous or allogeneic dendritic cells induce antitumor immunity. *J Immunol*. 2000;165(3):1705–11.

122. Koido S, Nikrui N, Ohana M, et al. Assessment of fusion cells from patient-derived ovarian carcinoma cells and dendritic cells as a vaccine for clinical use. *Gynecol Oncol*. 2005;99(2):462–71.

123. Kalos M, June CH. Adoptive T cell transfer for cancer immunotherapy in the era of synthetic biology. *Immunity*. 2013;39(1):49–60.

124. June CH, Riddell SR, Schumacher TN. Adoptive cellular therapy: a race to the finish line. *Sci Transl Med*. 2015;7(280):280ps287.

125. Wright SE, Rewers-Felkins KA, Quinlin IS, et al. Cytotoxic T-lymphocyte immunotherapy for ovarian cancer: a pilot study. *J Immunother*. 2012;35(2):196–204.

126. Dobrzanski MJ, Rewers-Felkins KA, Samad KA, et al. Immunotherapy with IL-10- and IFN-gamma-producing CD4 effector cells modulate "natural" and "inducible" CD4 TReg cell subpopulation levels: observations in four cases of patients with ovarian cancer. *Cancer Immunol Immunother*. 2012;61(6):839–54.

127. Spear P, Barber A, Rynda-Apple A, Sentman CL. NKG2D CAR T-cell therapy inhibits the growth of NKG2D ligand heterogeneous tumors. *Immunol Cell Biol*. 2013;91(6):435–40.

128. Zsiros E, Duttagupta P, Dangaj D, et al. The ovarian cancer chemokine landscape is conducive to homing of vaccine-primed and CD3/CD28-costimulated T cells prepared for adoptive therapy. *Clin Cancer Res*. 2015;21(12):2840–50.

129. Kandalaft LE, Powell DJ, Jr., Coukos G. A phase I clinical trial of adoptive transfer of folate receptor-alpha redirected autologous T cells for recurrent ovarian cancer. *J Transl Med*. 2012;10:157.

130. Perales-Puchalt A, Svoronos N, Rutkowski MR, et al. Follicle-stimulating hormone receptor is expressed by most ovarian cancer subtypes and is a safe and effective immunotherapeutic target. *Clin Cancer Res*. 2017;23(2):441–53.

131. Chan WM, Rahman MM, McFadden G. Oncolytic myxoma virus: the path to clinic. *Vaccine*. 2013;31(39):4252–58.

132. Correa RJ, Komar M, Tong JG, et al. Myxoma virus-mediated oncolysis of ascites-derived human ovarian cancer cells and spheroids is impacted by differential AKT activity. *Gynecol Oncol*. 2012;125(2):441–50.

133. Hirasawa K, Nishikawa SG, Norman KL, Alain T, Kossakowska A, Lee PW. Oncolytic reovirus against ovarian and colon cancer. *Cancer Res*. 2002;62(6):1696–701.

134. Jennings VA, Ilett EJ, Scott KJ, et al. Lymphokine-activated killer and dendritic cell carriage enhances oncolytic reovirus therapy for ovarian cancer by overcoming antibody neutralization in ascites. *Int J Cancer*. 2014;134(5):1091–101.

135. Galanis E, Atherton PJ, Maurer MJ, et al. Oncolytic measles virus expressing the sodium iodide symporter to treat drug-resistant ovarian cancer. *Cancer Res.* 2015;75(1):22–30.

136. Cubillos-Ruiz JR, Baird JR, Tesone AJ, et al. Reprogramming tumor-associated dendritic cells in vivo using miRNA mimetics triggers protective immunity against ovarian cancer. *Cancer Res.* 2012;72(7):1683–93.

137. Scarlett UK, Rutkowski MR, Rauwerdink AM, et al. Ovarian cancer progression is controlled by phenotypic changes in dendritic cells. *J Exp Med.* 2012;209(3):495–506.

138. Clark CA, Gupta HB, Sareddy G, et al. Tumor-intrinsic PD-L1 signals regulate cell growth, pathogenesis and autophagy in ovarian cancer and melanoma. *Cancer Res.* 2016;76(23):6964–74.

139. Svoronos N, Perales-Puchalt A, Allegrezza MJ, et al. Tumor cell-independent estrogen signaling drives progression through mobilization of myeloid-derived suppressor cells. *Cancer Disc.* 2017;7(1):72–85.

INDEX

Tables and figures are indicated by an italic *t* and *f* following the page/paragraph number.